FLAGLER COLLEGE LIBRARY
KING STREET
ST. AUGUSTINE, FLORIDA 32084

The Multihandicapped Hearing Impaired:
Identification and Instruction

Contributors

Clark Brannan, Ph.D.
Department of Education
McMurry College
Abilene, Texas 79604

Ruth Seth Funderburg, Ph.D.
Assistant Professor
Department of Education
Gallaudet College
Washington, D.C. 20002

Carmella Ficociello Gates, M.Ed.
University of Northern Colorado
Greeley, Colorado 80631

Edwin Hammer, Ph.D.
University Affiliated Center
University of Texas Health Science Center
  at Dallas
Dallas, Texas 77219

Ann Reilly Harris, M.Ed.
Communication Disorders/Speech and
  Hearing Clinic
Southern Methodist University
Dallas, Texas 75275

Corrine E. Kass, Ph.D.
Department of Education
Calvin College
Grand Rapids, Michigan 49506

Robert Lennan, Ed.D.
Superintendent
California School for the Deaf
Riverside, California 92506

Marya Mavilya, Ed.D.
Executive Director
Fort Lauderdale Oral School
Fort Lauderdale, Florida 33315

Kathryn P. Meadow, Ph.D.
Director, Child Development Research
Kendall Demonstration Elementary School/
  Model Secondary School for the Deaf
  Research Laboratory
Washington, D.C. 20002

Donald Moores, Ph.D.
Director
Center for Studies in Education and
  Human Development
Gallaudet Research Institute
Gallaudet College
Washington, D.C. 20002

Joan M. Moran, Ph.D.
Associate Professor in Physical Education
Texas Woman's University
Denton, Texas 76204

Doris Naiman, Ph.D.
Director of Graduate Program
Deafness Research and Training Center
New York University
New York, New York 10012

Anne Rutledge Powers, Ed.D.
Division of Communication Disorders
Speech and Hearing Clinic
Southern Methodist University
Dallas, Texas 75275

Lillian C. R. Restaino, Ph.D.
Division of Curriculum and Teaching
School of Education at Lincoln Center
Fordham University
New York, New York 10023

Ramon Rodriguez, M.A.
Assistant Professor
Department of Education
Gallaudet College
Washington, D.C. 20002

Charlotte H. Shroyer, Ph.D.
Assistant Professor
Department of Special Education
University of Maryland
College Park, Maryland 20740

Edgar H. Shroyer, Ph.D.
Assistant Professor
Department of Communication and Theater
University of North Carolina at Greensboro
Greensboro, North Carolina 27412

Kathleen Stremel-Campbell, M.A.
Teaching Research Division
Oregon State System of Higher Education
Oregon College of Education
Monmouth, Oregon 97631

Larry G. Stewart, Ph.D.
Executive Director
Texas Commission for the Deaf
Austin, Texas 78711

David Tweedie, Ed.D.
Dean, School of Communication
Gallaudet College
Washington, D.C. 20002

McCay Vernon, Ph.D.
Professor
Department of Psychology
Western Maryland College
Westminster, Maryland 21157

The Multihandicapped Hearing Impaired:
Identification and Instruction

David Tweedie and Edgar H. Shroyer,
Editors

Gallaudet College Press
Washington, D.C.

Published by the Gallaudet College Press
Kendall Green, Washington, D.C. 20002

Library of Congress Catalog Card Number 81-84511

All rights reserved. No part of this book may be reproduced in any form or by any method without permission in writing from the publisher.

Copyright © 1982 by Gallaudet College
Washington, D.C. 20002

Gallaudet College is an equal opportunity employer/educational institution. Programs and services offered by Gallaudet College receive substantial financial support from the U.S. Department of Education.

Text and cover design by Donna Lee Simons. Cover photographs by Peter J. Moran.

ISBN 0-913580-74-0

Contents

Preface   ix

Acknowledgments   xiv

Introduction   1

I Understanding the Population

1 Multihandicapped Deaf Children: Types and Causes   *McCay Vernon*   11

2 A Survey of Programs and Services to Hearing-Impaired/Mentally Retarded Children   *Clark Brannan*   29

3 Factors in the Educational Placement of the Multihandicapped Hearing-Impaired Child   *Robert Lennan*   37

4 The Effects of Public Law 94-142 on Programs for Multihandicapped Hearing-Impaired Children   *Ramon Rodriguez*   43

II Providing Comprehensive Programming

5 A Model of Behavior Management with Multihandicapped Hearing-Impaired Children   *Edgar H. Shroyer*   53

6 The Role of the Classroom Teacher in the Assessment of the Learning-Disabled Hearing-Impaired Child   *Ruth Seth Funderburg*   61

7 Physical Education and Recreation Movement Experiences for Hearing-Impaired Mentally Retarded Children   *Joan M. Moran*   75

8 Remedial Strategies for Age-Related Characteristics of Learning Disability   *Corinne E. Kass*   85

9 Early Intervention with Multihandicapped Children   *Carmella Ficociello Gates*   95

10 Working with Parents of Multihandicapped Children   *Kathryn P. Meadow*   103

III Developing the Curriculum

11 Assessment, Curriculum, and Intervention Strategies for Hearing-Impaired Mentally Retarded Children   *Marya Mavilya*   113

12 Developing the Curriculum for Severely Disturbed Hearing-Impaired Students   *Larry G. Stewart*   124

13 Assessing and Remedying Perceptual Problems in Hearing-Impaired Children   *Charlotte Shroyer*   135

14 Educational Programming for Hearing-Impaired Mentally Retarded Adolescents   *Doris Naiman*   148

15 A Curriculum Development Project for the Multihandicapped Hearing-Impaired Child Ten Years Later   *Lillian C. R. Restaino*   162

IV Developing Language and Communication Strategies

16 Structuring the Communication Program for the Needs of Multihandicapped Hearing-Impaired Children   *David Tweedie*   185

17 The Development of Language in the Deaf-Blind Multihandicapped Child: Progression of Instructional Methods   *Edwin Hammer*   193

18 The Language of Hearing-Impaired Mentally Retarded Children   *Donald Moores*   201

19 The Development of Language in the Mentally Retarded Hearing-Impaired Child: Instructional Methods   *Kathleen Stremel-Campbell*   211

20 Strategies for Teaching Language- and/or Learning-Disabled Hearing-Impaired Children   *Ann Rutledge Powers, Ann Reilly Harris*   249

Preface

Dedicated teachers who have experienced considerable frustration, but manifested dogged determination, in their attempts to educate multihandicapped hearing-impaired (MHHI) children provided the impetus for this text.

The editors of this text were both actively involved in setting up possibly the first MHHI specialization certified by the Council on the Education of the Deaf. This MHHI specialization was in the Department of Education, Teacher Training Program at Gallaudet College, Washington, D.C. In addition to the coursework requirements for this specialization, a student teaching practicum lasting for a ten-week period with MHHI children was required. This requirement afforded the editors many opportunities to visit a wide variety of MHHI programs throughout the country while supervising the student teaching practicum. It quickly became evident that teachers in these programs were genuinely concerned about the welfare of their MHHI children but were often unable to "reach" them. This inability to "reach" them was generally due to the teachers' lack of knowledge about and training with MHHI children. This lack, in turn, was due to a dearth of materials and inservice training regarding this population.

The editors, viewing this need in person, came up with the idea of a summer symposium which would bring together teachers of MHHI children and experts in the field to share some of the frustrations and, hopefully, to resolve some of the problems being encountered. The first symposium, held during the summer of 1976, was an immediate success. However, it was felt that the material covered in the first symposium, "The Multihandicapped Hearing-Impaired Child," was too general in scope. Subsequent symposia focused on specific disabilities of MHHI children, i.e., mental retardation and learning disability. A monograph was generated from each of the summer symposia (Monographs I, III, and IV), and another from a special seminar held for the graduate students in the MHHI specialization at Gallaudet (Monograph II). It was felt that each monograph individually was meeting a specific need of teachers, but, at the same time, the information was being presented in a fragmented way. It was also known that many people could not avail themselves of the summer symposia; many were not aware of the monographs; and others could not obtain a copy of each symposium monograph. Thus, the idea of a specific text dealing with a wide range of critical issues about MHHI children was conceived.

This text is organized to meet the needs of a diverse group of people—students, teachers, parents, and administrators—who may deal with MHHI populations. It is divided into four major sections. Each section contains contributions from professionals who have demonstrated considerable expertise in their fields.

Section I: Understanding the Population provides a comprehensive picture of MHHI children. It begins with Vernon's chapter in which he discusses the etiologies of deafness and the sequelae of each. This information is important in determining not only academic and mental health needs but also vocational expectations of each child. It represents invaluable information not only for teachers and administrators but for parents as well. Brannan then presents his findings on the mentally retarded hearing-impaired population, its program needs, and staff requirements. He succinctly points out the need for special programming for this population, programming which it is not receiving presently. (How to meet these special programming needs is presented in definitive terms in the other sections of the text.) The third chapter in Section I appeals mostly to parents and teachers. Written by Lennan from an administrator's point of view, the chapter explains the procedures used in accepting MHHI children into his program. The referral process and the need to communicate effectively with other professionals are the main themes in his chapter. Opening these avenues of communication may obviate some of the conditions found in Brannan's survey. In the last chapter, Rodriguez describes the effects and legal ramifications of Public Law 94-142. Rodriguez discusses what can and cannot be done under the law in the educational process involving MHHI children. What Lennan has said from an administrative standpoint is substantiated by Rodriguez.

Section II: Providing Comprehensive Programming deals with specific programs, activities, and procedures for MHHI children. The first chapter, by E. Shroyer, should serve as a basic framework or model within which all other activities take place. In order for children to learn, they have to be ready. They have to attend, perform certain tasks, and have certain experiences. Past practice with MHHI children has shown that activities have to occur in a structured environment if significant learning is to happen. Children must know what is expected of them and know that they will be reinforced when tasks are performed successfully. In Chapter Six, Funderburg stresses the importance of specific diagnostic/prescriptive procedures which should be undertaken by the classroom teacher. Her well-documented chapter provides strong support for continuous, ongoing assessment in the classroom. Naturally, a structured classroom situation makes these procedures occur with more positive results. Moran, in Chapter Seven, provides teachers and parents with a sound theoretical foundation for the importance of physical education and recreation movement. Too frequently, teachers become so involved in the academic side of instruction, they neglect motor development related to playing, walking, running, and other physical activities. Moran's chapter should be of considerable interest to everyone involved with MHHI children.

Assessment of MHHI children is also critical. Kass' chapter, "Remedial Strategies for Age-Related Characteristics of Learning Disabilities," provides the reader with a way to identify some critical deficits by developmental function. Then strategies for treatment are given for each deficit. After reading this chapter, the reader can better appreciate Gates' Chapter Nine. Gates emphasizes a "total child" approach in educating MHHI children. She emphasizes the importance of designing activities which incorporate several different behaviors in a realistic setting. She then "walks" the reader through the whole learning process using a step-by-step procedure with several charts which complement the written procedure. Kass looks at specific deficit areas, while Gates suggests how these areas may be integrated in working with MHHI children. The final chapter in Section II, by Meadow, is of considerable value in that it provides information on a critical dimension in working with MHHI children, a dimension which is often overlooked—the parents. Written specifically for professionals working with MHHI children, it discusses the needs of parents and how to provide the necessary support for them. However, parents who read this chapter will gain insight into potential problems they may encounter. Thus, being forewarned, parents can cope better with the inevitable problems that their MHHI child may present them and that they may present their MHHI child.

Section III: Developing the Curriculum should prove to be the section that most teachers embrace with great joy. An unpublished survey undertaken by one of the editors verified the great need for this section. A questionnaire regarding curricula was sent to approximately 150 agencies which reported having educational programs for MHHI children. The list of the MHHI programs was taken from a list of all programs for the hearing impaired in the United States completed by the Office of Demographic Studies, Gallaudet College, Washington, D.C. Well over half of the respondents indicated that they used no curriculum in their MHHI program; of the remaining respondents, a small number had either adapted or adopted an existing curriculum for use; and only a very, very small number had developed a curriculum specifically for their MHHI program. However, the chapters in Section III are not intended individually or collectively to serve as a curriculum, but instead to illustrate or highlight features to be included in a flexible curriculum.

Chapters by Stewart and Naiman deal generally with older MHHI children, specifically older, severely disturbed, and mentally retarded hearing-impaired students. These are important chapters which describe programs and curricula for an MHHI population which is not frequently covered in the literature. C. Shroyer and Mavilya have geared their chapters more toward younger MHHI children. Mavilya presents many resources in the area of assessment along with curricular suggestions. C. Shroyer's and Funderburg's chapters provide the teacher with procedures and resources for all hearing-impaired children who may exhibit learning problems. According to Vernon (Chapter One), " . . . a significant amount of the language disability found among deaf children is due, in part, to organically caused aphasoid disorders, not just deafness. The same is true of other types of learning disabilities." So these two chapters, Thirteen and Six, would also be helpful for the teacher of "normal" deaf children. This section ends with Restaino's chapter in which she presents the findings from a project titled Cooperative Research Endeavors in the

Education of the Deaf (CREED). This lengthy chapter provides the reader with some new and significant findings in the areas of cognition, visual analysis, and long- and short-term memory. The chapter appendix provides the assumptions inherent in the CREED project. They strongly reinforce what has already been covered on MHHI children with learning problems.

The final section of the text, Section IV: Developing Language and Communication Strategies, contains five chapters devoted to language development, an area recognized by everyone as perhaps the most crucial and difficult in working with all hearing-impaired children. While the chapters in this section deal with language development for MHHI children in specific areas of disability—deaf-blindness, mental retardation, and learning disability—they offer a wealth of information regarding language for teachers of hearing-impaired children in general. Tweedie's chapter compares the relative merits of sign language systems, depicting them on a communication continuum from which one should judiciously select the communication method(s) to employ with MHHI children. He uses deaf-blind children as an example in demonstrating the selection process. In reality, as he points out, one seldom selects a single sign system on the continuum. Rather, teachers utilize specific attributes from each system, whichever ones meet the communication needs of their children. This is the most efficacious use of the continuum. Hammer's chapter complements much of the information in Tweedie's chapter while going into more detail about instructional methods with deaf-blind children.

For MHHI children who exhibit problems which preclude the use of any form of manual communication, in Chapter Eighteen Moores presents alternative communication models. A creative teacher might easily employ several of these models individually or collectively to determine which models would most benefit his or her MHHI children. The models could also be employed as supplemental learning activities. Many possibilities are available for the creative teacher.

A wealth of information is also available in Stremel-Campbell's chapter on the mentally retarded child. The charts, tables, and activities presented help to crystallize the teaching process. If the readers of the text desire additional information on specific activities, they can rely on the last chapter by Powers and Harris. After presenting a basic framework for the various approaches and strategies to be employed, the authors provide a table of 17 references for the readers. These references are marked according to the particular strategy—motor, visual, written language, etc.—that they cover. Everyone who is concerned with exceptional children will find this resource invaluable.

Although a considerable amount of information was presented at the symposia, the editors have attempted to organize it in a logical, sequential way in this text. Granted, there is some overlap in some areas, and the reader may even notice some contradictions among authors. However, the editors decided that this multiplicity was a positive rather than negative feature of the text, and they made no significant changes for the sake of ideological conformity. The purpose of the text is not to present a cookbook approach to working with MHHI children, but to offer suggestions and techniques which teachers can think about, implement, and then apply. The editors' intent was to give something immediately useful to those working with this population, and, at the same time, to suggest a wealth of resources to which the reader can turn for additional information. There are by far too many variables in working with this population for one text to attempt to provide all the answers. However, progress is continually being made in the many different attempts to educate MHHI children. It is the hope of the editors that this text will provide the reader with a better understanding of MHHI children and the procedures used to educate them in order to continue the progress being made.

E.H.S.
D.T.

Acknowledgements

The editors wish to thank the contributors of this text for their time, expertise, and energy. Their combined efforts have made this significant text on MHHI children possible. Special thanks are in order for Virginia Torabi who, through her extraordinary organizational abilities and her dedication to the project, made the completion of this text possible.

Introduction

The history of the education of the deaf in America goes back to 1817, when the first institution for the education of the deaf, The American Asylum for the Deaf and Dumb in Hartford, Connecticut, was established. It appears fitting that one of the first documented attempts to educate a multihandicapped hearing-impaired (MHHI) child was at that school. It is on record that in 1844, 27 years after the school was founded, teachers at the school worked with a deaf "idiot" (Gearheart & Litton, 1975).

Unfortunately, that bit of history is indicative of the documented progress which has been made towards educating MHHI children in America. What has happened in the 123 years since the first attempts at Hartford? Dr. Powrie V. Doctor sums up our progress in deaf education and gives us a charge in a statement made in 1959 at the Convention of American Instructors of the Deaf:

The frontier in the field of deafness in the latter part of the 20th century lies in the field of the multihandicapped. The 19th century saw the establishment of schools for the deaf, the beginning of teacher training on a professional basis, and the establishment of definite patterns of teaching the deaf. The first part of this century saw the establishment of electronic amplification in our schools. The problem now, as I see it, is in the area of deafness with additional handicaps.

(Doctor, 1959)

The historical chronology of MHHI education shows that only in the last 20 years have MHHI children received any formal recognition:

Pre-1954
Very little information on MHHI children is available in the literature.

1954
Formal recognition was given to the problem of MHHI children when the Conference of Executives of American Schools for the Deaf (CEASD) authorized the *American Annals of the Deaf* to publish a list of schools and classes for MHHI children as a separate section in the statistical issue of the *Annals*.

1956
Elwood Stevens, Superintendent of the California School for the Deaf at Berkeley, presented a paper at the Conference of Executives of American Schools for the Deaf meeting in which he defined the problems that schools for the deaf faced with growing numbers of MHHI children. He also stated that schools should begin to recognize their responsibility in this field.

1957
Conference of American Instructors of the Deaf (CAID) established a section for consideration of multihandicapped individuals; however, the papers presented did not really touch upon the subject of MHHI children.

1959

Workshops held at the CAID meeting included sections concerned specifically with hearing-impaired children who had additional handicapping conditions, such as emotional disturbance, blindness, mental retardation, and aphasia.

1961

The Illinois School for the Deaf established a program for MHHI children whose additional handicapping condition was other than mental retardation. The school had already set up a program for mentally retarded hearing-impaired children.

1965

The Babbidge Report stated one of the major problems in the education of the deaf is the education of MHHI children. Some schools were providing special classes, but too often on an improvised and makeshift basis. The committee's study had been unable to discover any data which fully revealed the dimension of the problem, yet it did find indications that the problem warranted research.

1966

The California School for the Deaf at Riverside established a program for emotionally disturbed deaf boys. Also that year, McCay Vernon completed his doctoral dissertation on the causes and nature of learning disabilities, behavioral disorders, and physical defects in a sample of 1,468 deaf children (Brill, 1974).

1968

The Office of Demographic Studies at Gallaudet College did the first comprehensive study of MHHI children in the United States.

1969

Public Law 91-230 established the Centers and Services for Deaf-Blind Children. The Regional Centers have had a profound impact on the development of services to the MHHI student in all settings.

1975

Public Law 94-142, the Education for All Handicapped Children Act, had a significant impact on all hearing-impaired children, specifically on MHHI children.

1975

Gallaudet College, Department of Education, started MHHI specializations in the Teacher Training Program, Education of the Deaf.

Identification and recognition of the needs of the MHHI population was a slow process; however, this is not meant to imply that nothing was being done to provide services to MHHI children. State schools and hospitals, private agencies, some school districts, and residential schools were providing modest services to MHHI children, but their endeavors and the needs of this population were not brought to the attention of the special education profession as a whole (Stewart, Obstacle 5).

Who is considered an MHHI child? The problem of defining an MHHI child is extremely difficult because of the variables that are involved. That, in turn, makes the incidence and prevalence rates difficult to ascertain. The definitions used in one place may differ from that used in another area. Definitions also typically reflect the current sociocultural standards of a given society, and those are subject to constant change. The orientation of the person making the judgment of an additional handicapping condition must also be considered. Is the person's orientation medical, psychological, educational, or legal? The Office of Demographic Studies (ODS) uses a generic definition of the MHHI child because of the varying backgrounds of the professionals answering their surveys. Therefore, since the data on MHHI children presented are from ODS, their definition of the MHHI child is presented: "For the purpose of the Annual Survey, 'Additional Handicapping Condition' is defined as any physical, mental, emotional, or behavioral disorder that significantly adds to the complexity of educating a hearing-impaired student." (*Annual Survey of Hearing-Impaired Children and Youth,* 1973)

The degree of severity of an additional handicapping condition (mild, moderate, severe) is also important. This type of information was not indicated in earlier reports, but it was available in the 1973 *Annual Survey*. The 1973 *Annual Survey* showed that for all additional handicapping conditions, in terms of educational significance, 14.2% were reported as severe, 33.6% moderate, and 43.4% mild. No report was given on degree of severity for 8.8% of the conditions. These data refer to MHHI children in educational programs; more severely handicapped children are probably institutionalized or at home, and not included in the statistics given.

To provide an orientation to the prevalence of MHHI children, the most recent data available from the Office of Demographic Studies, are presented here. Table 1, Summary of Data on Additional Handicapping Conditions (*Annual Survey of Hearing-Impaired Children and Youth,* 1973), shows that the number of students included in the survey has risen since the initial survey in 1968, and now represents approximately 80% of the hearing-impaired children attending programs. While the prevalence (numbers) of MHHI students has increased, the incidence (percentage) of students reported as having an additional handicapping condition has not increased significantly when compared with the total deaf student population.

Table 2 is a Summary of Data by Types of Additional Handicapping Conditions. The prevalence of each additional condition appears to remain fairly constant over the years that the surveys were done. The most prevalent handicapping conditions are visual disorders (16.9%), emotional or behavioral problems (17.4%), and mental retardation (17.7%). Vernon's data, relative to the five major etiologies of deafness—heredity, meningitis, rubella, prematurity, and Rh factor—show that the high percentage of visual disorders are mainly results of prematurity and rubella; mental retardation is the result of meningitis and prematurity (Vernon, Chapter One).

The Office of Demographic Studies through surveys has identified approximately 300 programs that now provide educational services to MHHI children in the

Table 1

Summary of Data on Additional Handicapping Conditions for Seven School Years: United States, 1968–1975

	School Year	
	1968–1969	1974–1975
Total subjects enrolled in participating programs	25,363	47,235
Number of subjects by number of additional handicapping conditions		
None	14,685	27,981
One or more	6,445	13,737
Not reported	4,233	5,517
Percent of subjects by additional handicapping condition		
None	57.9	59.2
One or more	25.4	29.1
Not reported	16.7	11.7
Percent of subjects by additional handicapping condition, omitting subjects for whom no data were reported		
None	69.5	67.1
One or more	30.5	32.9
Total number of handicapping conditions reported	8,871	20,809
Number of conditions per 100 subjects for whom data were reported	42.0	49.9
Number of subjects with visual defects	883*	3,558
Percent of all conditions reported as visual defects	10.0	17.1
Number of conditions per 100 subjects for whom data were reported, omitting visual defects	37.8	41.4

* Reporting form asked for the reporting of "severe" visual handicaps.

United States. Several factors, all of which are interrelated, contributed to this tremendous growth over a relatively short period of time.

1. Litigation and judicial interpretations that make education the right of all children. The most publicized legal cases are Parents' Association of Retarded Children vs. the Commonwealth of Pennsylvania (1972) and Mills vs. the Board of Education of the District of Columbia (1972).
2. A shift in federal funding priorities to more severely multihandicapped children in general.

Table 2
Summary of Data by Types of Additional Handicapping Conditions for Seven School Years: United States, 1968–1975

	School Year					
	1972–73		1973–74		1974–75	
	Number	Percent	Number	Percent	Number	Percent
All types	19,040	100.0	19,033	100.0	20,809	100.0
Brain damage	1,537	8.1	1,455	7.6	1,571	7.5
Cerebral palsy	1,294	6.8	1,299	6.8	1,395	6.7
Epilepsy	411	2.2	414	2.2	469	2.3
Heart disorders	1,159	6.1	1,159	6.1	1,309	6.3
Mental retardation	3,373	17.7	3,325	17.5	3,735	17.9
Orthopedic disorders	774	4.1	797	4.2	903	4.3
Perceptual motor disorders	1,993	10.5	2,004	10.5	2,189	10.5
Emotional or behavioral problems	3,451	18.1	3,360	17.7	3,457	16.6
Visual disorders	3,202	16.8	3,219	16.9	3,558	17.1
All other	1,846	9.7	2,001	10.5	2,223	10.7

3. Parental pressure through advocacy groups.
4. School districts being held responsible and accountable for the education of all children.
5. Educational Amendment of 1974 (PL 93-380), which was later amended (PL 94-142) in 1975, Education for All Handicapped Children Act.

Since educational programs for MHHI children have come into existence relatively suddenly, the profession has endeavored to fill the voids that have existed so long; the task is a formidable one. Stewart (1971) cites several obstacles that impede the work being done with MHHI individuals.

1. Vague nomenclature—The term multihandicapped is vague and does not communicate the problem.
2. Inadequate description—The physical basis of the multihandicapped is alluded to in the term multihandicapped, but the term does not indicate the sociocultural and family interaction variable.

3. Inconsistent treatment—Although behavioral modification techniques reportedly produce successful results, such techniques have not been implemented widely. A stern disciplinarian approach is still taken.
4. Insufficient media—There exists a serious lack of materials for low verbal and low functioning deaf persons.
5. Poor dissemination—Education and rehabilitation programs for severely multihandicapped persons have gained knowledge of the problems and the needs of these people, but only minimal attempts have been made to share the information.

A sixth obstacle should be added to Stewart's list:

6. Insufficient personnel—There exists a lack of trained personnel to deal successfully with the problems presented by MHHI children.

It appears that this sixth obstacle has a definite bearing on the first five. More college and university training programs and inservice programs are needed to prepare individuals to work with this unique population. At the present time, colleges and universities offering teacher training programs in the area of exceptional children are tending to be more and more non-categorical. They are preparing teachers to work with a wide cross section of exceptional children; however, the major emphasis of none of these programs is with MHHI children. Several fine teacher training programs in the education of the deaf have added an MHHI specialization option to their programs. This addition has greatly improved MHHI children's overall education.

Only recently has more attention been focused on inservice training for teachers working with the MHHI population. It was through the Bureau of Education of the Handicapped funding that several symposia and workshops were held specifically to address the needs of teachers working with MHHI children. More state and local school districts are providing funds for workshops and consultants to reeducate their teachers regarding the particular and unique problems they may encounter while working with MHHI children. Significant progress is being made.

This volume cannot overcome all the obstacles which Stewart mentions, but it will provide the reader with immediate information which will be helpful in working with MHHI children. Certainly, Stewart's obstacle number five will be addressed. The editors and authors want to compensate for the benign neglect of MHHI children in most of the literature. Vernon et al. (1980) listed over 20 publications devoted exclusively to deafness, and they annotated the interest areas for each publication. Not once was MHHI listed as an interest area. Although most professionals in deafness know that publications occasionally have articles on MHHI children, the interested lay person and other professionals may not.

The educational future of MHHI children is considerably brighter today than it was as few as three or four years ago, in spite of the many needs still unmet. As residential schools, day schools, and other educational institutions continue to establish programs staffed with well-trained and qualified personnel to serve this population, we will see more postsecondary and vocational training programs developing to foster the MHHI person's independence and productivity in our society. The authors who contributed to this book hope to further that recent progress.

E.H.S.

Bibliography

Babbidge, H. D. *Education of the deaf: A report to the Secretary of Health, Education, and Welfare by his Advisory Committee on the Education of the Deaf.* Washington, D.C.: U.S. Government Printing Office, 1965.

Brill, R. G. *The education of the deaf.* Washington, D.C.: Gallaudet College Press, 1974.

Doctor, P. V. Workshop on multiple handicaps. *Proceedings of the 39th Convention of American Instructors of the Deaf, Colorado Springs, Colorado.* Washington, D.C.: U.S. Government Printing Office, 1959.

Gearheart, B. R., & Litton, F. W. *The trainable retarded: A foundations approach.* St. Louis: C. V. Mosby Co., 1975.

Office of Demographic Studies. Additional handicapping conditions among hearing-impaired students, United States: 1971–72. *Annual survey of hearing-impaired children and youth.* Washington, D.C.: Gallaudet College, 1973.

Office of Demographic Studies. Reported causes of hearing loss of hearing-impaired students, United States: 1970–71. *Annual survey of hearing-impaired children and youth.* Washington, D.C.: Gallaudet College, 1973.

Stewart, L. G. Problems of severely handicapped deaf: Implications for educational programs. American Annals of the Deaf, 1971, *116*(3), 362–368.

Vernon, M. *Multiply handicapped deaf children: Medical, educational, and psychological considerations* (research monograph). Washington, D.C.: Council for Exceptional Children, 1969.

Vernon, M., Bair, R., & Lotz, S. Journals relevant to the field of deafness and profound hearing loss: A list and description. *American Annals of the Deaf,* 1980, *125*(4), 499–504.

I

Understanding the Population

1

Multihandicapped Deaf Children: Types and Causes

McCay Vernon

Dr. McCay Vernon discusses the leading causes of deafness—maternal rubella, complications of the Rh factor, prematurity, meningitis, and certain genetic syndromes—and indicates why these causes are likely to lead to other handicapping conditions as well.

Appropriate education and rehabilitation for multihandicapped deaf children represent the most discussed, yet least acted-upon problem in the area of deafness today. Evidence of this is that from 15 to 35% of deaf youth, the overwhelming majority with multiple disabilities, are either not accepted into educational programs for the deaf or else are dropped out at or before 16 years of age (Boatner, Stuckless, & Moores, 1964; Kronenberg & Blake, 1966; and Vernon, 1969).

When Dr. Tjerle Basilear, the noted Norwegian psychiatric authority, visited facilities in the United States, he inquired of educators how they served multihandicapped deaf children. The answer given was that nothing was done for them. The irony of the United States spending millions of dollars on esoteric research projects in deafness while hundreds of these deaf children in need of education or treatment were literally being dumped back into the community was striking to Dr. Basilear. This is not to condemn research, but to indict the gross lack of service. Educators in schools for the deaf have the frequent and grisly responsibility of informing the parents of many of these young people that not only can their child not be accepted or kept in a regular school for deaf youth, but that there is absolutely no place for parents to go where they might get help for the multihandicapped deaf child. To fail to provide some sort of constructive program or opportunity for a child who already has the obstacles of deafness and other handicaps is to doom him or her to insurmountable odds in the struggle for even a chance at basic life satisfaction and human dignity.

Causes of Multiple Disabilities among Deaf Children

To approach the problem of multiple disabilities among deaf children constructively, it is essential to know the causes of the problem. Such information forms the basis for prevention, it contributes to predictions about the number of such children to be expected, it leads to an understanding of the kinds of problems the children may have, and it yields clues to diagnoses and therapy.

The research reported here examines certain of the leading causes of deafness because it is known that these etiologies also result in other disabilities. By establishing the prevalence of deaf children with other disabilities in these large etiological groups and then determining the nature of their handicaps, some picture of the magnitude and types of problems multihandicapped deaf children have will result.

The etiologies to be studied are prenatal rubella, complications of Rh factor, meningitis, genetics, and premature birth. As indicated in Table 1, they cause a significant amount of the deafness which occurs in school-age children. With the exception of about 10%, the remaining deafness is of unknown etiology.

The point to be made from presenting these data is that the multiple handicaps associated with the five etiologies under study probably represent a major share of such handicaps which are to be found among deaf school-age children.

Nature of the Etiologies

Before presenting additional research data, cursory background information about the etiologies to be investigated will be provided. This is important in understanding their role as a cause of multihandicaps.

MATERNAL RUBELLA Due to the 1963–1965 rubella epidemic and the ones projected for the future, there is going to be a huge increase in the number of postrubella children in schools. Estimates vary, but based on available statistics, the best guess is that there will be at least 4,500 children (Vernon, 1967) from 1963-65 alone. Reports indicate that two-thirds of the children who entered school in 1969 had prenatal rubella. A recent report by Chicago's Xavier College stated that 25 of the 30

Table 1
Prevalences of Major Etiologies of Deafness (1,468 Cases)

Etiology	Range of prevalence	
	From	To
Five etiologies studied in this research		
Genetics	5.4%	26.0%
Maternal rubella	8.8%	9.5%
Meningitis	8.1%	8.7%
Prematurity	11.9%	17.4%
Rh factor	3.1%	3.7%
Total	37.3%	65.3%
Other etiologies		
Unknown	30.4%	30.4%
Other	9.4%	32.3%
Total	39.8%	62.7%

This table is presented primarily to illustrate the prevalence of the five etiologies presented in this chapter. For a more complete report of etiological factors in 1,468 cases, refer to the original report (Vernon, 1969, pp. 42–50).

children in the preschool deaf program were rubella babies. Fragmented as these data may be, they clearly indicate an influx of rubella children of far greater numbers than has ever occurred before—even in the epidemic of 1943 when rubella had approximately a 20% incidence among the causes of deafness (Vernon, 1969). With this evidence illustrating the huge number of postrubella children entering schools, the question of the effects of rubella assume major importance.

Rubella is a viral infection which, when contracted by a mother during pregnancy, is often passed on to the fetus. The pathogenic organisms then attack developing organs of the embryo, rendering them defective. The major sequelae are eye defects, heart disease, deafness, microcephaly, mental retardation, abnormal behavior patterns, motor disabilities, and failure to thrive (Campbell, 1961; Jackson & Fisch, 1958; Lunstrom, 1962; Manson, Logan, & Roy, 1960, 1961; Montagu, 1962, p. 282; Signurjonsson, 1963; Skinner, 1961). Estimates of the percentage of postrubella children having at least one serious congenital defect vary from as low as 4.5% (Lunstrom, 1962; Manson, et al., 1961) to as high as 80% (Berger & Melnick, 1961, pp. 314-315), with the consensus being that from 12 to 19% of these children have major anomalies (Silverman, 1961, p. 277). See Table 2. Preliminary reports from Johns Hopkins (Hardy, 1965; Monif, Hardy, & Sever, 1966;

Table 2
Major Sequelae and Their Causes in Postrubella Children

Causes

Viral infections and damage to tissue during embryonic development.

Anoxia

Sequelae

Brain damage
    Cerebral palsy
    Epilepsy

Mental retardation and/or lowered intelligence level

Behavior disorders:
    Psychoses
    Learning disability
    Strauss Syndrome (hyperactivity, etc., with emphasis on impulse disorders)

Physical disabilities:
    Microcephaly
    Microphthalmus
    Deafness
    Cardiac defect
    Visual pathology (cataract, chorioretinitis, nystagmus, etc.)
    Dental pathology
    Premature birth
    Failure to thrive
    Orthopedic defect

and Hardy, Monif, & Sever, 1966) may cause an upward revision of these figures. Of all defects, hearing loss is probably the greatest risk (Campbell, 1961; and Jackson & Fisch, 1958).

Recent medical advances have resulted in a rubella vaccine which should eliminate this disease just as polio has been. However, the huge number of youth infected and deafened in the 1963–1965 and future epidemics will remain an educational and rehabilitative challenge for many years to come (Buynak, et al., 1969).

COMPLICATIONS OF RH FACTOR Certain combinations of parental blood type which involve Rh factor incompatibility can result in the mother's blood destroying the Rh blood cells of the fetus. As a consequence, the brain and central nervous system are often damaged. Eighty percent of children who survive kernicterus, a major complication of Rh factor incompatability, have complete or partial deafness (Cohen, 1956; Flower, Viehweg, & Ruzicka, 1966). Cerebral palsy, mental retardation, epilepsy, and behavior disorders are other prominent sequelae (Blakely, 1959; Brain, 1960, p. 216; Clarke & Clarke, 1958, pp. 143–144; Cook & Odell, 1957, p. 605; Grinker, Bucy, & Sahs, 1960, p. 1153; and Vernon, 1967d). See Table 3. Perhaps the most important factor about deafness and Rh factor is that aphasoid disorders and central nervous system lesions are often present in addition to hearing loss (Cohen, 1956; Hannigan, 1956; Myklebust, 1956; Rosen, 1956; and Vernon, 1967).

Table 3
Major Sequelae and Their Causes in Children Born with Complications of Rh Factor

Causes

Actual causality is not clear. Factors involved are:
Anoxia
Jaundice
Nuclear masses of the brain and central nervous system

Sequelae

Brain damage
    Cerebral palsy (very common)
    Epilepsy

Mental retardation and/or a lowered intelligence level

Behavior disorders
    Learning disability, especially aphasia
    Strauss Syndrome and chronic brain syndrome

Physical disability
    Deafness
    Visual pathology
    Orthopedic defect

Complications of Rh factor are now preventable with good prenatal care. Soon this condition may also cease to be a major cause of deafness (Clarke, 1968).

MENINGITIS Meningitis has long been the leading postnatal cause of deafness (Robinson, 1964; Vernon, 1967c). Other sequelae which result from the disease are hydrocephalus, paralysis, cortical blindness, mental retardation, epilepsy, cranial nerve palsy, learning disorders, and psychiatric symptoms (DeGraff & Creger, 1963, p. 249–255; Ford, 1960, pp. 544–550; Kelley, 1964, p. 36; Nelson, 1959, p. 428; and Swartz & Dodge, 1965a, 1965b). Estimates of the percent of cases having major neurological sequelae range from 15 to 71 (DeGraff & Creger, 1963, p. 243; Kelley, 1964, p. 36; Mackay, 1964, pp. 38–39; and Swartz & Dodge, 1964). See Table 4.

Table 4
Major Sequelae and Their Causes in Postmeningitic Deaf Children

Causes

Inflammation of tissue around the brain

Intracranial pressure

Hematomas

Rupturing of cranial blood vessels

General hemorrhaging

Accumulation of exudate

Cortical abscess

Abnormalities in body physiology and biochemistry

Sequelae

Brain damage
    Hydrocephalus
    Paralysis (hemiplegia, diplegia, etc.)
    Cortical blindness
    Epilepsy

Mental retardation and/or lowered intelligence level

Behavior disorders
    Learning disability, especially aphasia
    Psychoses
    Strauss Syndrome (hyperactivity, distractibility, etc., with an emphasis in some cases of difficulty controlling hostile impulses)

Physical disability
    Deafness
    Cranial nerve palsy

The important new consideration with regard to meningitis is that it responds favorably to the antimicrobal therapies developed in recent years. Consequently, a great change has occurred in the nature of the postmeningitic deaf population. Today those who contract the disease after the age of three or four generally recover with no loss of hearing (Vernon, 1967c & 1969).

The premature and newborn, who are especially susceptible to the disease and in whom it is most difficult to diagnose and treat, are now surviving, whereas in past years they almost invariably died (Ford, 1960, p. 537; Kelley, 1964; Nelson, 1959, p. 344). This means that today's postmeningitic deaf child is likely to be both prelingually deafened and to have other sequelae of the disease.

In years past, postmeningitic deaf children generally had naturally acquired language and no other disabilities. They comprised about one-third of the deaf youth who went to college, and from this group were drawn many of the academically capable students who were able to function successfully in day schools and classes and in competition with the normally hearing. Now that postmeningitic children are primarily a prelingually deafened group and have a high prevalence of multihandicaps, programs of higher education and programs that expect deaf children to compete in educational settings with hearing children are going to find that there will be fewer qualified students unless the educational level of present-day students is raised.

PREMATURITY Prematurity is approximately four times more prevalent in the deaf school-age population than among hearing children (DeHirsch, Jancky, & Langford, 1966; Vernon, 1976b). Related to this is the fact that more infants born prematurely are now surviving, but often with severe physical and psychological residua (Hardy & Paula, 1959; Kelley, 1964, p. 42; Nesbitt, 1959; Lubcheno, et al., 1963; Vernon, 1976b).

Conditions of prematurity which lead to these sequelae are numerous. One is that the weaker blood vessel walls of the premature infant lead to intracranial hemorrhage caused by mechanical trauma and/or the fragility of the tiny blood vessels (Brennemann, 1937, p. 40; Silverman, 1961, p. 301). Another condition is anoxia which, apart from the condition of the cranial blood vessels, is relatively frequent among prematures and can cause serious brain destruction (Montagu, 1962, pp. 370–386).

Consequently, cerebral palsy, epilepsy, mental deficiency, reading problems, degenerative brain conditions, visual pathology, other physical defects, and behavioral anomalies are more prevalent among prematurely born children (Douglas, 1956a, 1956b, 1960; Kelley, 1964, p. 42; Knobloch, et al., 1956; Weiner, 1962). Those prematures who are also deaf have an especially high prevalence of these conditions (Vernon, 1969a). See Table 5.

Table 5
Major Sequelae and Their Causes in Children Born Prematurely

Causes

Intracranial hemorrhage

Anoxia

Mechanical trauma

Sequelae

Brain damage
    Cerebral palsy
    Epilepsy
    Degenerative conditions of the brain

Mental retardation and/or lowered intelligence level

Behavior disorders
    Schizophrenia
    Learning disability (aphasia, reading problems, and others)
    Strauss Syndrome (hyperactivity, distractibility, restlessness, etc.)

Physical disabilities
    Visual pathology
    Deafness
    Hernia
    Cryptic orchidism
    Liver and kidney defects
    Stomach ruptures
    Failure to thrive

GENETIC DEAFNESS As a group, children deafened by heredity seem to be relatively free of other disabilities. However, one-third of genetic deafness is associated with some other trait, the Waardenburg syndrome and Usher's syndrome being the most common (Vernon, 1969b). The latter is particularly disabling as it involves congenital hearing loss, progressive blindness, and central nervous system lesions (Vernon, 1969b). All told there are some 30 known syndromes involving deafness, ten of which have ear, eye, and central nervous system pathology.

It is clear from this cursory medical picture of these five etiologies of deafness that among children having these causes of hearing loss are many who are multihandicapped. The balance of the chapter will address itself to the prevalence and nature of these multiple disabilities as they were distributed among the 1,468 children who entered or applied for admission to the California School for the Deaf at Riverside over the 11-year span following the school's opening in 1953. Although other etiologies, such as polio, maternal flu, head injury, mumps, etc., are also associated with multihandicaps, this report restricts itself to the five already discussed because it is felt they account for the major share.

Prevalence of Physical and Psychological Anomalies

Table 6 presents the prevalence of major types of physical and psychological anomalies in the deaf children of the five etiological groups under consideration. It is these groups which cause most major disabilities. The data will be discussed in terms of the categories of Table 6.

CEREBRAL PALSY AND/OR HEMIPLEGIA Cerebral palsy has a prevalence rate of from 0.1 to 0.6% in the general population (Nelson, 1959, p. 1138). Among this sample of deaf children, the rate is 15.8% or about a hundred times greater. Of particular note is the fact that over half of the children deafened by Rh factor are cerebral palsied. This figure is approximately 80% if marginal cases are included which involve clear problems of motor coordination but not gross palsy. A prevalence of almost one in five prematures with cerebral palsy also deserves attention in view of the increasing prominence this etiology is playing in deafness (Vernon, 1967a). With prematures, it is among those of the lowest birthweight categories that there is the most cerebral palsy. Hemiplegia, rather than what is generally considered cerebral palsy, accounts for the cases in the meningitic group. Fortunately, in view of the recent rubella epidemic, the prevalence of cerebral palsy among those children was low. Recent medical advances reducing the main causes of the clinical phenomena of deafness and cerebral palsy will result in fewer children with this double handicap in the future (Vernon, 1970).

MENTAL RETARDATION Approximately 2.2% of the general population is mentally retarded (IQ below 70). The rate for this sample of deaf children was about six times greater (12.2%). The highest prevalence was among the premature (16.5%) and the meningitic (14.1%) samples. The existence of about four times the normally expected rate of mental retardation among the postrubella children is an ominous sign in view of the expected influx of these children into schools within the next few years.

APHASOID DISORDERS The presence of aphasia or aphasoid disorders among the deaf is a rarely mentioned and little understood subject, probably because of the difficulty of making the diagnosis. However, it is logical to assume that etiological conditions resulting in nerve deafness and a higher than average prevalence of chronic brain syndromes, such as cerebral palsy and exogenous mental retardation would frequently cause lesions to the brain tissues involved in language functions. This would be especially true of cases of so-called central deafness because the areas of the brain where auditory and linguistic operations occur are close together; damage to one increases the probability of lesions to the other.

Table 6
Prevalence of Physical Anomalies in Four Etiologies of Deafness

	Etiologies											
	Rubella		Prematurity		Meningitis		Rh Factor		Total	
Physical anomaly	Total sample	Percent handicapped	Total sample	Percent handicapped	Total sample	Percent handicapped	Total sample	Percent handicapped	Total sample	Percent handicapped
Cerebral palsy and/or hemiplegia	104	3.8	113	17.6	92	9.7	45	51.1	354	15.8
Mental retardation (IQ below 70)	98	8.1	115	16.5	92	14.1	39	5.1	344	12.2
Aphasoid disorders	105	21.9	113	36.2	92	16.3	35	22.8	345	25.2
Visual defects	104	29.8	113	28.3	87	5.7	45	24.4	349	22.6
Orthopedic defects	104	4.8	101	8.9	92	5.4	45	2.2	342	5.8
Seizures	104	—	113	1.7	92	3.2	45	6.6	354	1.9

Differences in sample sizes for the various etiological groups, depending on the handicap reported, exist because it was not always possible to obtain valid diagnoses of the presence or absence of each of the six physical anomalies on every child.

The obvious conclusion from this medical knowledge is that a significant amount of the language difficulty experienced by many deaf children is in all probability due not only to the absence of hearing but is, in part, the result of brain lesions affecting language development. The problem of establishing this prevalence is tremendously difficult diagnostically. This research did not solve the problem, but approached it by using the best method available.

Classroom teachers and departmental supervising teachers were given the age, IQ, hearing loss, age of onset of deafness, and chronological age of the children in their class or, in the case of supervising teachers, their departments. Using the criterion for aphasia of "a marked difficulty with language greater than that expected due to deafness or level of intelligence," the school faculty were asked to indicate those children they thought to be aphasic. Only in cases where both the classroom teacher and the supervising teacher agreed on the diagnosis was a child classified aphasic. On behalf of this technique, it should be pointed out that the faculty of the California School for the Deaf at Riverside is outstanding, the classes are small, and many of the staff have had training or experience at the Central Institute for the Deaf and other centers specializing in aphasia.

The results as shown in Table 6 indicate that one-fourth of the children were judged to be aphasic using this criterion. When this criterion was applied to the genetically deaf where there is relatively little basis for suspecting brain damage, only 1.5% were judged aphasic (Vernon, 1969).

The professional literature has referred to aphasoid disorders associated with Rh factor complications (Cohen, 1956; Myklebust, 1956; Rosen, 1956; Vernon, 1967), but actual prevalences have not previously been established. However, until recent publications on rubella (Vernon, 1967a), prematurity (Vernon, 1967b), and meningitis (Vernon, 1967c), neither the presence of aphasia nor its prevalence had previously been reported among deaf children having these etiologies of hearing loss.

Extensive effort has been devoted to the discussion of aphasia as a second handicap in deafness for several reasons. First, language is the crucial educational variable in the life of a deaf child. Any condition affecting it must be diagnosed and therapies developed if the deaf child is to progress satisfactorily educationally and psychologically. Second, aphasoid involvements are almost invisible in deaf children despite their extreme importance. Greater attention must be focused upon their recognition, prevention, and treatment.

VISUAL DEFECTS In Table 6, the number of cases having visual defects includes all children who had refractory errors requiring glasses or who had other medically diagnosed pathologies of the visual system. Among the 113 prematures, 28% wore glasses, 4 were legally blind, and 6 had strabismus (Vernon, 1967b). The only other cases of blindness were postrubella children. Strabismus was found among them and those with complications of Rh factor. The meningitic represented primarily refractory problems.

These findings on vision are based on the number of children recommended by the school ophthalmologist for glasses and on visual defects noted in the child's general physical examination. They, therefore, reflect only a cursory survey of the visual anomalies of the sample.

ORTHOPEDIC DEFECTS Orthopedically, it is the premature infant who exhibited the greatest amount of pathology. Most conditions were congenital and included a case of only two toes on each foot, one bilateral dislocation of the hips, missing fingers and arm bones, rib cage anomaly, etc. Among the postrubella children were found spine curvatures, missing appendages, and structural defects of the legs, chest, and arms.

SEIZURES Seizures were not a major problem in any group except those deaf due to complications of Rh factor, where the prevalence was 6.6%. These cases involved a combination of marked athetoid cerebral palsy, abnormal EEG's, along with the seizures. Worthy of comment is the fact that, of the 104 postrubella cases, none were known to have seizures.

PSYCHOLOGICAL ADJUSTMENT Not contained in Table 6, but a part of the original report (Vernon, 1969a, pp. 69–74), are data on the amount and degree of emotional disorder present. Highest prevalences of psychological disturbance were noted among prematures and postrubella children. Here the rates of psychosis were 5 to 7% and emotional disturbance was present in from 25 to 30% of cases. The postmeningitic group had slightly less disturbance, and among the cases of complications of Rh factor only 12% were behavior disorders.

Bender-Gestalt response and administration of the Diagnostic Screening Forms for the Detection of Brain Injury in Deaf Children (Vernon, 1961) indicate extensive brain damage among all four of the etiological groups (Vernon, 1966, pp. 102–117). It is felt that this accounts for much of the mental illness found, particularly the impulse disorders noted in this sample and reported in other deaf populations by Rainier and Altshuler (1966, p. 142).

EDUCATIONAL ACHIEVEMENT A number of approaches were taken to determine the relationship of various aspects of educational achievement to the four etiologies, or, more specifically, to the central nervous system pathology associated with them. Written language skill, achievement test scores, academic records, etc., were all examined with the conclusion being that, as a group, children having maternal rubella, complications of Rh factor, meningitis, or premature birth as a cause of deafness did more poorly than deaf children having a genetic etiology where brain damage was not suspected (Vernon, 1969, pp. 85–89). The postrubella children had the greatest prevalence of educational failures and had an overall below-average academic achievement. They were followed in this respect by the prematures and those having complications of Rh factor. The meningitic group having a number of cases of postlingual deafness showed great variability in academic achievement.

Multiple Handicaps

Since the nature and prevalence of various physical anomalies were given in Table 6, this section approaches the same basic problem somewhat differently by examining the prevalence of multihandicapped deaf children and the number and type of disabilities which they have in addition to deafness.

The data of Table 7 are rather striking in that over two-thirds of deaf children having prematurity complications of Rh factor as etiologies have at least one other major disability in addition to deafness, as do over half of postrubella cases. Among the postmeningitic, more than one-third had secondary disabilities.

In order to place these data in some perspective, it is helpful to recognize that among genetically deaf children there are very few who are multihandicapped. For example, those of deaf parents have only a 6.5% prevalence of other disabilities. Most of this is accounted for by a single genetic syndrome (Vernon, 1969a, pp. 90–98). Incidentally, the same criteria of multihandicapped were applied to this genetic sample as had been used in establishing the prevalences for the other five etiological groups.

It is important to know the types as well as the number of secondary disabilities associated with the various causes of deafness. Those multihandicapped with an etiology of complications of Rh factor generally have cerebral palsy or aphasoid disorders alone, in combination with each other, or in combination with mental retardation and emotional disturbance. Of the Rh children having four or more major handicaps, cerebral palsy and aphasia are almost always present (Vernon, 1969a, pp. 109–110).

The premature children, in contrast to the Rh factor cases, have a broad spectrum of disabilities. Aphasia, cerebral palsy, mental retardation, visual pathology, and emotional disturbance all occur frequently as the second handicap. Cerebral palsy and mental retardation are almost always present among the prematurely born children who had four or more disabilities.

Postrubella children have a 53.8% prevalence of multiple handicaps. Aphasia and emotional disturbance are the most common conditions. Heart defects, cataracts, cerebral palsy, and orthopedic conditions are noted in severely disabled cases, and a high rate of psychoses is found (Vernon, 1969a, pp. 90–98).

Postmeningitic children have a 38.0% rate of secondary disabilities. Only 8.6% have more than one handicap in addition to deafness. This second handicap is generally aphasia, followed in frequency by mental retardation, emotional

Table 7
Distribution of Multiple Handicaps Among the Four Etiological Groups

Multiple handicaps: Cerebral palsy, mental retardation, aphasia, blindness or strabismus, orthopedic defect, or emotional disturbance	Etiologies									
	Rubella (104 Cases)		Prematurity (115 Cases)		Meningitis (92 Cases)		Rh Factor (45 Cases)		Total (356 Cases)	
	Handicapped	Percent	Handicapped	Percent	Handicapped	Percent	Handicapped	Percent	Handicapped	Percent
Deafness and one other handicap	31	29.8	38	33.0	26	28.3	16	35.6	111	31.1
Deafness and two other handicaps	18	17.3	31	27.0	4	4.3	12	26.7	65	18.2
Deafness and three other handicaps	4	3.8	9	7.9	4	4.3	4	8.9	21	5.8
Deafness and four other handicaps	3	2.9	—	—	1	1.1	—	—	4	1.1
Totals	56	53.8	78	67.8	35	38.0	32	71.1	201	56.4

In order to present these data in a two dimensional table, it was necessary to use a constant N for each etiological group in computing the percentages. As noted from Table 6, data with regard to some disabilities were not available on all cases. Consequently, certain prevalences stated in percentages are slightly higher than Table 3 indicates (Vernon, 1969, pp. 167–168).

disturbance, and cerebral palsy. When the age of onset of meningitis is early, the danger of multiple involvements is much higher (Vernon, 1969, pp. 107–109).

Conclusions

The data reported here provide factual information about the magnitude and nature of the problem of the multihandicapped deaf child. This information has great theoretical and practical importance.

Theoretically, it is now apparent that behavior noted as characteristic of deaf children cannot be explained primarily as a reaction to deafness, as has been done in the past (Vernon & Rothstein, 1968). It is instead often an interactional effect of both the loss of hearing and of other central nervous system lesions associated with the condition causing the deafness. For example, a significant amount of the language disability found among deaf children is due, in part, to organically caused aphasoid disorders, not just deafness. The same is true of other types of learning disabilities.

The impulse disorders, psychoses, and general behavioral disorders found in the deaf population can also be accounted for in part by the central nervous system pathology present. For example, Rainier and Altshuler (1963, 1966) report symptoms among some deaf mentally ill that are similar to the Strauss syndrome found to characterize brain-injured people.

From a practical viewpoint, an understanding of the kinds of disabilities and their prevalence provides a description of the educational, vocational, and mental health problem which is to be met. With the increasing complexity of our society, the greater productivity demands being made upon workers, and the fewer simple manual tasks available on the job market, the past educational policy in the United States of eliminating multihandicapped deaf children from school at an early age, or else not admitting them at all, is no longer tenable. Whereas there used to be agricultural or other routine tasks that offered these people job opportunities, this is no longer true. Today uneducated multihandicapped deaf adults and children are forced to stay at home, unemployed and out of school, living with their parents until the parents will not or cannot provide for them any longer. At this time, these individuals frequently are sent to state hospitals for the mentally ill or the retarded or, in some instances, they get into difficulty with the law and are placed in penal institutions. The tendency toward custodial institutionalization is further accentuated by the current lack of emphasis on strong family ties in our society, a trend contingent in part on the increase in mobility of our population and its greater urbanization.

This kind of management of the multihandicapped deaf is morally wrong and grossly inexpedient. What is needed are educational training programs for these individuals when they are young and vocational services for them as adults. The schools serving them would have to offer flexible, experimental approaches to teaching because the answers about how to educate these youths are not available.

Certainly, efforts to adapt existing materials developed in the area of learning disabilities to the deaf children would be a minimal first step. Vocational services should consist not only of the existing programs of the Division of Vocational Administration, but terminal workshops (Chouinard & Garrett, 1956, p. 7) and transitional workshops (Gellman & Friedman, 1965; Usdane, 1959).

The multihandicapped deaf person's dilemma today is that he or she faces a high probability of receiving little or absolutely no educational opportunity. Following this, he or she is asked to compete as a worker in the contemporary job market in spite of being functionally illiterate and deaf with one or more other major disabilities. When failing to do this successfully, he or she faces either institutionalization as mentally ill or mentally retarded or else custodial dependency upon the family. This is an indictment of public education and vocational services, and it abrogates the rights of multihandicapped deaf persons to a fair opportunity in our society.

Bibliography

Berger, E., & Melnick, J. L. (Eds.). *Progress in medical virology.* New York: Hafner Publ. Co., 1961.

Blakely, R. W. Erthroblastosis and perceptive hearing loss: Response of athetoids to tests of cochlear function. *Journal of Speech & Hearing Disorders,* 1959, *2,* 5–15.

Boatner, E. B., Stuckless, E. R., & Moores, D. F. *Occupational status of the young adult deaf of New England and demand for a regional technical-vocational training center.* West Hartford, Conn.: American School for the Deaf, 1964.

Brain, R. *Clinical neurology.* New York: Oxford University Press, 1960.

Brennemann, J. *Brennemann's practice of pediatrics.* Hagerstown, Md.: W. F. Prior, 1937.

Buynak, E. B., Weibel, R. E., Stokes, J., & Hilleman, M. R. Combined live measles, mumps, and rubella virus vaccines. *Science,* 1969, *207,* 2259–2262.

Campbell, M. Place of maternal rubella in the aetiology of congenital heart disease. *British Medical Journal,* 1961, *1,* 691–696.

Chouinard, E. L., & Garrett, J. F. (Eds.). *Workshops for the disabled: A vocational rehabilitation resource.* U.S. Office of Vocational Rehabilitation. Washington, D.C.: U.S. Government Printing Office, 1956.

Clarke, A. M., & Clarke, A. D. B. *Mental deficiency: The changing outlook.* New York: The Free Press, 1958.

Clarke, C. A. The prevention of "Rhesus" babies. *Science,* 1968, *219,* 46–48.

Cohen, P. Rh child: Deaf or "aphasic"? 2. "Aphasia" in Kernicterus. *Journal of Speech & Hearing Disorders,* 1956, *21,* 411–412.

Cook, R. E., & Odell, G. B. Perinatal factors in the prevention of handicaps. *Pediatric Clinics of North America,* 1957, 595–609.

DeGraff, A. C., & Creger, W. P. *Annual review of medicine.* Palo Alto: George Banta Co., 1963.

DeHirsch, K., Jansky, J., & Langford, W. S. Comparisons between prematurely and maturely born children at three age levels. *Journal of Orthopsychiatry,* 1966, *36,* 616–628.

Douglas, J. W. B. The age at which premature children walk. *Medical Officer,* 1956 (a), *95,* 33–35.

Douglas, J. W. B. Mental ability and school achievement of premature children of eight years of age. *British Medical Journal,* 1956 (b), *1,* 1210–1213.

Douglas, J. W. B. Premature children of primary school. *British Medical Journal,* 1960, *1,* 1008–1013.

Flower, R. M., Viehweg, R., & Ruzicka, W. R. The communicative disorders of children with Kernicteric Athetosis, Part I. Auditory disorders. *Journal of Speech & Hearing Disorders,* 1966, *31,* 41–59.

Flower, R. M., Viehweg, R., & Ruzicka, W. R. The communicative disorders of children with Kernicteric Athetosis, Part II. Problems in language in comprehension and use. *Journal of Speech & Hearing Disorders,* 1966, *31,* 60–68.

Ford, F. R. *Diseases of the nervous system in infancy, childhood and adolescence* (4th ed.). Springfield, Ill.: Charles C. Thomas, Publisher, 1960.

Gellman, W., & Friedman, S. B. The workshop as a clinical rehabilitation tool. *Rehabilitation Literature,* 1965, *26,* 23–38.

Grinker, R. R., Sr., Bucy, P. C., & Sahs, A. L. *Neurology* (5th ed.). Springfield, Ill.: Charles C. Thomas, Publisher, 1960.

Hannigan, H. Rh child: Deaf or "aphasic"? 3. Language and behavior problems of the Rh child. *Journal of Speech & Hearing Disorders,* 1956, *21,* 413–417.

Hardy, J. B. Viral infections in pregnancy: A review. *American Journal of Obstetrics & Gynecology,* 1965, *93,* 1052–1065.

Hardy, J. B., Monif, G. R., & Sever, J. L. Studies in congenital rubella, Baltimore, 1964–1965, II. Clinic and Virologic. *Bulletin of the Johns Hopkins Hospital,* 1966, *118,* 97–108.

Hardy, W. G., & Pauls, M. D. Atypical children with communicative disorders. *Children,* 1959, *6* (1), 13–16.

Jackson, A. D. M., & Fisch, L. Deafness following maternal rubella. *Lancet,* 1958, *2,* 124–144.

Kelly, V. C. (Ed.). *Practice of pediatrics* (Vol. 4). Hagerstown, Md.: W. F. Prior, 1964.

Knobloch, H., Rider, R., Harper, P., & Pasamanick, B. Neuropsychiatric sequelae of prematurity. *Journal of the American Medical Association,* 1956, *161,* 581–585.

Kronenberg, H. H., & Blake, G. D. *Young deaf adults: An occupational survey*. Washington, D.C.: Vocational Rehabilitation Administration, Department of Health, Education & Welfare, 1965.

Lubcheno, L. O., Horner, F. A., Reed, L., Hix, I. E., Metcalf, D., Cohig, R., Elliott, H. C., & Bourg, M. Sequelae of premature birth. *American Journal of Diseases of Children*, 1963, *106*, 101–115.

Lunstrom, R. Rubella during pregnancy. *Acta Pediatrica*, 1962, *50*, Suppl. 133.

Mackay, R. P. (Ed.). *The yearbook of neurology, psychiatry, and neurosurgery*. Chicago, Ill.: Yearbook Medical Publishers, 1964.

Manson, M. M., Logan, W. P. D., & Roy, R. M. Rubella and other virus infections during pregnancy. *Reports on Public Health and Medical Subjects* (No. 101). London: H. M. Stationery Office, 1960.

Manson, M. M., Logan, W. P. D., & Roy, R. M. Rubella and other virus infections during pregnancy. *Quarterly Review of Pediatrics*, 1961, *16*, 57–59.

Monif, G. R., Hardy, J. B., & Sever, J. L. Studies in congenital rubella, Baltimore 1964–1965. I: Epidemiologic and Virologic. *Bulletin of the Johns Hopkins Hospital*, 1966, *118*, 85–96.

Montagu, A. M. F. *Prenatal influences*. Springfield, Ill.: Charles C. Thomas, Publisher, 1962.

Myklebust, H. R. Rh child: Deaf or "asphasic"? 5. Some psychological considerations of the Rh child. *Journal of Speech & Hearing Disorders*, 1956, *21*, 423–425.

Nelson, W. E. *Textbook of pediatrics*. Philadelphia: W. B. Saunders Co., 1959.

Nesbitt, R. E. L., Jr. Perinatal casualties. *Children*, 1959, *6* (4), 123–128.

Propp, G. Chaff from the threshing floor. *Deaf American*, 1966, *20*.

Rainier, J. D., & Altshuler, K. Z. *Comprehensive mental health services for the deaf*. New York: Columbia University, 1966.

Rainier, J. D., Altshuler, K. Z., Kallmann, F. J., & Demings, W. E. (Eds.). *Family and mental health problems in a deaf population*. New York: New York State Psychiatric Institute, 1963.

Robinson, G. C. Pediatrics and disorders in communication. I. Hearing loss in infants and young preschool children. *Volta Review*, 1964, *66*, 314–318.

Rosen, J. Rh child: Deaf or "aphasic"? 4. Variations in auditory disorders of the Rh child. *Journal of Speech & Hearing Disorders*, 1956, *21*, 418–422.

Signurjonsson, J. Rubella and congenital deafness. *American Journal of Medical Science*, 1963, *242*, 712–720.

Silverman, W. A. *Dunham's premature infants* (3rd ed.). Springfield, Ill.: Paul H. Hoeber, 1961.

Skinner, C. W. The rubella problem. *American Journal of Diseases of Children*, 1961, *101*, 78–86.

Swartz, M. N., & Dodge, P. R. Bacterial meningitis: A review of selected aspects. II. Special neurologic problems, postmeningitic complications and clinopathical correlations. *New England Journal of Medicine,* 1965, *272* (18), 954–962.

Thompson, N. Z. Experimental evaluative instrument based on standards for sheltered workshops recommended by national institute on workshop standards. Washington, D.C.: National Institute on Workshop Standards, 1960, p. 5.

Usdane, W. Employability of the multiply handicapped. *Rehabilitation Literature,* 1959, *20,* 3–9.

Vernon, M. The brain-injured (neurologically impaired) child: A discussion of the significance of the problem. Its symptoms and causes in deaf children. *American Annals of the Deaf,* 1961, *106,* 239–250.

Vernon, M. Psychological, educational and physical characteristics associated with post-rubella deaf children. *Volta Review,* 1967 (a), *69,* 176–185.

Vernon, M. Prematurity and deafness: The magnitude and nature of the problem among deaf children. *Exceptional Children,* 1967 (b), *38,* 289–298.

Vernon, M. Meningitis and deafness. *Laryngoscope,* 1967 (c), *77,* 1856–1874.

Vernon, M. Rh factor and deafness: The problem, its psychological, physical and educational manifestations. *Exceptional Children,* 1967 (d), *38,* 5–10.

Vernon, M., & Rothstein, D. A. Prelingual deafness: An experiment of nature. *Archives of General Psychiatry,* 1968, *19,* 361–369.

Vernon, M. *Multiply handicapped deaf children: Medical, educational and psychological considerations.* Washington, D.C.: Council of Exceptional Children, 1969 (a).

Vernon, M. Usher's Syndrome—Deafness and progressive blindness. *Journal of Chronic Diseases,* 1969 (b), *22,* 133–151.

Vernon, M. The clinical phenomenon of cerebral palsy and deafness. *Exceptional Children,* 1970, *36* (10), 743–751.

Weiner, G. Psychologic correlates of premature birth: A review. *Journal of Nervous & Mental Disorders,* 1962, 129–144.

A Survey of Programs and Services to Hearing-Impaired/Mentally Retarded Children

Clark Brannan

In succinct terms, Dr. Clark Brannan explains why traditional programs either for the mentally retarded or for the hearing impaired cannot serve the hearing-impaired/mentally retarded population. He then reports the results of a survey of 212 facilities for the mentally retarded in order to assess the needs of and services to the hearing-impaired mentally retarded client.

Emerson once wrote, "What each of us needs is someone to make us do what we can." This is probably the most succinct statement which could be made on the philosophy undergirding all special education. This certainly speaks directly to those people involved in providing programs and services for the hearing-impaired/mentally retarded person.

The hearing impaired/mentally retarded (HI/MR) have been spoken of as aliens, not able to establish communication, not able to function on the same level in activities nor to have social experiences with the same degree of involvement and quality as their non-deaf retarded peers. The presence of more than one handicap in an individual produces a compounding effect which is greater than that expected singularly with each. In the case of the dual handicap of hearing impairment and mental retardation, this compounding effect is devastating because of the lack of communication skills which normally require the proper functioning of both sensory and cognitive faculties. This lack of communication is perhaps the major deterrent to the HI/MR client achieving his or her maximum potential. It is also the primary reason why the HI/MR person cannot usually benefit from traditional programming for the mentally retarded alone or the hearing impaired alone.

Background Information

A brief overview of past services, educational trends, and social concerns for the HI/MR person in the United States may assist the reader in understanding the magnitude of the problem.

There are two general types of special education services for the HI/MR individual. First are the special classes provided for the multihandicapped within state residential schools for the deaf. Deficiencies within programs for the mentally retarded at residential schools for the deaf were exemplified by the neglect of the severely mentally impaired individual (Hall & Talkington, 1970).

The reasons for this neglect become apparent when the basic philosophy of many of these schools is expressed. The student at a school for the deaf is expected to conform to the normative behavior of the hearing-impaired student with normal intelligence. The schools for the deaf, in bidding for academic respectability, have, at times, worked to the detriment of the multihandicapped person. Need the reader be reminded that the history of education of the deaf has been a struggle by the hearing impaired to free themselves from the fallacious conception that all, or most all, deaf people are idiots, feebleminded, mentally deficient, or whatever term any particular period of time happened to give those members of the human society who deviate from the average? Educators of the deaf are, therefore, sometimes reluctant to accept more inclusiveness. It is perceived as impairing their image, regardless of its merit.

The second kind of special educational service provided the HI/MR, and the kind with which this research was primarily concerned, are specialized educational and/or training programs established within facilities for the mentally retarded. Personal observations suggested that programs for the HI/MR provided by the facilities for the mentally retarded are relatively recent, few in number, and vary considerably in the range of services offered. A review of the literature confirmed this observation.

The HI/MR client does require something extra to achieve individual success. Because of these extra requirements, multidisabled people of any nature constitute complex management problems for the facilities of which they are clients.

Objectives

The task of planning for the HI/MR client must begin with a knowledge of the scope of the problem (i.e., population, program needs, staff requirements). Individual facilities cognizant of HI/MR clients within their total population find scant data to assist them in planning.

There was, therefore, a need for a valid comprehensive survey of programs and services available to HI/MR persons. Such a survey was undertaken with the vital assistance of the Research and Training Center in Mental Retardation at Texas Technological University.

The ultimate goal of this research was the advancement of the total services available to the HI/MR person through positive identification of educational problem areas.

The specific objectives of this nationwide study were to:
1. Determine the number of HI/MR clients in state institutions for the retarded.
2. Provide preliminary descriptive information about the characteristics of HI/MR clients.
3. Determine how the HI/MR client is identified and evaluated.
4. Determine what special equipment, programming, and staff are currently available to the HI/MR client.

Survey Procedure

With the aid of several organizations concerned with the hearing impaired and/or the mentally retarded, the HI/MR Survey was constructed and mailed to 212 facilities listed in the directory of the National Association of Superintendents of Public Residential Facilities for the Mentally Retarded. After the initial mailing and two rounds of follow-up inquiries to nonrespondents during a period from July 1973, to April 1974, 181 or 85% of the facilities responded in one fashion or another. Seventy-five percent of the 181 returned were usable surveys.

Population Finding

According to population figures provided by respondents, 9.53% of the institutionalized population is hearing-impaired, with 7.24% of the population falling in the hard of hearing category and 2.29% classified as deaf.

Definition of Terms

For the purpose of this study, functional definitions of hearing impairment and deafness were employed.

A *hard of hearing/mentally retarded* (HOH/MR) person was defined as a mentally retarded person who has a hearing loss but can use residual hearing to understand speech (with a hearing aid if necessary). The HOH/MR person may use oral receptive and expressive language as the primary means of communication.

A *deaf/mentally retarded* (DEAF/MR) person was defined as a mentally retarded person with a severe hearing loss who cannot hear or understand speech even with a hearing aid. The DEAF/MR person may use some form of manual receptive and expressive language as the primary means of communication.

Analysis and Evaluation

The validity of these incidence figures was jeopardized by varying definitions of hearing impairment, approximate census figures, and incomplete survey data. Percents of hearing-impaired clients varied considerably from institution to institution, though more so with respect to the hard of hearing than with respect to the deaf. The figures are in accord with other survey results and suggest that the HI/MR population is a significant one.

Characteristics of the HOH/MR and DEAF/MR populations were compared to those of the general institutionalized population. The ages of HI/MR clients, whether they were deaf or hard of hearing, were distributed much like those of the total institutionalized population. Approximately two-thirds of hearing and hearing-impaired clients were reportedly over the age of 18. Similarly, the two hearing-impaired groups appeared to be no more or less retarded than the general institution population. Approximately two-thirds of them fell in the severe and profound ranges of retardation.

At least part of the variability in estimates of the size of the HI/MR population is probably attributable to variations in diagnostic procedure. Most facilities used a variety of audiological testing procedures.

Only 48% of the respondents indicated that they had a distinct program for the hard of hearing. A comparison of living arrangements for the HOH/MR and DEAF/MR showed them to be almost identical. Approximately 95% of the living arrangements for the HI/MR clients are not separated from the institution's general population.

Whether or not "distinct" programs were available, institutions appeared to offer a wide range of educational services.

Most facilities used more than one communication method with the hearing impaired. Comprehensive, or total, communication was the most frequently cited means of receptive and expressive language used by the reporting programs, although 96 programs for the HOH/MR and 36 programs for the DEAF/MR stated that oral communication was predominant.

Although 13% of the facilities apparently offered no specialized hearing therapies, roughly 70% of them did offer regular hearing therapy to the HI/MR client.

As for classroom instruction, approximately 80% of the facilities indicated that capable clients spent at least some time in an instructional setting each day. The amount of daily instruction varied widely. Pupil-teacher ratios also varied widely, in part because so many facilities did not operate distinct programs for HI/MR clients and had difficulty providing estimates. Some reported ratios of six or fewer pupils per teacher. Overall, tutorial instruction was available in slightly less than half of the institutions.

HI/MR clients often had access to additional services which were presumably offered to hearing residents as well. Roughly two-thirds of the institutions indicated that sheltered workshops and volunteer services were available to HI/MR clients. Slightly less than half of the facilities offered foster homes, group homes, or various community programs. These figures, of course, do not reveal how many HI/MR clients actually benefit from these services.

This basis of availability was seemingly true of Vocational Rehabilitation (VR) programs as well. Whatever VR services were available to the facilities as a whole were likewise available to the HI/MR client. There was, however, a fallacy in the conclusion one might draw from these statements, too.

With respect to vocationally-oriented programs such as a special rehabilitation counselor, prevocational training, and work-study, 23% of the respondents apparently did not provide any such services for the hard of hearing client and 34% apparently did not do so for the deaf/mentally retarded client. Prevocational instruction was the only vocational program reportedly available in a majority of institutions. However, the vast majority of HI/MR clients are not clients of Vocational Rehabilitation agencies.

Some HI/MR clients who could potentially benefit from individual hearing aids do not have them. Approximately 10% of the HI/MR clients wore hearing aids personally prescribed for them. The majority of respondents claimed that HI/MR clients have difficulty caring for hearing aids. Approximately two-thirds of the facilities have access to a soundproof testing booth, but only 35% have at least one room equipped with a group auditory training unit.

There is a dearth of information regarding the characteristics of the staff available for serving the HI/MR in specialized programs. At the time of this study, populations working with the HI/MR client could not be separated from the general faculty and staff of the responding facility because of overlapping of duties even when specific programs for the HI/MR had been established.

While data on the number and characteristics of the HI/MR program worker were not available, other pertinent facts were. A percentage calculation regarding the in-service training provided the person working with the HI/MR client showed that 41% of the facilities responding to the question did not offer any special orientation to the direct care personnel.

A very important aspect of the findings occurred in relation to the number of facilities with college or university affiliations regarding their programs for the HI/MR client. It was reported that more than half (56%) of the participating facilities for the mentally retarded did not have any college or university ties in this area of specialization. The primary institution contact with the university was through student practicums. Only 22 facilities reported any research activities being conducted by the institutions of higher learning.

Conclusions

A comprehensive study of the programs for the HI/MR based on a national survey of facilities for the mentally retarded offers the concerned professional much needed baseline information. Until a target population is defined, the profession cannot know the magnitude of the specific problem. Hence, requests for legislative action, realistic fiscal support, and personnel cannot be made at any level. It was the intent of the HI/MR Survey to establish initial groundwork for the later endeavors leading to fully implemented services for the HI/MR client.

The analysis and discussion of the data obtained from the survey of programs for the HI/MR ranged over a variety of problems and needs, but the following conclusions encompass the basic findings.

There is a substantial group of mentally retarded clients who suffer from the additional disability of hearing impairment.

There is a lack of special services designed to meet the needs of the large HI/MR client population over the age of 18.

Educators working with the HI/MR client are not separated from the general faculty and staff of the institutions.

The institutions for the mentally retarded are not fully utilizing research and training services that might be available through cooperative arrangements with colleges and universities.

A less objective conclusion is that the extremely varied HI/MR population indicates a serious problem in properly evaluating the hearing-impaired client.

This problem of variability is not nearly as critical for the DEAF/MR as it is for the HOH/MR. Respondents to the HI/MR Survey and diagnosticians in general seem to have reached some consensus as to what constitutes deafness. Consensus as to what constitutes lesser degrees of hearing impairment, however, simply does not exist.

It is truly important to develop ways of distinguishing those hearing-impaired clients who would benefit from special programming from those whose hearing loss does not constitute a significant disability in everyday functioning. Relying on the criterion of functional need is no cure-all, however. The whole concept of functional need must be clarified through a behavioral approach.

Criteria of hearing loss vary, even when a standard technique such as puretone audiometry is used. Consequently, diagnosis is difficult. Until consensus is reached regarding criteria of hearing impairment, the speech and hearing specialist can only attempt to conduct thorough and periodic evaluations of clients by using the most sophisticated procedures available, by using criteria which appear to have more wide-spread acceptance than others, and by carefully documenting the procedures actually selected.

Recommendations

At present, most HI/MR clients are not receiving special programming; rather, they are an invisible group within institutions. Apparently, they receive services which are appropriate to hearing clients of the same general level of intellectual functioning. Once hearing-impaired clients are identified, they should be placed in special programs. They should have access to classroom instruction under the direction of a teacher knowledgeable about programming both for hearing impairment and for mental retardation. In addition, they should have access to a well planned sequence of physical, occupational, and speech-language therapy.

Cottage personnel must be incorporated into the master plan. A critical problem in most institutions for the retarded, as well as schools for the deaf, is coordinating the educational program with the dormitory program. The HI/MR Survey suggests that most HI/MR clients spend relatively little time in instruction and therapy. Since training of cottage personnel is minimal, it may be inferred that HI/MR clients are not receiving total programming. If the special requirements of the HI/MR client are to be met, staffing and staff training must become a priority. Colleges and universities might also play a stronger role in staff development as well as preparing professionals for successful work in the area of this dual disability.

Finally, there is a need for more sharing of information about HI/MR persons and programs for them.

It appears from the material collected by this survey that future planning involving the HI/MR client should be twofold. First, there is a need to look closely at HI/MR assessment procedures. There are many indications that misdiagnosing of the HI/MR client does indeed occur. Assessment and diagnosis must be realistically viewed as continual processes which should be included in the continuum of services for all ages. The second task is to devise techniques and methods for assisting the HI/MR individual that has been identified.

Once proper diagnostic tools have been developed, it becomes the responsibility of the special education professional to provide the appropriate remediation to meet the needs of the population.

Bibliography

Anderson, R. M., & Stevens, G. D. Policies and procedures for admission of mentally retarded deaf children to residential schools for the deaf. *American Annals of the Deaf,* 1970, *115,* 30–36.

Brannan, A. C. *Programs for the hearing impaired in state facilities for the mentally retarded.* (Doctoral Dissertation, Texas Technological University, 1974).

Brannan, A. C., Sigelman, C. K., & Bensberg, G. J. *The hearing impaired/ mentally retarded: A survey of state institutions for the retarded.* Lubbock: Texas Technological University Research and Training Center in Mental Retardation, 1975.

Bricker, D. D., Bricker, W. A., & Larsen, L. A. *Operant audiometry manual for difficult-to-test children.* Nashville, Tenn.: Institute on Mental and Intellectual Development, George Peabody College, 1968.

Costello, P. The Dead End Kid. *Volta Review,* 1966, *68,* 639–643, 714.

Darnell, W. T. *Comprehensive programming for the deaf retarded within New York State: A survey and proposal.* Albany, N.Y.: New York State Temporary Commission to Study Problems of the Deaf, 1971.

Hairston, E. Instructional media for mentally retarded deaf children. In L.G. Stewart (Ed.), *Deafness and mental retardation: Proceedings of a special study institute.* New York: New York University Deafness Research and Training Center, 1972, 35–39.

Hall, S. M., & Talkington, L. W. The Redwood Project. *The Training School Bulletin,* 1972, *69,* 10–12.

Healey, W. C., & Sontes, M. A. *Project for the hearing impaired.* Washington, D.C.: American Speech and Hearing Association, 1973.

Hirshoren, A., & Lloyd, L. L. *Bibliography on the dual handicaps of hearing impairment and mental retardation.* Washington, D.C.: American Speech and Hearing Association, 1973.

Monaghan, A. Educational placement for the multiple handicapped hearing-impaired child. *Volta Review,* 1964, *66,* 383–387.

Stewart, L. G. Identification of mentally retarded deaf children. In L. G. Stewart (Ed.), *Deafness and mental retardation: Proceedings of a special study institute*. New York: New York University Deafness Research and Training Center, 1972, 3–9.

Vernon, M. *Multiply handicapped deaf children: Medical, educational, and psychological considerations*. Washington, D.C.: Council for Exceptional Children, 1969.

Vernon, M., & Kilcullen, E. Diagnosis, retardation, and deafness. *The Rehabilitation Record*, 1972, *13*(2), 24–27.

3

Factors in the Educational Placement of the Multihandicapped Hearing-Impaired Child

Robert Lennan

Dr. Robert Lennan explains the factors that affect admission of multihandicapped children to typical educational programs. He offers case histories to illustrate his points about the difficulties of accurate assessment, appropriate placement, and successful retention of students in such a program.

This chapter reviews the variables that affect the admission, placement, and retention of multihandicapped hearing-impaired children in various types of programs and suggests administrative procedures that might be applied to deal with them.

The issue of educational placement of multihandicapped hearing-impaired children is a subject of great interest and concern among educators of the deaf in the United States today. Over the past several years attempts have been made to provide services for multihandicapped hearing-impaired children in specialized educational programs in response to the impact of the rubella epidemic of 1964–65, the increased militancy of parents of these children in their efforts to ensure their constitutional right to an education, and the passage of Public Law 94-142 which constitutes a Bill of Rights for handicapped children.

One of the major provisions of Public Law 94-142 is the requirement it carries for identification of handicapped children who are not receiving educational services and of those who are receiving inadequate educational services. The law further requires that each school district or school for the deaf submit a formal plan for providing comprehensive educational services to these children.

A concurrent development has been the national trend away from custodial institutionalization toward community placement for children who are mentally retarded and/or have severe emotional or behavior problems. This trend has resulted in increasing requests for educational placement in local school programs and in residential schools for hearing-impaired children. Previously, these children were placed in community care facilities.

These factors have brought increasing pressure on educational programs serving hearing-impaired children to provide educational services for multihandicapped hearing-impaired children. The issue of educational placement of these children can be considered from three perspectives:
1. Referrals from community agencies and state hospitals.
2. Transfers from programs for multihandicapped hearing-impaired children to so-called "regular" programs for hearing-impaired children.
3. Transfers from "regular" programs for hearing-impaired children to programs for multihandicapped hearing-impaired children.

One of the basic problems in the placement of multihandicapped hearing-impaired children is the lack of a common frame of reference among professionals in the various agencies that serve these children. Perhaps the best way to illustrate this is to cite three examples of this problem.

I received a telephone call some time ago from a psychiatric social worker at a nearby state hospital for the mentally retarded. She was anxious to have a teenage girl, one of her clients from the ward she was assigned to, evaluated for admission to our Deaf Multi-Handicapped Unit. She was convinced that this young lady was functioning much too high to remain in the state Hospital. This opinion was based on her personal observation of the girl's attempts at speech and her apparent ability to speechread in social situations with adults in the ward setting.

An appointment was made to evaluate the young lady. Our school psychometrist and I went to the hospital to conduct the evaluation. The girl earned a score of 35 on the Leiter International Performance Scale. She had no concept of verbal communication. She was echolalic and nodded and smiled when in the presence of hearing people who were speaking, but she had no understanding of what was said. Since she was already 15, we felt that the prognosis for significant educational achievement in our Unit was poor. Ironically, the girl had been attending school at the state hospital and was enrolled in a class with other deaf students taught by a deaf teacher. The charge nurse on her ward had refused to let her continue to attend the class because she felt that the use of manual communication would have an adverse effect on the development of the girl's oral skills.

In this situation, the social worker's referral was made on the basis of her valid perception that a deaf client was functioning at a higher level than the other residents on the ward. However, the social worker lacked knowledge and understanding of deafness and of our program.

The lesson we learned from this and other similar experiences was that we needed to establish better lines of communication with referring agencies. To achieve this end, we now provide the agencies a printed description of our program and our admissions criteria. We also invite their staff members to visit our Unit. These visits include classroom observations and an orientation conference with the principal and the supervisor of our residence hall program. We find this to be an effective orientation for personnel from other agencies. We also try to establish a working relationship with those agency personnel who are knowledgeable about our program so that they can serve as the liaison between their agency and our Unit.

These efforts have helped to clarify for referring agency personnel the role of our Unit and the population we serve. The clarification has resulted in more appropriate referrals.

From time to time teachers in our Deaf Multi-Handicapped Unit question the appropriateness of the educational placement of one of the students in their class and make a recommendation for transfer to a "regular" class. This value judgment is made on the basis of the teacher's comparison of the other students in the class. Since almost all of the teachers in our Unit come to us directly from a teacher training program, their perceptions of deaf children are limited to their experiences in working with the multihandicapped hearing impaired.

To help our teachers maintain their perspective, we arrange observations for them of classes in which there are children of comparable age to their own students. This affords them the opportunity to see the level of academic work being done and the behavioral expectations in other departments of the school. These observations also help our teachers in developing goals for students in our Unit who appear to have potential for eventual admission to a so-called "regular" class. Recently we have also been able to arrange voluntary teacher exchanges between our Unit for younger multihandicapped hearing-impaired children and the elementary department at our school for periods of two to three days. We feel that these exchanges can have a significant effect on teacher perspectives, on their attitudes, and on our relationship with other departments in this school.

Just as teachers in our Unit occasionally feel that their students are inappropriately placed, teachers in other departments in our school, from time to time, feel that one of their students would be more appropriately placed in the Deaf Multi-Handicapped Unit. Generally, these students are those who present behavior problems. While they function at a lower academic level than their classmates, they generally function at a much higher level than children of comparable age in our Unit. It has been our impression that many of these children have learning problems that cause them to fall further and further behind their classmates in achievement.

For these children, school is a continual failure experience, and their frustration eventually results in avoidance and/or attention-getting types of behavior. When we bring these children into the Unit for an extended evaluation, we find that they resond quite well in a highly structured classroom environment. By highly structured we mean an environment where behavior modification principles are applied and where there is a great deal of emphasis on individualized instruction with particular attention to remediation of learning problems.

The three examples I have cited indicate the lack of a common frame of reference among professionals in their conceptualization of multihandicapped hearing-impaired individuals. This undermines our ability to provide appropriate placement and services. There is ample evidence of this problem in articles by Anderson and Stevens (1970), Power and Quigley (1971), Stewart (1974), and Jensema and Trybus (1975). Further evidence can be obtained by reviewing the data on the incidence of additional handicapping conditions reported by educational programs for the hearing impaired in the April directory issues of the *American Annals of the Deaf*. The wide variance in reported incidence among programs of comparable size leads one to question reliability of the data and the conceptual commonality of those providing it.

If further evidence is required, I would suggest a simple experiment, one that this author has conducted in many settings across the United States. Ask any group of educators of the deaf to write a concise definition of mental retardation or of any of the other additional handicapping conditions listed in the Office of Demographic Studies questionnaires. The typical wide range of responses will provide ample evidence of a general lack of understanding of basic terminology used in referring to multihandicapped hearing-impaired children.

How can we expect teachers of the deaf to operate as objective professionals in their identification, assessment, referral, and educational programming of the hearing-impaired child with special needs when we fail to provide them with a common frame of reference for the basic terminology we employ? We cannot afford to continue the dangerous and inexcusable practice of labeling children on the basis of arbitrary decisions made by those who lack the basic professional terminology related to additional handicapping conditions or the professional qualifications to make such a diagnosis. This practice will continue to have an adverse effect on the attitudes and expectations of teachers and on the future of children who have been branded with the labels we unjustifiably apply to them.

Obviously, a consensus on terminology is only a beginning step in resolving the problem that confronts us. There is a critical need for psychologists who have the necessary competence to work with multihandicapped hearing-impaired individuals and with the other professionals who work with the children.

Levine (1974) presents a sobering description of the current state of affairs in this regard. For teachers of the deaf to function most effectively with multihandicapped hearing-impaired children, they will require the help of competent psychologists working as psychoeducational consultants to assist in assessment, diagnosis, prescription, remediation, and evaluation as required by Public Law 94-142.

Very few teacher preparation programs provide specific course work designed to prepare their graduates to work with multihandicapped children. This, despite the fact that 30% of school-aged hearing-impaired children are presently classified as being multihandicapped, according to the Office of Demographic Studies. Nor has there been much developed in the preparation of veteran teachers of the hearing impaired to help them develop the skills necessary to enable them to deal more effectively with these children with special needs.

In summary, then, it would appear that there are two basic problems that will continue to have a negative influence on the placement and education of multihandicapped hearing-impaired children.

The first of these is our lack of a common frame of reference in the diagnosis and identification of these children. Without such a frame of reference, we will continue to apply labels unjustly, labels which will have a far-reaching influence on the future of these children. Without some common frame of reference we will also lack the basis for coordinated planning of appropriate education services for these children.

The second problem is a lack of trained personnel: trained psychologists who can function effectively as psychoeducational consultants to teachers of the hearing impaired; and prepared teachers of the hearing-impaired themselves who can work effectively with hearing-impaired children with additional handicapping conditions.

From the administrative point of view, there is a need for criteria on the educational placement of multihandicapped hearing-impaired children in specialized programs. This requires an objective assessment of the capabilities and limitations of the program and the development of an admissions policy that clearly communicates its basic mission. No single program can serve the broad spectrum of multihandicapped hearing-impaired children effectively. Consequently, the parameters of the population that can be reasonably served with the financial and human resources available must be clearly defined. This, of necessity, implies the need for coordination among agencies that can or should serve multihandicapped hearing-impaired children. Within a given locality or geographic region, there should be a cooperative board to coordinate services for multihandicapped hearing-impaired individuals and to serve as a clearinghouse for dissemination of information concerning available programs and services. However, a lack of communication and coordination among agencies appears to be endemic in the United States.

In line with the requirement for annual evaluation of student progress and periodic review of educational placement under Public Law 94-142, it is essential to develop criteria and procedures for obtaining alternate placements of multihandicapped hearing-impaired children as the need arises. Such alternatives will help to ensure the continued growth and development of these children in the most appropriate educational setting through close communication and coordination among cooperating programs.

I have attempted to outline briefly some of the factors that affect the educational placement of multihandicapped hearing-impaired children in our nation today and to suggest some administrative procedures that might be brought to bear on them. The mandate of Public Law 94-142 to provide equitable services to these children is clear, and we, as a profession, are being called upon to meet this new challenge.

Bibliography

Anderson, R. M., & Stevens, G. D. Policies and procedures for admission of mentally retarded deaf children to residential schools for the deaf. *American Annals of the Deaf,* 1970, *115,* 30–36.

Jensema, C., & Trybus, R. J. *Reported emotional/behavioral problems among hearing-impaired children in special educational programs: United States, 1972–73.* Washington, D.C.: Office of Demographic Studies, Gallaudet College, 1975.

Levine, E. S. Psychological tests and practices with the deaf: A survey of the state of the art. *Volta Review,* 1974, *78*(5), 298–319.

Power, D. J., & Quigley, S. P. *Problems and programs in the education of multiply disabled deaf children*. Urbana: Institute for Research on Exceptional Children, University of Illinois, 1971.

Stewart, L. We have met the enemy and he is us. *American Annals of the Deaf,* 1974, *119*(6), 706–715.

4

The Effects of Public Law 94-142 on Programs for Multihandicapped Hearing-Impaired Children

Ramon Rodriguez

What are the implications of Public Law 94-142 for multihandicapped hearing-impaired children? In layman's language, Mr. Ramon Rodriguez outlines the purpose and stipulations of this landmark legislation.

The regulations to implement Public Law 94-142 were first proposed on December 30, 1976, and adopted on August 23, 1977, with considerable public participation and input. The major issue addressed by many individuals concerned the amount of detail and the degree of specificity necessary to implement the new law. Teachers of multihandicapped hearing-impaired children must become knowledgeable about the legislation and attuned to numerous interpretations and precedents that will be adopted in the coming months. This chapter provides a summary outline of some of the major features of this landmark legislation.

Specifically, this chapter will present: (1) a statement of finding and purpose; (2) an overview of basic features of PL 94-142; (3) a description of an individualized education program; (4) a review of personnel development; (5) an outline of procedural safeguards or due process; and (6) some implications for the education of multihandicapped hearing-impaired children.

Child accounting surveys—conducted by the U.S. Office of Education: Bureau for the Education of the Handicapped, reported to Congress, and cited from Section 601 of PL 94-142 Regulations—indicate:

1. There are more than eight million handicapped children in the United States today;
2. The special education needs of such children are not being fully met;
3. More than half of the handicapped children in the United States do not receive appropriate educational services which would enable them to have full equality of opportunity;
4. One million of the handicapped children in the United States are excluded entirely from the public school system and will not go through the educational process with their peers;
5. Many handicapped children participating in regular school programs throughout the United States endure handicaps which are undetected;
6. Because of the lack of adequate services within the public school system, families are often forced to find services outside the public school system, often at their own expense;
7. Developments in the training of teachers, in diagnostic procedures, and in instructional methods have advanced to the point that, given appropriate funding, state and local educational agencies can and will provide effective special education and related services to meet the needs of handicapped children;

8. State and local educational agencies have a responsibility to provide education for all handicapped children, but present financial resources are inadequate to meet the special educational needs of handicapped children; and
9. It is in the national interest that federal government assist state and local efforts to provide programs to meet the educational needs of handicapped children in order to assure equal protection of the law.

It is the purpose of PL 94-142 to assure that all handicapped children have available to them, within the time periods specified in Section 612 (2)(B), a free appropriate public education which emphasizes special education and related services designed to meet their unique needs, to assure that the rights of handicapped children and their parents or guardians are protected, to assist states and localities to provide for the education of all handicapped children, and to assess and assure the effectiveness of efforts to educate handicapped children. (Public Law 94-142 and Deaf Children, 1977.)

Public Law 94-142: An Overview

The Education for All Handicapped Children Act was signed into law by President Ford on November 29, 1975, and was implemented on October 1, 1977. This legislation contains extensive amendments to the Education of the Handicapped Act (EHA), particularly Part B, which provides assistance to states in the initiation, expansion, and improvement of programs for the education of handicapped children.

PL 94-142 was designed to assure that all handicapped children have available to them: (1) a *free,* appropriate public education; (2) special education and related services to meet their unique needs; (3) assurance that children's and parents' rights are protected; (4) assistance from states and localities; and (5) assurance of program accountability.

FREE APPROPRIATE EDUCATION A free appropriate public education refers to special education and related services which: (a) are provided at public expense under public supervision and direction, and without charge; (b) meet the standards of the state education agency (SEA); (c) include preschool, elementary school, or secondary education; and (d) conform with an individualized education program.

RELATED SERVICES Related services mean transportation and such developmental, corrective, and other support services as are required to help a handicapped child benefit from special education. These include speech pathology and audiology, manual and oral interpreting services, psychological services, physical and occupational therapy, early identification and assessment of handicapped conditions in children, school social work services, counseling services (including parent counseling and training, providing parents with information about child development, and assisting parents in understanding the special needs of this child), and medical services for diagnostic or evaluation purposes.

STATE RESPONSIBILITY To obtain assistance, states must submit an annual program or state plan. This plan must assure a free appropriate public education for all handicapped children within the prescribed timelines, and it must give assurances relating to such items as public participation, types of facilities, personnel and services, confidentiality of personally identifiable information, procedural safeguards, least restrictive alternatives, monitoring procedures, and numerous other stipulations.

LOCAL RESPONSIBILITIES For local education agencies (LEA) to receive payments under the Act, they must submit an application to the state education agency (SEA). Each local application must include provisions relevant to:
- Confidentiality of personally identifiable information;
- Assurance of full educational opportunity goals;
- Personnel development;
- Parent involvement in plan development;
- Handicapped participation in regular education programs in the least restrictive alternative;
- Assurance that federal dollars are used for excess cost;
- Public accessibility to records and information;
- Individualized educational plans; and
- Procedural safeguard guarantees.

Each state and local education agency must take steps to insure that handicapped children have available to them the variety of programs and services available to nonhandicapped children, including art, music, industrial arts, home economics, vocational education, physical education, nonacademic services, and extracurricular activities.

There are two priorities, the first being those handicapped children who are not receiving any education, and secondly, those children who are "underserved." That includes those children within each disability with the most severe handicaps who are receiving some, but not all, of the special education and related services as specified in the individualized education programs of those children.

Individualized Education Programs (IEP)

The regulations require that the local education agency develop or revise, whichever is appropriate, an individualized education program (IEP) for each handicapped child at the beginning of the school year, and review (or if appropriate, revise) its provisions periodically, but at least annually. The IEP is a written statement describing educational objectives and services to be provided for each child. Educational objectives and services include both instructional and related services required to meet the unique needs of the handicapped child. They are derived from a careful evaluation of the child and his or her environment.

The elements included in the plan are: (a) statement of the child's present level of educational performance; (b) statement of annual goals, including short-term instructional objectives; (c) statement of specific educational services to be provided; (d) statement regarding the extent to which the child will be able to participate in regular programs; (e) projected dates for initiation and anticipated duration of such services; and, (f) appropriate objective criteria and evaluation procedures for determining, at least on an annual basis, whether instructional objectives are being met.

IEP PLANNING CONFERENCE The IEP is developed in a planning conference, which the local education agency is responsible for initiating. For a handicapped child who is currently receiving special education, a planning conference must be held early enough so that the IEP is developed by the beginning of the next school year. For a handicapped child who is *not* currently receiving special education, an individualized planning conference must be held within 30 days of a formal determination that the child is handicapped.

IEP CONFERENCE PARTICIPANTS Local education agencies shall insure that an individualized planning conference includes, at the minimum, the following participants:
- A representative of the local education agency (other than the child's teacher) who is in the field of school administration, supervision, or special education and meets state certification requirements;
- The child's teacher(s), special or regular;
- Other specialists (e.g., psychologist, social worker, resident advisor, etc.) as needed;
- One or both of the child's parents; and
- Where appropriate, the child.

PARENT PARTICIPATION IN THE IEP PROCESS Each local education agency must take steps to insure that one or both parents are present at the planning meeting or are afforded the opportunity to participate. Opportunity entails scheduling the meeting at a mutually agreed upon time and place. If neither parent can attend, the local education agency must use other methods to insure parent participation, including individual or conference telephone calls. Furthermore, the local education agency will take whatever action necessary to insure that the parent understands the proceedings, including making arrangements for interpreters for parents who are deaf or those whose native language is other than English.

Planning conferences may be held without parents if: (a) a parent furnishes a written waiver of both parents' right to participate; or (b) the local education agency is unable to convince the parents that they should attend. In this case, the local

agency must record its attempts to arrange a mutually agreed upon time and place. Such a record includes:
1. Detailed records of telephone calls made or attempted and the results of those calls;
2. Copies of correspondence sent to the parents and any responses received; and
3. Detailed records of visits made to the parents' home or place of employment and the results of those visits.

Personnel Development

One of the unique features of the law is that it provides for a comprehensive system of personnel development via the state's annual program plan. That plan must include a description of programs and procedures used to develop and implement such a system. The plan must include the inservice training of general and special education personnel for instruction and support. It lists detailed procedures to insure that all personnel necessary to carry out the purpose of the Act are appropriately and adequately prepared and trained. The plan also enumerates effective procedures for acquiring and disseminating information to teachers and administrators of programs for handicapped children to assist them in providing an appropriate education.

The proposed regulations stipulate that the state's annual program plan must provide for the use of incentives to insure participation by teachers, such as release time, payment for participants, options for academic credit, salary credit, certification renewal, or updating professional skills.

Procedural Safeguards and Due Process

Due process—once a term used only by lawyers—is beginning to be a part of our everyday lives and vocabulary. Due process means the principles and practices which insure that every person is treated fairly. It refers to the procedures which protect the rights of every person. Due process has a special meaning for educators and for parents of handicapped children. In education, due process is necessary when and if significant changes are made or even proposed in a child's educational placement. It is a safeguard for everyone involved—the child, the parents, and the schools.

There are a number of specific procedures written into the law and expanded in the regulations. These safeguards include: (a) due process; (b) nondiscriminating testing; (c) least restrictive alternative; (d) native language; (e) confidentiality; and (f) the right to representation.

The parents of a handicapped child must be afforded the opportunity to obtain an independent educational evaluation. If the parents initiate the evaluation procedure, the education agency is not required to pay for the evaluation. However, the results of such an evaluation must be considered by the education agency in any decision made with respect to the child's education and may be presented as evidence at a hearing regarding the child.

If the parents request that an independent evaluation be provided by the local or state education agency, and if the agency grants the request, then the cost must be at public expense. However, if the agency does not grant the parents' request, and if the parents present a complaint, then the question of an independent evaluation at public expense may be subject to a hearing regarding the child.

Written notice must be given to parents of a handicapped child before the education agency (a) proposes to initiate (or refuses to initiate) a change in the identification, evaluation, or educational placement of the child, or (b) proposes any changes in the provision of a free, appropriate public education. Parental consent must be obtained before a formal evaluation is conducted.

The prior notice must give details of the proposed action and reasons for it. In the event of a refusal by the education agency, the agency must be prepared to identify the evaluation procedures, texts, records, or reports on which the refusal is based, and it must inform the parents of their right to a hearing to challenge the proposal or refusal. Furthermore, the notice must be in the native language of the parents, unless it is clearly not feasible to do so.

A formal evaluation must be conducted before any action is taken with respect to: (a) the initial placement or denial of a handicapped child in a special education program, or (b) the transfer or denial of transfer of a child from a special education program to full-time, regular class placement. Furthermore, any change in a child's special education placement (e.g., self-contained special class to resource room) must be based on: (a) the child's current individualized education program, (b) any other information relating to the child's current educational performance, and (c) existing formal evaluation information which is not more than two years old.

The interpretation of the evaluation data and the subsequent determination of the child's educational placement are made by a group of persons knowledgeable about the child, the meaning of the evaluation results, the placement options, and the personnel available to provide special education and related services. In a November 17, 1977, letter, U.S. Office of Education: Bureau of Education for the Handicapped (BEH) Deputy Commissioner Edwin W. Martin clarified the intent of the statement of specific special education and related services to be provided to the child. "It does *not* mean that a handicapped child gets only those services which are currently available in the district." According to regulations in PL 94-142, public education agencies *must* provide handicapped children the services they *need*. Martin also stated that other interpretations would violate the rights of handicapped children under both PL 94-142 and Section 504 of the Rehabilitation Act of 1973.

Each state education agency shall insure that to the maximum extent appropriate, handicapped children are educated with children who are not handicapped and that special classes, separate schools, or other removal of handicapped children from the regular educational environment occur only when the nature or severity of the handicap is such that education in regular classes with the use of supplementary aids and services cannot be achieved satisfactorily.

Implications for the Education of Multihandicapped Hearing-Impaired Children

The major focus of PL 94-142 is to increase acceptance of handicapped children by local public school systems. The law describes the wide range of programs and services which should be available to all handicapped children. For educating multihandicapped hearing-impaired children, these programs and services are invaluable in determining appropriate placement.

Assessment is a crucial issue because it yields information upon which the IEP and placement will be determined. The IEP cannot be designed until the child's current functioning level and learning styles are known. The accomplishment of this task requires qualified and competent personnel. Furthermore, the law is explicit about testing and evaluation.

The tests and materials must be validated for the specific purpose for which they are used; they must be used for the specific purpose recognized by the producer; and they have to be conducted in the child's native language or preferred mode of communication, unless it is clearly not feasible to do so. No one test or type of test or other means of evaluation can be used as the sole criterion for placement, according to PL 94-142.

The law and regulations require that individuals who administer the tests be certified, competent, and experienced in testing multihandicapped hearing-impaired children. Furthermore, "the interpretation of the evaluation data and the subsequent determination of the child's educational placement must be made by a team or group of persons knowledgeable about the child, his handicapping condition, the meaning of the evaluation results, the placement options, and the personnel available to provide special education and related services" (Pappanikou et al., 1974).

Teachers working with multihandicapped hearing-impaired children have a responsibility to insure that every consideration mandated by PL 94-142 is implemented. Teachers are encouraged to take an active role in meeting this responsibility.

Bibliography

Adilman, H. Teacher education and youngsters with learning problems. *Journal of Learning Disabilities,* 1972, *5,* Oct., 467–483, Nov., 25–31, Dec., 593–604.

Coffing, H., & Copper, J. Continuity in teacher education. In Devault and Associates (Eds.), *Competency based teacher education.* Berkeley: McCutchan Publishing Corp., 1973.

Connor, F. P., & Cohen, M. J. (Eds.). *Leadership preparation for educators of crippled and other health-impaired multiply handicapped populations*. New York: Teachers College, USOE Report (OEG-0-72-4121), 1974.

Jones, R. Labels and stigma in special education. *Exceptional Children,* 1972, *38,* 553–564.

Meyer, J. The efficacy of special day schools for EMR pupils. *Mental Retardation,* 1976, 3–10.

National Education Association. *Mainstreaming.* Washington, D.C.: NEA, 1976.

Pappanikou, A. J., Kochanek, T. T., & Reich, M. L. Continuity and unity in special education. *Phi Delta Kappa,* April 1974, 546–548.

Pronovost, W., Bates, J., Clasby, E., Miller, N. E., Miller, N. J., & Thompson, R. Hearing-impaired children with associated disabilities: A team evaluation. *Exceptional Children,* May 1976, *42*(8), 439-443.

Public Law 94-142 and deaf children. Washington, D.C.: Gallaudet College Alumni Association, 1977.

Public Law 94-142: The Education for All Handicapped Children Act Implementing Rules and Regulations. *Federal Register,* August 23, 1977, *42*(163), 42474–42518.

Rauth, M. *Mainstreaming: A river to nowhere or a promising current.* (Task Force Special Report) Washington, D.C.: American Federation of Teachers, 1978.

Report to Congress. Public Law 94-142: The Education for All Handicapped Children Act. August 1979.

Whitehead, A.N. *The aims of education and other essays.* New York: New American Library, 1949.

Yates, J. Model for preparing regular classroom teachers for mainstreaming. *Exceptional Children,* 1972, *39,* 471–473.

II

Providing Comprehensive Programming

A Model of Behavior Management with Multihandicapped Hearing-Impaired Children

Edgar H. Shroyer

Dr. Edgar H. Shroyer describes classroom procedures that have proven effective in educating multihandicapped hearing-impaired children. The detailed directions he offers to teachers are readily adaptable by parents in the home.

A major concern facing teachers today is that of discipline. It seems that every year the new students are much less disciplined than those of the previous year. Teachers of the multihandicapped hearing-impaired (MHHI) also have the same concerns, but the causes of discipline problems are more complex. Vernon, in his chapter, has shown that the major etiologies of deafness result in physical sequelae, e.g., brain damage, aphasic disorders, and mental retardation, which contribute to deviant behavior. With significant medical advances being made, more and more children with multiple disabilities—those who would have died in the past—are now being saved. These children present enormous problems to teachers. Another factor contributing to deviant behavior among MHHI children is their inability to manipulate their own environment effectively. Still another factor is the treatment that MHHI children receive in their environment. This treatment is often due to ignorance on the part of the significant others in the child's world: parents, teachers, and childcare workers. These individuals are just not educated appropriately to deal with the phenomenon of the MHHI child.

Many of the suggested procedures for reducing or eliminating deviant behavior are extremely effective with the normal deaf child but often less effective with the MHHI child. This difference may occur because the teacher is not knowledgeable enough about the procedures. Sometimes the classroom is not structured sufficiently well for the procedures to be effective. In order to offset such problems, two procedures that have proven effective with MHHI children will be presented with some examples (both appropriate and inappropriate). Then a suggested procedure which provides considerable structure will be presented in detail.

Overcorrection

Overcorrection was developed by Foxx and Azrin (1972) as an alternative to procedures which may involve punishment or other less effective efforts to modify inappropriate or deviant behavior. The general objective of the overcorrection procedure is to educate the individual to assume full responsibility for the disruption caused by his or her behavior. This is done by requiring the child after a disruptive activity (1) to restore the environment to an acceptably improved state, and (2) to practice correct forms of relevant appropriate behavior (Gardner, 1977).

Examples of restoring the environment to an improved state would be: having a child who marks with crayon on the walls to wash all the walls in the area (not in the whole school); having the child who breaks a pencil to display frustration sharpen 10 to 15 pencils (not to break 10 or 15 more pencils); having the child who throws articles on the floor pick up all the articles on the floor in the room and/or hall (not to throw more on the floor).

The positive practice overcorrection approach has the child who committed the error or disruptive action practice the correct manner of behaving. For example, the child who makes an obscene gesture in class would be required to recite several times that he or she broke a rule and will obey all the rules from now on.

The overcorrection procedure is a powerful way to reduce and eliminate inappropriate behaviors. It can be used in conjunction with the more structured procedure described later. In that procedure, the child is rewarded with primary or secondary reinforcers immediately after environmental restoration or positive practice has been completed.

Time-Out

Gardner (1977) defines time-out as "a procedure of temporarily removing the child from a reinforcing situation, following inappropriate behavior, to a location in which reinforcement is minimal or unlikely to occur."

Gardner's rules for what the teacher should do to establish time-out are presented below with brief descriptions pertinent to the MHHI child.

ADMINISTER IT IN A MATTER-OF-FACT, NONEMOTIONAL MANNER. There should be no dialogue between child and teacher other than directions for him or her to go to time-out. Some MHHI children will do everything possible to avoid time-out. In fact, they are getting attention that they want by acting out prior to and while being directed to time-out. When the child comes out of time-out, he or she is praised for good behavior and given a primary or secondary reinforcer.

INSURE THAT REMOVAL FROM A SITUATION OR LOCATION IS IN FACT UNPLEASANT TO THE CHILD. The teacher's knowledge of the MHHI child is critical in using time-out. A child removed from a reinforcing situation in the classroom into the time-out area, which should be nonreinforcing, must *want* to be and *enjoy* being in the classroom. For example, the day-dreaming or shy child would not be a good candidate for time-out. Neither would the child who is too challenged by the academic work. He or she may be acting out in order to be put into time-out to avoid academic work. However, with the detailed procedure explained later, this, hopefully, will not be a big problem.

BE CONSISTENT IN THE TIME-OUT PROCEDURE. "The procedure should be continued until sufficient time has elapsed to evaluate its effectiveness. If the child's misbehavior is reinforced on occasion, this reinforcement may well offset the suppressive effects of more frequent time-outs" (Gardner, 1977, p. 362).

CHOOSE THE PLACE FOR TIME-OUT JUDICIOUSLY. The physical location of the time-out period must be carefully evaluated to insure that the time-out area is void of sources of positive reinforcement.

Often, the most advantageous time-out area for the MHHI child is in the classroom. A specific time-out area in the classroom should be void of all reinforcement, not an area where the child can look out the window. Also, in the classroom, he or she is not entertained by individuals who are walking the hallways or people coming and going into the principal's office. In the classroom, he or she may feel a part of the ongoing activities. It also provides the teacher with an opportunity to observe his or her behavior in time-out.

KEEP THE TIME-OUT PERIOD RELATIVELY SHORT. Time-out can easily be abused by the teacher, who, by putting the disruptive child in time-out, is relieving herself or himself of a problem. Instances have been reported of children being placed in time-out for a half hour to several hours. This excess is not at all beneficial for the child. Usually, two to ten minutes is the maximum time a child is placed in time-out. The teacher is the best judge. All too often, a child will resist going to time-out by crying, kicking, attacking the environment, etc. However, the length of time in time-out does not actually begin until the child is in the time-out area.

REINFORCE ALTERNATIVE BEHAVIORS. Time-out does not teach appropriate behaviors; it is only used to eliminate inappropriate behaviors. For all other appropriate behavior in the classroom, the MHHI child should be reinforced using primary and secondary reinforcers.

INFORM THE CHILD OF THE BEHAVIORS WHICH RESULT IN TIME-OUT. With some MHHI children, describing which inappropriate behaviors will result in time-out is impossible because their level of communication is not adequate. In these cases the teacher firmly tells the child his or her behavior is inappropriate and places the child in time-out. An aide is usually necessary in the beginning to keep the child in the time-out area. Therefore, with the child who may not understand why he or she is placed in time-out, considerable social and primary reinforcement is needed when the child leaves time-out and has exhibited appropriate behavior. The child who poses no communication problem should be informed of the classroom rules and advised that an infraction of the rules will result in time-out. Before being placed in time-out, he or she is told why as matter-of-factly as possible.

These two practices—overcorrection and time-out—are described in order to provide some alternative behavior management techniques to implement the detailed procedure presented below. The process of using primary and secondary reinforcers is detailed from a very simple activity to a more complex activity applying reinforcement. All are described in what is considered normal stages of development with MHHI children. The teacher has considerable flexibility in operating the system but must remember that consistency in the system's application is paramount.

In-Seat Behavior

As trite as it may seem, the first objective of any teacher working with an MHHI child should be to have the child sit appropriately in a seat, assuming the child is physically able to do so. Needless to say, it is extremely difficult, if not impossible, to teach a child while he or she is lying on the floor or walking around the room. The following is one method of achieving appropriate in-seat behavior.

One area of the room should be designated as a "work area" with a table and chairs for teacher and child. The child needs to be taken to the area on a regular basis, every half hour or hour, throughout the day. The child is put or told to sit down in his or her chair. Any approximation of "sitting" is acceptable; one leg on the side of the chair, one leg in the front, hands on the chair back, etc. The minute in-seat behavior occurs, the child is "sitting," and the teacher reinforces the behavior by giving the child some primary reinforcer (usually something edible) that the child likes. In the beginning, reinforcers should be given quite frequently over a span of several minutes. The length of time the child is sitting should increase while successive approximations of appropriate sitting improve: for example, feet on the floor, in front of chair, etc. During this time the frequency of reinforcers given should be decreased. A very important fact for all teachers to heed is that they set the parameters for sitting. They should stick to the precise behavioral objective and criterion levels established. The child, under no circumstances, should decide when to terminate his or her in-seat behavior or how he or she will sit. That decision is solely the teacher's. If the child does not respond, then the reinforcer being used is not powerful enough. A minute timer is often helpful for teacher and child to see. Records should be kept to insure time increments are gradual and consistent.

Eye Contact

Once the child is exhibiting appropriate in-seat behavior for short periods of time on a consistent basis, the next step can begin. Teacher-pupil eye contact is important in all learning situations, but especially between teacher and the MHHI child. Construction paper hands made child-size are taped on the table in front of the child. The child is taught to put his or her hands on the paper hands and reinforced for leaving his or her hands there. This may be achieved over a very short period of time with appropriate approximations and reinforcers.

When the child is displaying appropriate in-seat behavior, with hands on paper hands, eye-contact shaping may begin. The edible reinforcer is used to get the attention of the child. When the child looks at the reinforcer, it is moved towards the teacher's eyes and given to the child immediately upon eye contact. Approximations of eye contact by the child are always reinforced. The teacher has to be careful not to reinforce a skill level below the higher level already attained. For example, a distance of ten inches from the teacher's eyes should not be reinforced if the child was looking at a distance of five inches away earlier. These eye-contact activities are then coupled with imitative activities.

Imitative Activities

Upon achieving appropriate in-seat behavior and eye contact, the teacher establishes imitative behavior as the next objective. The child is still reinforced for appropriate responses. The reinforcers are given either to the child immediately after an appropriate response or put into a small container near the child to be consumed later. The teacher is the best judge as to how quickly the reinforcers can be put into the container, but this is one of the objectives that should be accomplished as quickly as possible. Very simple imitative behaviors are first introduced, such as touching nose, eye, mouth; sticking out tongue; blinking, etc. All activities around the face reinforce eye contact with the child. Before initiating any imitative behavior, the child should have his or her hands on the table, make eye contact, do the activity, and then return hands to table in preparation for the next activity. The beginning imitative activities should be simple and table-oriented. The activities should follow the hands-on-table, eye-contact, activity, hands-on-table sequence. Of course, the sequence must be followed by appropriate reinforcers.

All of the behavioral objectives established and the activities to achieve them must be done in a consisent manner. Very often there is no logical sequence to activities presented to the child because the teacher has not carefully thought through the activity using a task analysis approach based on specific behavioral objectives. These two teacher responsibilities—setting objectives and analyzing tasks—along with accurate and consistent record keeping are paramount for any MHHI child to succeed. They also guarantee that the behavior will be present again at a later date if taught correctly. How often have teachers said, "I just taught that to him yesterday, and he has forgotten already."

Concept Development

At this point, it is particularly relevant to discuss effective teaching which results in some type of behavior change in the child's learning. The above procedures may or may not be exciting activities for teacher and child to plod through, but they are certainly prerequisites for any concept development that will occur within the child. When individuals learn, they do so generally in bits and pieces which are built on other bits and pieces previously learned. How much and how quickly the new bits and pieces can be learned depends a great deal on how many bits and pieces have already been learned, and how well new bits and pieces can be integrated. In other words, if there is nothing, or very little to build on, new material should be presented in small pieces again and again until it is mastered. Then the teacher adds something else which is related in the same manner.

To delve into a little learning theory, a psychologist would say that we have developed a concept when we are able to discriminate between classes for that particular concept. A child who is learning colors is often frustrated by the normal approach taken. He or she is shown several colors and told what their names are. Then he or she is required to regurgitate the name back to the teacher. In contrast, learning theorists would say to show the child several blue objects while asking, "What color is this?" Every time the child gives the right answer, he or she is reinforced for the correct response. The teacher does not point to the objects, saying, "This is blue; this is green, etc." After the child says or signs blue for all the blue objects, the teacher introduces a non-blue object and accepts the response of "not blue." Red, orange, green are not identified because the child is working on only one concept—blue; everything else is "not blue." The child is shown shades of blue and a variety of blue objects both large and small, distant and near, in order not to attribute shape or texture to the concept blue. The child is learning to generalize among objects that have nothing else in common except blueness. The teacher then introduces another color, red, and accepts "blue," "red," and "not red" from the child in developing the red concept. The process may seem tedious at times, but the child is learning concepts, the ability to *generalize* within classes (of all blue) and *discriminate* among classes (red, blue, white). The teaching of any concept should follow this basic approach.

Independent Work

It is impossible for any teacher to provide individualized attention to five or six MHHI children throughout the entire day. Therefore, a very high priority is to get the students working independently in specific areas of the room while the teacher and one child are in the "work area." This will not happen overnight, in several weeks, or sometimes even in months, but it is a worthwhile goal. Two very important prerequisites are necessary before independent work can be achieved: (1) the child has to be "hooked" on the reinforcement system, and (2) the child has to enjoy a considerable amount of success at his or her independent activity.

Up to now, the child has been reinforced with primary reinforcers for all appropriate behavior, immediately at first (right into the mouth) and then, later, the reinforcers are placed into a container to be consumed later. By now, the teacher should also have a very good idea as to which primary reinforcers are favorites of each child.

The reinforcement system can now take on a new dimension. Secondary reinforcement is introduced to serve as immediate reinforcement rather than the edible primary reinforcement. When the child leaves the "work area," he or she is given a check card with his or her name at the top and 100 blank spaces to take to his or her own desk, next area, or wherever he or she goes. When the child reaches the area and sits down, either the teacher or aide goes immediately to the child giving him or her social praise for sitting, in addition to three checks on the card, making sure the child sees them administered, and the child is given an edible reinforcement. The teacher or aide makes routine visits to each child who is sitting, giving each social praise, three checks, and an edible reinforcement. With some older children, there have been incidents where the teacher or aide spent the entire day rewarding students with checks for staying in their seats. When a child gets out of his or her seat, the child is told to return or is ushered back to the seat, is told to sit down, and then is praised; the child also receives three checks and an edible reinforcement. If the edible reinforcement is something the child values, then he or she will remain in the seat in order to get some more checks which lead to the reinforcement.

Paralleling the "hooking" of the child on the reinforcement system, which will result in appropriate in-seat behavior, is the success factor needed to make the whole system work. As already mentioned, the biggest problems encountered with the MHHI child are disciplinary, mainly due to constant "failure" in school. The child reacts to not achieving like others much more than he or she does to his or her disability. Therefore, it is incumbent upon the teacher to provide success rather than failure. Teachers often forget that their job is to teach, and the children's job is to learn. Teachers should do everything possible to insure success. They can do this by using programmed instruction materials or techniques; by never giving anything completely new to the child without also giving something that he or she already knows how to do (this is especially true with written work; the teacher should know that the child will achieve better than 60% mastery); by never putting X's on work that is wrong (leaving it without a C for correct tells the child what you want); and by never letting a child become frustrated over a task (either give the child help or move the child to another area).

The teacher's goal is to move the MHHI child slowly off of any kind of primary or secondary reinforcement, eventually resorting only to social praise. On the check card the child may have to get 10 checks before being given primary reinforcement: three for in-seat behavior, three for beginning work, and four for finishing (*not* for right or wrong). This may be increased to 20, then 30, and so forth. The target behaviors may also change, and this will change the number of points given. If the child exhibits appropriate in-seat behavior all the time, you may want to stop him or her from making guttural noises, banging on the desk, or tripping students who walk by. All of these have to be prioritized, and then a decision must be made as to which is the most harmful or annoying. Thus, it becomes the target behavior or the concept to be dealt with. The primary reinforcement may need changing from time to time. One class of emotionally disturbed deaf boys got to the point that 450 checks at the end of the week meant they would get a quarter for pop at the student lounge. In the beginning, they were reinforced every 15 minutes with primary reinforcement.

These techniques have proven effective and useful both individually and collectively. For more detail regarding the techniques, the reader is referred to the bibliography.

Bibliography

Benoit, R. B., & Mayer, G. R. Timeout: Guidelines for its selection and use. *Personnel and Guidance Journal,* 1975, *53*(7), 501–506.

Foxx, R. M., & Azrin, N. H. Restitution: A method of eliminating aggressive-disruptive behavior of retarded and brain-damaged patients. *Behavior Research and Therapy,* 1972, *10,* 15–27.

Gardner, W. I. *Learning and behavior characteristics of exceptional children and youth.* Boston: Allyn and Bacon, Inc., 1977.

Gerber, B. M., & Goldberg, H. K. Psychiatric consultation in a school program for multihandicapped deaf children. *American Annals of the Deaf,* 1980, *125,* 579–585.

Haag, R. F. A residential program for deaf multi-handicapped children. *American Annals of the Deaf,* 1978, *123,* 475–477.

Hewett, F. M., & Forness, S. R. *Education of exceptional learners* (2nd ed.). Boston: Allyn and Bacon, Inc., 1977.

Mindel, E., & Vernon, M. *They grow in silence.* Silver Spring, Md.: National Association of the Deaf, 1971.

Naiman, D. W. Educating severely handicapped deaf children. *American Annals of the Deaf,* 1979, *124,* 381–396.

Withrow, F. B., & Nygren, C. J. *Language, materials and curriculum management for the handicapped learner.* Columbus, Ohio: Charles E. Merrill Publishing Co., 1976.

The Role of the Classroom Teacher in the Assessment of the Learning-Disabled Hearing-Impaired Child

Ruth Seth Funderburg

What are learning disabilities—their causes, their manifestations? How are they assessed in a hearing-impaired child? How can the classroom teacher identify a hearing-impaired child with learning disabilities? Dr. Ruth Funderburg addresses these questions and cites the limitations of conventional diagnostic procedures with respect to the learning-disabled hearing-impaired child.

It is difficult to believe that there are so few in-depth studies of the learning-disabled hearing-impaired child. But a review of the literature on the subject of the LDHI child reveals a paucity of information on this topic. There may be, however, many studies and viable programs that have not yet been described or reported in the literature.

At the same time, many of the practitioners in the education of the deaf child have not been trained in detecting or exposed to remedies for learning disabilities in our hearing-impaired population. This is not an indictment of teacher preparation programs, that, because of time and program constraints, must limit required coursework as a result of the many classes already required for certification. It is a simple statement of regrettable fact.

Many problems which are generally attributed to the sensory impairment of the deaf child are, in fact, also characteristic of learning disabilities. These learning problems that an LDHI child exhibits are present in any cross-section of any given classroom. However, persistence of the problems and a high degree of dysfunction distinguish a learning disability. Erratic performance or an overall poor performance may indicate clusters of learning deficits. These dysfunctions are manifested in certain cognitive, psychomotor, and affective behaviors. As with any handicapped population, however, this is not a homogenous group. Rather, each child is unique with his or her own individual manifestations of problems somewhere on a continuum from mild to severe dysfunction.

Identification

According to Moores (1978), as a group, multihandicapped hearing-impaired children have suffered from a lack of systematic identification and investigation. Moores also states that procedures for defining, classifying, and categorizing the multihandicapped hearing impaired have tended to be imprecise, inconsistent, and frequently inappropriate.

Research has found that classroom teachers have been the major source of referrals and identification of children with learning "problems." In a self-contained classroom of hearing-impaired children, there are always those children that cause the teacher to ponder why the methods and materials used with the other children do not appear to produce results with these particular children. Teachers are also aware that there are some children in the classroom who are underachieving, but they are at a loss to explain why. Once the teacher has identified and referred the problem child, most administrators are at a loss as to a course of action for proper programming and placement. The pertinent psycho-educational evaluation of the child poses a particular difficulty.

The problems of these underachieving students are manifest in many ways:

1. *Memory problems,* e.g., Johnny demonstrated mastery of a task yesterday, but today he acts as if he has never before seen the material.
2. *Uneven skills,* e.g., Mary shines in arithmetic computational skills but cannot put a straight sentence together or comprehend a math language problem.
3. *Perceptual problems,* e.g., Susie cannot copy letters and words from the blackboard, but she can tell you the name of the letters and read the words.
4. *Motor problems,* e.g., George is constantly bumping into things, tripping, or playing awkwardly on the playground, yet in activities that require fine eye-hand coordination he may be outstanding.
5. *Language problems,* e.g., James obviously has quite a bit of usable hearing, according to his audiogram, but his expressive skills are poor. He is echolalic; that is, he repeats a lot of what you say rather than expressing his own ideas. He answers questions inappropriately. He can decode a basal reader but shows little or no comprehension about the material itself.
6. *Attention and hyperactivity problems,* e.g., Sam seemingly could learn far more if he weren't so boisterous and if he would only pay attention and settle down more often.

These are some of the enigmas teachers face in the classroom. Teachers are also aware that there are some children in the classroom who utilize unique learning strategies; who require a different pace of instruction; who learn at a different rate from their peers; who need frequent repetition to retain learning; who, in short, need different approaches to learning.

Etiology

Before we discuss diagnosis and assessment, we should consider etiology. The cause of a disability cannot be altered or reversed; only the behavioral symptoms can be dealt with. However, understanding the etiology does aid in choosing appropriate assessment and intensive remedial procedures. We need not study cause nor effect specifically, but in most cases, knowing the cause of the problem may help us understand the effects which are so plainly seen in the child's observable classroom behavior. In many cases, it also gives insight as to the direction of remediation.

Twenty to thirty years ago, the major causes of hearing impairment were very different. We had large numbers of children who were deafened (postlingually deaf), or who were genetically deaf (inherited deafness, mostly without major secondary handicaps). There has been a shift in incidence, time of onset, and etiology in the population. By the early 1970s, more than 66% of the population in schools for the deaf were prelingually deaf and multihandicapped (Vernon, 1969). There are more today. Neurological, behavioral, emotional, and learning disorders are significantly more common among hearing-impaired individuals than in the past. Vernon (1969), Clements (1969), Zwirecki et al. (1976) indicate that prenatal rubella, premature birth, complications of the RH factor, various pre-, peri-, and postnatal insults to the developing child, and meningitis are some of the major causes of sensorineural hearing impairment. Furthermore, these maladies cause other major physical, behavioral, and learning anomalies as well. Rubella, for example, has been linked to many auditory, visual, and haptic-perceptual problems. The rubella child's language dysfunction has been described widely in many research articles as being either *aphasoid* or *autistic-like*. In many instances, the insult to the fetus by the rubella virus not only caused the hearing impairment, but also contributed to central nervous system damage resulting in visual defects, cerebral palsy, orthopedic problems, learning disabilities, and other concomitant problems. Any one of these problems can contribute to altered, distorted, or compensatory learning skills.

Over 90 different terms have been used to describe a child with learning problems (Fass, 1976). The child with a learning handicap, with concomitant language and communication problems, has been called slow, language-delayed, aphasic, brain-damaged, or neurologically impaired, to name a few. Labels are not our primary concern. The major concerns are identifying, screening, and assessing those hearing-impaired children who are also learning-disabled. These tasks are of special concern since one handicap compounds the other and affects the entire child.

Defining Learning Disabilities for Identification

Over the years, several definitions of learning disabilities have been formulated. Most of them describe children with developmental imbalances or those who manifest educationally significant discrepancies between expected and actual achievement. The disorders are described in terms of the learning processes related to education (reading, writing, speech, mathematics, and spatial orientation). Most definitions add that the learning disability results from possible cerebral dysfunction. However, nearly all of the accepted definitions have exclusion clauses that specify that the learning disability is *not* the result of, nor primarily the result of, *sensory loss,* mental retardation, nor severe emotional disturbance (National Advisory Committee, 1966; Kass and Myklebust, 1969; Gallagher, 1966; Johnson and Myklebust, 1967; Kirk, 1962; and Bateman, 1965). We need to be more knowledgeable about learning disabilities in order to find valid ways of identifying these children so that the remediation or intervention (which is an integral part of diagnostic teaching) is carried through in a meaningful way, in a way that meets the needs of the individual child.

Hearing Children and Learning Disabilities

Environmental conditions, psychological factors, and physiological factors have been described as contributing to or being related to learning disabilities in hearing children (Kirk, 1972).

ENVIRONMENTAL FACTORS Research is continually turning up evidence linking inadequate nutrition to deficient learning (Cott, 1972; Fiengold, 1976). It is felt that inadequate nutrition may cause a child to have general lethargy, little motivation, short attention span, and poor task application. Other health-related problems, such as allergies (Cook, 1974) and chronic respiratory problems, may also be involved. Wallace and McLaughlin (1979) report that histories of falls, brain injury, and head trauma are also found in clinical records of children with learning disorders. Many more cases of child abuse with resulting severe head injuries (brain damage) and emotional trauma are being recorded as a cause of multihandicaps. Other environmental factors may include a lack of stimulation, poor teaching, insufficient variety of teaching methods, and unstable emotional and social development. Because of these environmental factors, there is a deleterious effect upon the child's emotional and social development. This deleterious effect is reflected in school learning. For example, many learning-disabled children are anxious, insecure, impulsive, and withdrawn because of an inadequate school and home environment.

PSYCHOLOGICAL FACTORS Chalfant and Scheffelin (1969), Kass (1975), Kirk (1972), and many others emphasize that learning-disabled children exhibit disorders in the basic psychological functions of perception, memory (recall, recognition, reproduction, imagery), and concept formation. In those children, sensory information is not processed appropriately nor in an integrated fashion. The feedback mechanism can also be affected. The psychological faculties are closely associated with learning and cognition, yet we still know little about these functions.

PHYSIOLOGICAL CONDITIONS Brain dysfunction (whether severe or minimal) and damage to the central nervous system have been described in reams of literature by Strauss and Lehtinen, Hallahan and Cruickshank, Myklebust, Clements and others, as a primary or basic cause of learning disabilities. Levy (1973), in his book *Square Pegs, Round Holes,* describes how the alteration of the structure and normal chemical balance of the body results in distorted, disturbed, disordered, and confused activity, behavior, thought, and learning.

Diagnosis

FUNCTION The functions of diagnosis, as it is practiced, are threefold, according to Bryan and Bryan (1975). The first function is to *categorize* within specified dimensions in order to stimulate further research about individuals who share the defining characteristics. The second is to gain a generic viewpoint of the larger population or *group* to which the individual belongs. This grouping, in turn, aids in better understanding of the individual and situational constraints. Third, diagnosis may also serve to *identify* the desirability or undesirability of certain behaviors in the individual. "The criteria used to judge the adequacy of diagnosis will vary according to the function the diagnosis serves" (p. 244). Educationally, diagnosis must be the forerunner of educational programming.

SEQUENCE The diagnostic sequence for the LDHI child in a school setting usually starts with a teacher but could be initiated by anyone who comes in contact with the child. Learning disability is an invisible handicap until behavior or learning problems begin to surface in the academic milieu. Learning is intimately tied to developmental levels, as described by Piaget's theory of hierarchical cognitive development (1950). Consequently, learning, for the most part, is an age-related function; children who do not fit the norm are quickly detected by an earnest teacher.

Lerner (1971, 1976) described the diagnostic-prescriptive process as a clinical teaching cycle comprised of five separate processes which are sequential. She lists these processes as diagnosis (which includes identification and assessment), planning of the teaching task, implementation of the teaching plan, evaluation of student performance, and modification of the diagnosis. Teaching is testing; testing is teaching. You cannot teach without testing to see how much, how well, and in what way the child has learned.

CHARACTERISTICS AND TERMINOLOGY Identifying symptomatic characteristics of children exhibiting learning problems is like identifying physical symptoms for the medical doctor. The classroom teacher is usually alert to learning-related areas in which problem behaviors occur even though her descriptors may not be in psychological jargon. Describing observable behaviors concisely is important because in diagnostics, one works with an ever-widening assortment of professional people. When a multidisciplinary team is utilized, it becomes more and more critical to describe children's learning skills and weaknesses in precise and meaningful language. Otherwise, the information may be too vague and may be interpreted differently according to the professional orientation of the specific interpreter. Behavior that arouses a teacher's concern should consequently be described as specifically as possible (Wallace & McLaughlin, 1970).

Johnson and Morasky (1977) list 12 related areas in which problem behaviors occur. They are as follows:
1. Attention—Problems related to focus of attention, distractibility, and hyperactivity.
2. Curiosity—Problems of undeveloped, reduced, restricted, or limited exploratory and investigative behavior.
3. Motivation—Problems of disinterest, lack of persistence, low enthusiasm.
4. Memory—Problems of retention, recall, and learning of memory strategies.

5. Imitation—Problems of poor mimicking, identifying relationships, basic imitating behaviors.
6. Transfer—Problems of generalization and extension of learning.
7. Incidental learning—Problems of failure to profit from nonstructured or unplanned experiences.
8. Learning facilitation—Problems resulting from behaviors which compete with or disrupt the learning task through avoidance behavior or competing responses.
9. Frustration tolerance—Problems related to inability to tolerate failure or to delay gratification.
10. Independence—Problems of restricting dependency upon others.
11. Activity level—Problems of apathy, inactivity, and limited emotional reactions.
12. Rate of learning—Problems related to the pace at which new behaviors are acquired and become part of the behavior repertoire.

It is the contention of this writer that a thirteenth must be added:

13. Language and communication—Problems in this area can be pervasive throughout the other 12 areas.

Clements (1966), in his classic research for the *Learning Disability Task Force*, sifted through hundreds of terms that were used to describe symptoms attributed to children with learning disabilities. Many were too broad or too general. Others were too parochial or judgmental. Most checklists used today contain some modification of the categories of signs and symptoms which he distilled into the following nine characteristics:

1. Hyperactivity.
2. Perceptual-motor impairment.
3. Emotional problems.
4. General orientation defects.
5. Disorders of attention (e.g., short attention span, distractibility).
6. Impulsivity.
7. Disorders of memory and thinking.
8. Specific learning disabilities in reading, writing, spelling.
9. Disorders of speech and hearing.

Kass and Wissink (1975), described learning disabilities in terms of age-related dysfunctioning. They list 40 component disabilities with the learning process and the function with which each is identified. The 40 components were refined and reduced to:

1. Sensory orientation—Physiological and functional readiness to respond.
2. Memory—Function by which experience is stored and recalled for awareness or response.
3. Reception—Acquisition of personal meaning from internal stimuli.
4. Expression—Communication of meaning.

5. Integration—Coordination of the separate components for the foregoing processes into internal representations.

One of the most important cautions about describing a child's dysfunctions using any of these terms is that any or all of these behaviors can also be found within a "normal" population. It cannot be emphasized enough that the behaviors of concern must be dealt with on a continuum of (1) frequency of occurrence, (2) duration of behavior, and (3) appropriateness of the behavior to the learning task or situation. Otherwise, the child may be wrongly labeled. The functional or developmental age of the child must also be considered. Appropriate behavior at one age may be completely inappropriate when the child is two or three years older. A relevant fact to remember is that many of these children may have a developmental delay or lag. Much of this labeling in diagnosis becomes subjective and judgmental labeling if not carried out in a systematic, professional way.

In order to carry out a meaningful assessment of a child, a functional evaluation must be made which would include the measurement of: (1) physical factors, (2) attentional factors, (3) preferred input channel, (4) preferred response channel, (5) level of cognitive development, (6) self-structuring behavior, and (7) reinforcement factors. The inclusion of all seven factors allows for a description of the LDHI child's specific characteristics which are typical, as well as those which may be atypical (Stellern, Vasa, and Little, 1976; Chalfant and Foster, 1969).

Formal Assessment

PROS AND CONS The major responsibility of assessing the specific behavior of the LDHI child should be the responsibility of the child's *teacher*. Because of the uniqueness of the MHHI child, it is difficult to assess the major handicap or the scope and breadth of the presenting problems without long-term observation (Funderburg, 1978).

The teacher, next to the parents, is the one who sees more of the child in a greater number of situations and in many different physical and emotional states, on a day-to-day basis, five hours a day, five days a week. The teacher has established rapport with the child and can work with the child in a familiar, non-threatening environment. The teacher's observations directly relate to the learning strategies the child uses: learning characteristics, attentional factors, information processing, and so on. The teacher can also describe events antecedent and consequent to the specific behaviors being observed or tested. The latter, many times, has a cause-effect relationship on the learning behavior. Lastly, the teacher is in a better position to communicate effectively with the student as he or she usually is *the one* who is teaching the child how to communicate!

Formal assessment, on the other hand, should consist of audiological, physiological, neurological, psychological, and some achievement testing carried out by highly trained, usually certified, competent professionals with expertise in specific areas. Formal assessment calls for interpretation of normative information with reliability and validity factors built in. Formal assessment also entails standardized and scaled scores.

Informal Assessment

The human organism is made up of cognitive, affective, and perceptual-motor domains. Distinct taxonomies have been written for each of these three areas; when you teach a child, however, you teach the whole child. The interaction of the parts becomes more than the sum of the parts: the child, the hearing-impaired child, the learning-disabled hearing-impaired child, the multihandicapped hearing-impaired child—the learner.

With the ever increasing numbers of LDHI students, the compounding effect of learning disabilities creates unique needs and requires specific educational services. We do not have a magical assessment tool at this time for this population. Hopefully, in the near future we will have a complete battery from which to choose.

For the reasons already mentioned, the teacher is responsible for the informal assessment of the LDHI child. It is the teacher who needs to judge which behaviors to observe; who must pick the tool or medium which best tests or measures the skills (strengths *and* weaknesses) of the child; who will collect and report facts which most accurately describe behavior and changes in each pupil; who assesses the course of each child's growth; and finally, through this baseline data, who assists in the decision-making for placement and programs which best meet the individual needs of the child.

PURPOSES OF INFORMAL ASSESSMENT There are many reasons why teachers need to assess a child (Salvia and Ysseldyke, 1978). Two of the major reasons are to justify placement and to establish instructional objectives based on diagnostic results.

TYPES OF EVALUATION Diagnosis might include one or more of the following: structured observation, probes, task analyses, formal standardized tests, achievement tests, criterion-referenced tests, case histories, interviews, and interest inventories (Wallace and Larsen, 1978).

Through the use of *observational techniques,* the measurement of behavior basically charts the child's performance in terms of quality, quantity, frequency, duration, and categories of behavior. Checklists, charts, graphs, and rating scales enable one to tally and date observations.

Teacher-made tests, sometimes called *probes,* can pinpoint learning progress and provide feedback in the reinforcement of learning. They can also identify and correct learning errors. Structured observations can supplement this approach. Many times when a child does poorly, a teacher might want to recheck results on formal subtests. This further testing could be carried out by utilizing classroom tasks where the skill is truly applied.

Task analysis is a widely used technique wherein the teacher breaks down a task into discrete steps. In other words, demands of the task itself are analyzed instead of the child's skills. Then the locking steps, rather than the product, aids the teacher in seeing at which stage of the task the child's skills are breaking down. Of course, tasks may be analyzed on different levels, such as introductory, mid-level, and refined. Task analysis also calls for a look at how the task is to be accomplished: with paper and pencil, orally, by demonstration, or through some other activity related to the task. For the LDHI population, it is oftentimes important to analyze the task in terms of the sensory demands made upon the child for processing the task. Quite often teachers unwittingly teach to the channel of information processing that is defective.

Achievement tests, though basically standardized items, are frequently administered by the teacher in a classroom of hearing-impaired children. Informally administered achievement tests can provide the teacher with some baseline information, particularly with a new student, or at the beginning of the year, or for placement purposes. They also describe the grade level of the skill which might not be a match to what is anticipated. The discrepancy between chronological age, functional age, and achievement age yields much information to the teacher.

Criterion-referenced tests can be readily adapted to identify specific skills because they describe pupil performance in terms of a specific domain (affective, cognitive, or perceptual-motor) reaching toward a specific goal. For example, "the student is able to add single-digit whole numbers," (Gronlund, 1976). The tests can be a perfect match with well-written, meaningful, appropriate behavioral objectives leaving little doubt as to whether or not the child met the criteria.

Case histories and interviews also assist assessment. Information derived from the cumulative folders or supplied by the parents directly to the teacher through parent interviews can be extremely important supplemental information. The environmental forces in the life of the child are reflected in classroom learning. Performance is obviously affected by competence, but the events and people in a child's life that the teacher is unaware of can also shape the learning behaviors of the child. The classroom performance of a child reflects the day-to-day changes in that child's life. At times, the teacher must reach beyond the classroom for understanding.

Keeping records is essential to accurate assessment. Keeping track of a child's progress is easier when records are filed on a regular basis. Many times, teachers are too close to the problems to see when progress has been made. Checking papers on a cumulative basis at regular time spans aids in measuring slow growth as well as great strides.

CATEGORIES OF TESTS Categories of tests related to their role in teaching are placement, formative, diagnostic, and summative evaluation.

Placement evaluation includes information about a student's knowledge and skills, current performance on selected measures, his or her preferred modes or most efficient modes of learning, and modes of instruction which best facilitate learning.

Formative evaluation monitors learning progress during instruction for both the teacher and the student. Teacher-made checklists are useful in monitoring and identifying learning progress. Prescriptions can be made for alternatives or modifications for teaching skills that have been found weak.

Diagnostic evaluation is more comprehensive and detailed. It determines the specifics of learning problems by more in-depth probing. It particularly focuses on problem areas while also pointing out strengths.

Summative evaluation is used at the end of a teaching unit or testing session(s) to test achievement. It summarizes in order to determine whether objectives have been met and whether to make revisions for treatment or placement. Summative evaluation is often used at the IEP meeting.

TASK ANALYSIS VS. FUNCTIONAL ANALYSIS There are two schools of thought about analyzing learning behaviors of children: (1) the ability training model or the skills sequence approach and (2) the task analysis model. Both have their merit, both some drawbacks. Chalfant and Foster (1967) propose a four-part model which includes situation analysis, product analysis, process analysis, and procedural analysis. This results in a functional analysis of the child by the teacher. The situational analysis is an on-the-spot study of how a child performs a given task; that is, approach to task, rate of work, avoidance techniques, environmental factors, and individual compensations. The process analysis (input, memory, meaning, output) investigates the child's learning circuits for tasks: how he or she analyzes, stores, synthesizes, and retrieves information from storage as well as how he or she conducts symbolic operations. The product analysis assesses the kinds of responses the child makes to a given task, such as patterns of response, their quality or consistency, their adequacy in meeting criteria, and so forth. In other words, a functional analysis provides a thorough picture of an evaluation.

Implications

The importance of informal classroom assessment for the LDHI child has been glossed over or misunderstood by educators of the hearing impaired. Teachers of the retarded, deaf-blind, emotionally disturbed, and others have employed diagnostic-prescriptive teaching (DPT) using various approaches in the classroom for a long time. It has been found necessary for securing baseline data and for planning educational programs.

With the advent of PL 94-142 and mainstreaming, the children who can function at the higher end of the academic continuum are moving out of self-contained classes and programs.

It has been prophesied that residential schools, in particular, will be left with the education of the hard core learning-disabled hearing-impaired and other MHHI children. These should not be classes of the past. We must update our preparation, teaching strategies, and evaluation skills in order to meet the needs of the LDHI individual more efficiently.

In many programs there is a diagnostic-prescriptive teacher who is not the homeroom teacher but who does all of the diagnosing and prescribing. This practice is reminiscent of training classroom teachers of the hearing impaired to teach speech and then having all of the speech sessions relegated to the speech therapist who works with the child outside the classroom without input from the classroom teacher. As emphasized throughout this chapter, the classroom teacher should be trained and competent to go through the clinical cycle. She or he is the "general practitioner" who treats the whole child. If the problem is serious enough to warrant more in-depth assessment, the "specialists" may be called in to aid in the re-evaluations and modifications in conjunction with and in cooperation with the primary teacher, who then would integrate the findings in the classroom.

Educational evaluation is as inevitable in teaching as it is in all fields of activities where judgments have to be made. It involves roles, attitudes, diagnosis, and communication skills. Unfortunately, evaluation in the classroom, as Gronlund (1976) describes it, is all too often being done as though it were extraneous to the main purpose of teaching. If diagnostic teaching or clinical teaching is viewed as a roadmap for more effective teaching and programming, as well as a catalyst for more effective learning, then the challenge has been met.

Bibliography

Altshuler, K. Z., Deming, W. E., Vollenweider, J., Rainier, J. D., & Tendler, R. Impulsivity and profound early deafness: A cross-cultural inquiry. *American Annals of the Deaf,* 1976, *121*(3), 331–345.

Anthony, J. Learning disabilities: Detection, diagnosis, remediation. *Proceedings of the 46th Meeting of CAID,* Indiana School for the Deaf. June 1973.

Bateman, B. An educator's view of the diagnostic approach to learning disorders. In J. Hellmuth (Ed.), *Learning disorders* (Vol. 1). Seattle: Special Child Publications, 1965, 219–236.

Birch, H. G., & Bortner, M. Brain damage: An educational category? In M. Bortner (Ed.), *Evaluation and education of children with brain damage.* Springfield, Ill.: Charles C. Thomas, Publisher, 1968, 3–10.

Brown, J. C. A communication model for evaluation and remediation. *Exceptional Children,* 1972, *38*(5), 385–394.

Bryan, T., & Bryan, J. *Diagnosis and educational assessment: Understanding learning disabilities.* Port Washington, N.Y.: Alfred Publishing Company, 1975, 242–322.

Cartwright, C., & Cartwright, G. P. Behavior tallying and charting. In *Developing observation skills.* New York: McGraw-Hill Co., 1974, 83–89.

Chalfant, J., & Scheffelin, M. Central processing dysfunctions in children: A review of the research. *N.I.N.D. Monograph No. 9*. Bethesda, Md.: U.S. Department of Health, Education and Welfare, 1967.

Charles, C. M. Cognitive styles. In *Individualizing instruction*. St. Louis: C. V. Mosby Co., 1976, 45–63.

Clements, S. D. Minimal brain dysfunction in children. *Public Health Services Publications No. 14.15*. Washington, D.C.: U.S. Department of Health, Education and Welfare, 1966.

Cook, W. Letters to the editor: Allergy, nutrition, and hyperactivity. *Journal of Learning Disabilities,* 1974, *7*(8), 524.

Cott, A. Megavitamins: The orthomolecular approach to behavioral disorders and learning disabilities. *Academic Therapy,* 1972, *7*, 235–257.

Cunningham, C. E. The role of academic failure in hyperactive behavior. *Journal of Learning Disabilities,* 1978, *11*(5), 274–279.

Divoky, D. Screening: The grand delusion. *Learning,* March 1977, *5*, 28–34.

Fass, L. A. *Learning disabilities: A competency based approach*. Boston: Houghton Mifflin Co., 1976.

Fiengold, B. F. Letter to the editor. *Journal of Learning Disabilities,* 1977, *10*(2), 122–124.

Funderburg, R. S. *Differential diagnosis for the multiply handicapped hearing-impaired child*. Paper presented to the International Leadership Group. Washington, D.C.: Gallaudet College, October 1978.

Funderburg, R. S. Informal assessment of the deaf-blind child. *Mid-Atlantic Caribbean Waves Newsletter*. Mid-Atlantic (North) and Caribbean Regional Center for Services of Deaf-Blind Children. Winter 1978–79, *1*(9), 2–8.

Gallagher, J. J. Children with developmental imbalance: A psychoeducational definition. In W. Cruickshank (Ed.), *The teacher of brain injured children: A discussion of bases of competency*. Syracuse: Syracuse University Press, 1966.

Gallagher, J. J., & Moss, J. W. New concepts of intelligence and their effect on exceptional children. *Exceptional Children,* 1963, *30*(1), 1–5.

Gardner, W. *Children with learning and behavior problems: A behavior management approach*. Boston: Allyn and Bacon, Inc., 1974.

Gearheart, W. R., & Willenberg, E. P. A tridimensional model for analysis and interpretation of assessment information. In *Application of public assessment information for the special education teacher*. Denver: Love Publishing Co., 1974, 91–97.

Gronlund, N. The role of evaluation in teaching. In *Measurement and evaluation in teaching*. New York: Macmillan, 1976.

Hammill, D. D., & Bartel, N. R. Teacher assessment of school-related problems. In *Teaching children with learning and behavior problems*. Boston: Allyn and Bacon, Inc., 1978.

Hardy, W. G., & Bordley, J. E. Problems in diagnosis and measurement of the multiply handicapped deaf child. *Archives of Otolaryngology,* 1973, *98,* 269–274.

Hewett, F. M. Student assessment according to developmental sequence of educational goals: Inventory. *American Annals of the Deaf,* 1970, *115*(4), 474–480.

Jensema, C. J. A note on the achievement test scores of multiply handicapped hearing-impaired children. *American Annals of the Deaf,* 1975, *120*(1), 37–39.

Johnson, D. J., & Myklebust, H. R. *Learning disabilities: Educational principles and practices.* New York: Grune and Stratton, 1967.

Johnson, S. W., & Morasky, R. L. Handling behavior problems accompanying learning disabilities. In *Learning disabilities.* Boston: Allyn and Bacon, Inc., 1977.

Kass, C., & Myklebust, H. Learning disabilities: An educational definition. *Journal of Learning Disabilities,* 1969, *2,* 377–379.

Kirk, S. A. *Educating exceptional children.* Boston: Houghton Mifflin Co., 1962.

Lerner, J. *Children with learning disabilities* (2nd ed.). Boston: Houghton Mifflin Co., 1976.

Levine, E. S. Psychological tests and practices with the deaf: A survey of the state of the art. *Volta Review,* 1974, *76*(5), 298–319.

Levine, E. S. *The psychology of deafness.* New York: Columbia University Press, 1960.

Levy, H. B. *Square pegs, round holes: The learning disabled child in the classroom and at home.* Boston: Little, Brown and Co., 1973.

Lovitt, T. Diagnosis. In *In spite of my resistance...I've learned from children.* Columbus, Ohio: Charles E. Merrill Publishing Co., 1977, 21–30.

Mayron, L. W. Ecological factors in learning disabilities. *Journal of Learning Disabilities,* 1978, *11*(8), 40–47.

McCormack, J. E. The assessment tool that meets your needs: The one you construct. Mass.: Massachusetts Center for Program Development & Evaluation, (n.d.).

McGrady, H. J. From diagnosis to remediation. *Proceedings of the Fourth Annual Conference of the ACLD: Management of the child with LD: An interdisciplinary challenge.* New York, March 9–11, 1967, 37–41.

McLaughlin, J. A., Hinojosa, V., & Trlica, J. Comprehension of statistical terms by special education students. *Exceptional Children,* 1973, *39*(5), 408–412.

Meier, J. *Developmental and learning disabilities: Evaluation, management and prevention in children.* Baltimore: University Park Press, 1976.

Meier, J. *Screening and assessment of young children at developmental risk.* The President's Committee on Mental Retardation. Washington, D.C.: D.H.E.W. Publications, No. O.S. 73–90, March 1973.

Moores, D. F. *Educating the deaf: Psychology, principles, and practices.* Boston: Houghton Mifflin Co., 1978.

Paine, R. Organic neurological factors related to learning disorders. In J. Hellmuth (Ed.). *Learning disorders* (Vol. 1). Seattle: Special Child Publications, 1965.

Piaget, J. *The psychology of intelligence.* N.Y.: Harcourt, Brace and World, 1950.

Quanty, C., & Davis, A. *Observing children.* Port Washington, N.Y.: Alfred Publishing Co., 1974.

Quick, M. A. Identification and operational dealings with language handicapped children in a school for the deaf. *Proceedings of the 43rd Meeting of CAID.* 1967, 263–294.

Riessman, F. Student's learning styles: How to determine, strengthen, and capitalize on them. *Today's Education,* September-October 1976, *65,* 94–98.

Richard, S. O. Learning disabilities: An introduction. *Proceedings of Third Annual International Conference of the ACLD: An international approach to learning disorders of children and youth.* Tulsa, Okla., March 3–5, 1966, 11–19.

Salvia, J., & Ysseldyke, J. *Assessment in special and remedial education.* Boston: Houghton Mifflin Co., 1978.

Schlesinger, H., & Meadow, K. The prevalence of behavior problems in a population of deaf school children. *American Annals of the Deaf,* 1971, *116*(3), 346–348.

Stellern, J., Vass, S., & Little, J. *Introduction to diagnostic prescriptive teaching and programming.* Glen Ridge, N.J.: Exceptional Press, 1976.

Stevens, R. P. Experiential deprivation: Another response. *American Annals of the Deaf,* 1976, *121*(5), 494–96.

Trybus, R., & Jensema, C. *Reported emotional/behavioral problems among hearing-impaired children in special education programs: United States 1972-73.* Washington, D.C.: Gallaudet College, Office of Demographic Studies, 1977.

Vernon, M. *Multiply handicapped deaf children: Medical, educational, and psychological considerations.* Washington, D.C.: The Council for Exceptional Children, Inc., 1969.

Vonderhaar, W. F., & Chambers, J. F. An examination of deaf students' Wechsler Performance subtest scores. *American Annals of the Deaf,* 1975, *120*(6), 540–544.

Wallace, G., & Larson, G. *Educational assessment of learning problems: Testing for teaching.* Boston: Allyn and Bacon, Inc., 1978.

Wallace, G., & McLaughlin, J. *Learning disabilities: Concepts and characteristics* (2nd ed.). Columbus, Ohio: Charles E. Merrill Publishing Co., 1979.

Wissink, J. E., Kass, C. E., & Ferrell, W. R. A Bayesian approach to the identification of children with learning disabilities. *Journal of Learning Disabilities,* 1975, *8*(3), 36–44.

Wunderlich, R. C. Treatment of the hyperactive child. *Academic Therapy,* 1973, *8,* 375–390.

Zwirecki, R. J., Stansberry, D., Porter, G., & Hayes, P. The incidence of neurological problems in a deaf school-age population. *American Annals of the Deaf,* 1976, *121*(4), 405–408.

Physical Education and Recreation Movement Experiences for Hearing-Impaired Mentally Retarded Children

Joan M. Moran

First describing the differences between play of the hearing-impaired child and that of others, then describing the differences between the play of mentally retarded children and that of others, Dr. Joan Moran suggests activities for hearing-impaired mentally retarded children to broaden their world and to prepare them for further education. Hearing-impaired mentally retarded children can be, in fact, must be taught to play, Dr. Moran argues, so that they may develop the same repertoire of play patterns for later learning as other children.

As each star differs in brightness, so do the children of man. Yet each serves its purpose in "one nation under god" and each is entitled to an opportunity to achieve his full potential—to adjust to his environment—to grow physically, emotionally, intellectually, socially, and spiritually.

(Molloy, 1963, p. 1)

Movement, a basic requirement of all living organisms, is the primary modality through which learning occurs in the infant and young child. Such early motor activity, or play, is natural, overt, purposeful behavior which facilitates the acquisition of neuromuscular, perceptual-motor, sensorimotor, and interpersonal skills. Play, perhaps in its purest form, can be observed in a young child who runs about shouting and laughing, jumping and dancing, seeming to be completely dominated by an irrepressible desire for noise and movement, using play purely for its functional pleasure.

All children, including the deaf retarded, engage in this natural phenomenon called play. The deaf retarded child's play patterns, however, are not performed with as much confidence or skill as those of the normal child.

Play Patterns of the Deaf

Research (Kretschmer, 1972) tends to indicate that the hearing-impaired child engages in little pure play. In fact, when compared to the play of normal children, the hearing-impaired child's play contains quicker motions and, when viewed in its entirety, more motor activity. It is less goal-directed in that tasks identified as "general scanning" or nonintentional movements occur frequently. Such general scanning movements use all of the sensory modalities, but primarily those involving the visual and tactile senses.

The mobility and space relationships of the hearing-impaired child may be very poorly developed. In addition, these children may exhibit fears, anxieties, or inhibitions about moving freely in space. Such feelings are frequently reinforced because of past motor errors, lack of experience, or lack of learning opportunities. Wandering behavior may frequently result from this lack of experience or learning opportunity. This lack may cause the child to wander about, seeming lost in the situation, and not knowing how to play. The end result may be a physical expression of frustration in the form of temper tantrums (Mindel & Vernon, 1971).

As a group, hearing-impaired children are immature in their exploratory techniques; they avoid free and spontaneous activity; and they tend not to use make-believe play or subject substitutions in their play. The child who has received early auditory training will, however, usually have higher levels of skill in constructive play and dramatic play as compared to the child who has not received such early training. Games with rules, especially when verbal concept skills are involved, may also be difficult for these children.

The hearing-impaired child's motor performance is significantly lower than that of normal children (Vance, 1968). Balance may be poor if damage has occurred in the semicircular canals, and swimming would be contraindicated if the child has had a fenestration operation.

As a group, hearing-impaired children are less cohesive and make fewer successful social contacts in their play than their normal counterparts, relying on gesturing as a communication device. They attempt less interaction with peers; they respond less often to peers; they vocalize less; and they are less self-directed and more self-attentive. This lack of socialization is directly proportional to the degree of hearing loss experienced by the child. Because hearing-impaired children may have fewer opportunities to learn through early experimental play with other children, they are frequently reluctant to enter group settings (Mindel & Vernon, 1971; Kretschmer, 1972).

Play Patterns of the Mentally Retarded

The mentally retarded child is not as creative or imaginative in play as his or her normal counterpart. The child cannot be turned loose and be expected to use equipment properly or to participate in normal activities with contemporaries of the same chronological age. The mentally retarded child's play may be slow-moving, clumsy, and sedentary, or extremely hyperactive. Frequently, his or her play patterns are random and unimaginative. Because of this lack of creativity in movement, he or she tends to follow set patterns of activity as prescribed by the play materials provided.

Mentally retarded children at play usually perform at an age level of complexity commensurate not with their chronological age but rather their mental age. This incapacity is reflected in both their play performance and social behavior. They may lack the ability to use toys appropriately, show little awareness of the function of each toy, and have no inventiveness or variety in the use of toys.

If the child's mental retardation is the result of brain damage, he or she may exhibit hyperactivity, perseveration, poor motor control, social ineptness, overreaction to minutiae, and a variety of speech difficulties. Some mentally retarded children are subject to excessive and useless movements, while others exhibit diminished mobility or muscular asthenia. The failure of these children to keep intellectual pace with their normal peers can contribute to personality maladjustment and to the development of undesirable behavior patterns. A lack of emotional stability is frequently exhibited in competitive play and in circumstances in which more is expected of them than they are capable of delivering. Such instability usually manifests itself in expressions of fear and aggression. Or aggression may be an attempt to cover weakness, to demonstrate worth, to attract attention, or to relieve tension. Rebellious acts and other undesirable behavior can be similarly motivated. Occasionally, the mentally retarded child may use the handicap as a protective shield or as a means of obtaining sympathy to compensate for the lack of social acceptance (Moran & Kalakian, 1977).

Play Patterns of the Deaf Retarded

When one analyzes the play patterns of the deaf or hearing-impaired child and those of the mentally retarded child, numerous similarities are evident. One can assume from these similarities that the deaf retarded child may lack adequate play experiences and may exhibit immature play patterns. These children may even lack the ability to play. Lack of cooperation and undesirable behavior may be exhibited in group situations. The play patterns of the deaf retarded child will, in all probability, develop at a slower rate than that of normal counterparts. Generally, the lower the child's IQ, the greater are the concomitant social and emotional problems. Such a child usually needs extensive stimulation for the development of both communication and motor skills.

The deviations exhibited in the play patterns of deaf retarded children will be directly related to the degree of hearing loss and mental retardation. In addition, because all of these children may differ widely in both degree of hearing loss and level of intelligence, no preconceived baseline of behavioral, developmental, or educational standards can be assumed. Consequently, a valid assessment of the child's functional level may be difficult. Each and every deaf retarded child must, therefore, be considered as a unique individual with a potentially variable developmental level.

These children must be taught, at as young an age as possible, how to play. They need to be taught the skills of individual play, parallel play, and especially group play. Such early play experiences, if they contain appropriate sensorimotor stimulation, can have a crucial and positively facilitating effect on the total development of the children, helping them acquire those skills needed for later integration into activity with nonhandicapped peers.

Instructional Considerations

If the play experiences taught to the deaf retarded child are to be beneficial, they must provide adequate auditory stimulation; they must be geared to the optimum arousal level of the child; and they must be appropriately structured to meet the physical, mental, social, and emotional development of the child. Program diversity and individualized goals that maximize physical achievement and produce immediate results are essential to insure that each child will have successful experiences. Play experiences should be highly structured, occur in an atmosphere that is genuinely warm and cordial, and contain the developmental activities needed by the child. Free play and socially centered programming should be avoided until the acquisition of social, physical, and behavioral skills by the child are adequate for enjoyable and successful participation in such activity. Because of their incomprehensibility, complex games should be avoided. If they are not, the deaf retarded child may display anger and aggressiveness in addition to unsportsmanlike conduct.

The child should be guided, encouraged, and motivated in activities that have meaning and importance to him or her. Interest should be aroused and maintained. Inactivity or boredom should be avoided by keeping the activity snappy and lively and by utilizing a wide variety of stimulation to all of the various sense modalities. Language should be paired with movement. Emphasis should be placed on utilizing the child's remaining sensory modalities. Simple auditory stimulation in the form of verbal phrases should be combined with visual, tactile, and kinesthetic movement cues to facilitate understanding on the part of the child. Activity choice should help the deaf retarded child learn to discriminate between and organize the various sensory stimuli used in instruction. It should be kept in mind that activity should be stopped at a high point of enthusiasm, before frustration or inability to perform occurs.

Firm discipline which the child is capable of understanding must be established, especially when a hazard is involved. The child should always know the limits imposed on his or her activity, and the teacher should be firm in this regard, especially when the child attempts to stretch these limits.

In addition to teaching to the child's needs, abilities, and level of readiness, the teacher must discover and utilize those methods which facilitate responses in the child. The tasks to be presented to the deaf retarded child must be analyzed carefully. Such tasks or play skills taught must be presented sequentially. In addition, each skill should be broken down into its smallest components. Much repetition will be necessary, and tangible or intangible rewards may be essential if learning is to be reinforced.

The teacher should keep in mind that misunderstanding can contribute to undesirable behavior on the part of the deaf retarded child. Play activities, therefore, should be selected and designed to channel any deviant behavior exhibited by the child. This is especially necessary for the child who exhibits defiance, aggression, hyperactivity, or boisterousness. With highly aggressive children, contact activity should be avoided. Appropriate behavior exhibited by the child should be reinforced, and inappropriate behavior should be ignored. If behavior modification is used, a consistent and total system should be used by all staff having contact with the child.

A developmental teaching approach geared to the functional and intellectual level of the child is ideal. Such an approach encompasses small, sequential, and concrete steps. In addition, the mental and emotional age of the child should be considered when toys and skills are selected for play. If toys are too fragile or the skills too refined for the child's chronological age and developmental level, success in play may be impossible without injury to the child or the toys. Sturdy equipment may, of necessity, have to be improvised for older, stronger, immature deaf retarded children to insure success.

The teacher should focus on the uniqueness, complexity, and developmental diversity of each child. The teacher must be aware of the child's inner world, emotional needs, and environmental problems. (See also Chapter 17, Hammer.) Teaching methods should be simple, open ended, and flexible. Methods must be constantly changing to meet the uniqueness of the child's current needs. They should reflect teacher sensitivity, adaptability, innovativeness, and creativity. Methods used should have a highly personal, artistic quality combining sound judgment, good taste, and individual intuition.

Methods of arousing interest and motivation might include the use of visual aids, such as simple, colorful pictures for the introduction of a new skill. Other stimuli that facilitate response on the part of the child to the environment should precede or accompany the activity. Praise should be offered generously for the child's efforts. Purpose should be given to movement, and the element of fun should be ever present. Careful demonstrations and clear, concise explanations should be used by the teacher, and she or he should face the child when speaking. These methods should be combined with patience and much repetition.

The teacher must possess patience, empathy, a sense of humor, and an appreciative commitment to the child as an individual of worth and dignity who can progress, achieve, and succeed. In addition, the teacher should rely only minimally on verbalization in promoting behavior change, especially in the initial stages. If verbal commands are used, comprehension on the part of the child is essential. To ensure understanding, it may be necessary to have the child repeat the command before he or she is expected to execute the movement. The results of such structured experiences will be wholesome, vigorous activity and its accompanying physical development and spirit of fun.

The Development of Play Skills

The first developmental level of play is classified as individual play in which the child amuses himself. This play is usually free, spontaneous, and solitary. It may be necessary to teach the deaf retarded child the simple skills of individual play involving visual exploration, grasping objects, manipulating objects, crawling, creeping, walking, and running.

VISUAL EXPLORATION, GRASPING, AND MANIPULATING OBJECTS Simple play toys, such as five- and six-piece animal puzzles, five- and six-piece color and shape recognition puzzles, hammer peg sets, creative building blocks, interlocking toys (such as Krazee Klowns), screwing toys (such as nuts and bolts or Kitty in the Kegs), and stack color and size sets, can be used to teach the child the basic skills of visual exploration, grasping, and manipulating objects. The child should be taught these skills on a one-to-one basis. Many deaf retarded children may need more than a demonstration in how to complete these tasks. It may be necessary to guide their hands through the skills, at least the first few times they are attempted.

The individual play skills of crawling, creeping, walking, and running are considered natural and alternate gross motor skills. They are used as transportation patterns by children to mobilize their exploration of space as they search and discover the environment.

CRAWLING AND CREEPING Crawling, or forward motion on the stomach, involves the entire body in contact with a surface. During creeping, the trunk is elevated, the child assumes a quadrupedal stance, and forward motion occurs on the hands and knees. Both crawling and creeping should involve smooth, coordinated, alternate movements, with the right hand and left leg working simultaneously, and the left hand and right leg following in the same manner.

Crawling precedes creeping developmentally. Prerequisite to crawling, the deaf retarded child must be able to raise his or her head and chest. Such elevation, if not present, can be facilitated by use of a padded barrel or similar device on which the child should be placed face down on his or her tummy, following the contour of the barrel. The hands will naturally fall forward away from the head and chest. This natural positioning stimulates the head and chest elevation position. For additional stimulation, the barrel should be rolled slowly forward and backward. As the barrel rolls forward the child will often initiate some head elevation in righting reflex fashion. To facilitate further head elevation, the child might be encouraged visually to spot some attractive stimulus placed on the floor in front of him or her. As the barrel rolls forward, the child is encouraged to elevate his or her head so as not to lose sight of that stimulus.

Once head and chest elevation has been achieved, the arm and shoulder strength and muscular coordination necessary for crawling must be developed. A scooter board can improve these capabilities in the deaf retarded child. The child should be placed stomach down on the scooter board with the arms forward in crawling position. Teacher assistance of holding alternately the child's left hand, then right hand, firmly to the crawling surface may be necessary. Such assistance serves the two-fold purpose of providing a kinesthetic cue and preventing the hand from slipping back toward the scooter board. With practice and decreasing assistance, the child will eventually be able to pull the scooter board forward in crawling fashion. When this feat has been mastered, the child is ready to crawl on the floor, with and without teacher assistance.

As trunk, arm, and leg strength develop, the child gradually moves from crawling into creeping. Practice in both of these skills can be achieved through the use of crawl tunnels. An obstacle course is another excellent device to add variety and challenge to the exercise of these skills.

WALKING Walking normally and naturally is an extremely vital skill for the deaf retarded child to learn. The public has stereotyped the ways in which it believes handicapped individuals are supposed to look. Unfortunately, the more deviant one looks, the less likely are one's chances of success among normal peers. The deaf retarded individuals whose posture or carriage fit the stereotype may find themselves encountering unwarranted discrimination and rejection.

A variety of techniques can be used to develop skill in walking. Rhythm can be developed by using a treadmill placed at a slight upward angle and run at a slow speed. A harness should be used to hold the child securely as he or she holds onto the handrails and practices walking.

Colored footprints with matching colored ribbons tied around the ankles can be used to develop skill in foot placement. This task can be made more difficult by placing a rope between the footprints for the child to lift his or her feet over. Or a ladder can be placed flat on the floor for the child to use as practice in lifting the feet. If necessary, colored footprints can be added to this task.

A coordinated arm swing can be developed by using long wands or broom handles. With the child in front of the teacher, both the child and teacher should hold opposite ends of a wand, one in each hand. The teacher can control the child's arm action by pushing the appropriate wand forward as the child walks.

RUNNING After the child has developed skill in walking, he or she should be taught to run. The tempo of the walk should be increased, with and then without the teacher assisting the child by holding one hand.

Because the stride of a run is greater than that of the walk, colored footprints placed an increasing distance apart may stimulate increasing the length of the child's stride. Manipulation of the arms and legs into the correct bent positions may be necessary. The child can be encouraged to run silently on the toes, or down an incline, with much teacher encouragement. Or the teacher can run behind the child and give frequent, small pushes on the back or arm to encourage faster motion.

Additional individual play skills which should be developed in the deaf retarded child as he or she is developing skill in the manipulation and exploration of the environment consist of imitative play, creative play, and fantasy play.

Imitative Play

Imitative play provides the deaf retarded child with opportunity to practice adult skills without excessive censure or fear of failure. It provides a socially acceptable outlet in which to act out anxieties and conflicts; it contributes to social maturity; and it promotes within the child an effective interaction with the environment. The proper selection of toys and play objects, combined with good demonstrations, can facilitate the development of imitative play skills. The child can learn to imitate animals, pretend to be a mother feeding her baby, talk on a play telephone, or imitate any other commonly observed activity in the environment. With patience, repetition, and practice, the deaf retarded child can and will learn to be imaginative in his or her play patterns.

Creative Play

Imitative play, the precursor of creativity, increases the child's insight and sensitivity, thus facilitating the development of creative play skills. Creative play or thoughtful, exploratory play with materials, objects, feelings, and ideas, occurs as the child manipulates these materials giving them meaning and purpose to convey or fulfill his or her intent. In addition, creative play encourages learning through exploration, experimentation, manipulation, and transformation as it develops curiosity, flexibility, improvisation, commitment, and the courage to risk. The creative process can be nurtured in the deaf retarded child if he or she is provided with rich and varied sensory input, sensory stimuli, and kinesthetic experiences. To encourage creative play, therefore, the child should be offered a stimulating and varied play milieu including easily accessible toys, raw materials, and physical objects which engage the senses. Additionally, the child should be provided meaningful contacts with accepting adults and then allowed private time to assimilate these experiences in solitary play.

Fantasy Play

The play acting of fantasy provides the deaf retarded child with concrete methods for the expression of fears, hopes, and needs. It is a safe and secure means for fulfilling those desires he or she cannot or dare not express in words, thus facilitating adjustment to difficult life experiences. Paints, clay, sand, and water are useful media for fantasy play. They can be used by the child symbolically as a means of expression. Teacher sensitivity and acceptance is an essential element in fantasy play if the deaf retarded child is to feel secure and unthreatened enough to express himself or herself fully. Ultimately, fantasy play should enable the child to be completely expressive without feeling ashamed or guilty, thus resolving interpersonal conflicts and emotional tensions in a socially acceptable manner.

Parallel and Group Play

As the deaf retarded child develops skill in isolated individual play, a socialization system develops, and parallel play skills begin to appear. Parallel play, or activity in which the child plays beside (rather than with) other children, sharing the same physical environment, but, for the most part, playing independently, is an important developmental forerunner of group play skills. If deaf retarded children are grouped for play experiences with any success, they should be of approximately the same developmental level mentally, physically, emotionally, and socially. Later play experiences can involve children of differing developmental levels if care is taken regarding the placement of destructive or highly emotional children.

Group, or interactive play, begins to emerge in the parallel play environment as the deaf retarded child begins to relate to his or her age mates. If the child lacks skill in group play, he or she should be taught how to share play items in a cooperative effort, first with only one child, and then in increasingly larger groups. After cooperative partner and group play skills are acquired, partner and then group competitive activities should be introduced.

Once the deaf retarded child has mastered those play skills, he or she is ready to begin participation in a number of increasingly difficult activities designed to provide wholesome development and the spirit of fun. The ultimate goal, of course, is integration of the child back into the mainstream of life with nonhandicapped peers.

Bibliography

Kretschmer, R. R. *A study to assess the play activities and gesture output of hearing handicapped pre-school children: Final report.* Cincinnati: Cincinnati Speech and Hearing Center, 1972.

Mindel, E. D., & Vernon, M. *They grow in silence: The deaf child and his family.* Washington, D.C.: National Association of the Deaf, 1971.

Molloy, J. S. *Trainable children: Curriculum and procedures.* New York: John Day Co., 1963.

Moran, J. M., & Kalakian, L. H. *Movement experiences for the mentally retarded or emotionally disturbed child* (2nd ed.). Minneapolis: Burgess Publishing Co., 1977.

Vance, P. C. *Motor characteristics of deaf children.* Unpublished doctoral dissertation, Colorado State College, 1968.

Suggested Readings

Anderson, R. M., & Stevens, G. D. Deafness and mental retardation in children: The problem. *American Annals of the Deaf,* 1969, *114,* 15–22.

Benoit, E. P. The play problems of retarded children. *American Journal of Mental Deficiency,* 1955, *60,* 41–55.

Francis, R. J., & Rarick, G. L. Motor characteristics of the mentally retarded. *American Journal of Mental Deficiency,* 1959, *63,* 792–811.

Leland, H., & Smith, D. *Play therapy with mentally subnormal children.* New York: Grune and Stratton, 1965.

McDermott, E. F. Free play—A pleasurable learning experience. *Volta Review,* 1970, *72,* 541–543.

Sessoms, H. D. The mentally handicapped child grows at play. *Mental Retardation,* 1965, *8,* 12–14.

Takata, N. The play history. *American Journal of Occupational Therapy,* 1969, *23,* 314–318.

Truax, C. B., & Carkhuff, R. R. *Toward effective counseling and psychotherapy: Training and practice.* Hawthorne, N.Y.: Aldine Publishing Co., Inc., 1967.

Wisher, P. R. Dance and the deaf. *Journal of Health, Physical Education, and Recreation,* 1969, 40–81.

Wisher, P. R. Status of physical education for the hearing impaired. In *Physical education and recreation for handicapped children: Proceedings of a study conference on research and demonstration needs.* Washington, D.C.: American Alliance of Health, Physical Education, and Recreation and National Recreation and Park Association, 1969.

Remedial Strategies for Age-Related Characteristics of Learning Disability

Corinne E. Kass

Dr. Corinne Kass defines learning disabilities as deviations from the norms for acquisition and use of symbols. Consequently, she asserts, learning disabilities can be treated as age-related developmental deficits. Her paper describes typical developmental deficits in multihandicapped hearing-impaired children and suggests remedies for these deficits.

Learning disability is characterized by extreme deviance in the acquisition and use of symbols in reading, writing, computing, listening, or talking. What separates learning disability from other handicaps is that the deviance is due to specific deficits in age-related developmental functions. These deficits require remedial techniques and may interact with environmental or other handicapping conditions.

The following paragraphs will describe some critical deficits by developmental function. Strategies for treatment are given for each deficit area.

Sensory Orientation Function

This function, which occurs from birth to 18 months of age, may be defined as the physiological or functional readiness of the child to respond to the environment. During this state, the child deals with the environment on a sensorimotor basis. After spoken language is acquired, the human being cannot return to this manner of interaction with the environment and be considered normal. Some deficits shown by the learning disabled are the following:

VISUAL PURSUIT This is the ability to follow stimuli with the eyes. Related to this is the discrimination of the familiar from the unfamiliar. Right from birth, it appears that infants with learning disability, while not blind, do not use their eyes as do normal infants. The learning disabled either look at anything and everything without really discriminating, or they drop their eyes often. It was noted in one study (Schnorr, 1976) that parents, when asked to remember what their learning-disabled children were like when they were babies, stated that they were not afraid of strangers. We can interpret this to mean that they did not recognize unfamiliarity.

Remediation should be initiated immediately when an infant does not study objects and people visually. The infant should be handled a great deal to establish physical contact, should be talked to eyeball to eyeball, and a flashlight, ball, or finger should be presented to the child to look at and then moved while the child is watching.

BODY BALANCE This is the ability to maintain equilibrium. In the infant, the vestibular system is closely related to oral and tactile sensations. Normally, the infant can tolerate much more movement than can the adult who may suffer motion sickness. Ayres (1968) suggests that lack of vestibular reflex is the basis of later school learning problems. While the normal baby, when held under the tummy, will arch up head and legs, some babies do not. Should this problem occur, remediation would include rocking the baby a great deal and swinging the baby inside a blanket held hammock-like.

AUDITORY DISCRIMINATION This is the ability to react differentially to sound stimuli. This deficit may be the basis for disturbances in attention commonly attributed to the learning disabled. There are some children who are not deaf, but who show abnormal reactions to sounds, including speech. These reactions are usually revealed in supersensitivity or passivity. The learning disabled appear to pick up enough from speech sounds so that they are able to score within the normal range on a verbal intelligence test. However, the affective aspect may be deficient during the early months when the parent-child relationship is the most important. Irritability, distractibility, and restlessness are symptoms which most probably interfere with normal auditory discrimination.

Remediation for auditory discrimination problems should focus on meaningful sounds (mainly speech). Make noises at various distances from the infant, and call for reactions such as looking, smiling, sudden turning of the head, or verbal responses. The infant's name should be used often to call attention to the person saying the name. Time should be given the infant for responding to sounds, since they usually do not respond while the adult is making sounds, but respond later. Watch for the latency period while the infant appears to be practicing internally, and encourage the final response. Babbling of the infant should be imitated by the adult as encouragement and for shaping the babbling into correct sounds. Simple directions, such as "come here," "take it," "eat it," "say ball," should be repeated again and again until the infant uses verbal directions for self-instruction. A proper foundation in auditory discrimination will lead to later phonic skills.

Memory Function

This function is present from 18 months to 8 years of age and is defined as the ability to reproduce sensory impressions when the stimuli which initially aroused the sensory impressions are no longer externally present. While memory is usually thought of as a process which undergoes developmental changes from infancy to adulthood, it is here defined only in its purest, or narrowest, form; that is, without the overlay of complex comprehension. After age eight, mnemonic aids and context are important. Before that age, memory appears to be more straightforward. It is well known that young children can acquire another language with more facility than older people. It is during this sensitive period that the symbol systems of letters and numbers are learned. The learning disabled have difficulty with this learning due to the following deficits:

HYPEREXCITABILITY This is the inability to control one's own reactions to stimuli, both external and internal. There is diminished input as a result. The hyperexcitability of the learning disabled appears to be internal noise, and what triggers this noise is not obvious from the external situation. In fact, while normal children can "work off steam" by running around a bit, the learning disabled seem merely to become more "revved up." Because of this deficit, the learning disabled often cannot pay attention. Their behavior is irrelevant.

Remediation requires competing with the internal stimulation of the child. Whatever we wish the child to attend to must be of such an intensity as to capture the attention. In the past, it was typical to take all extraneous stimulation away (Strauss & Lehtinen, 1947; Cruickshank, 1967). The teacher was not to wear colorful clothes, and no jewelry; there were to be no pictures on the walls, and children were placed in cubby-holes with only the immediate task before them. This treatment is still used with adaptations, but treatment of hyperactivity has more recently centered on the use of drugs.

Remediation which may be as successful as diminution of stimulation or as successful as drugs is that of providing close personal experiences with care-taking adults. A learning-disabled child is often supersensitive to stimulation, frequently not focusing long enough for input to enter through the senses and to be recalled later. Much repetition and verbal reassurance about experiences are needed. Before school age, an adult should almost always be with the child who is hyperactive. The nurturing adult should be constantly pointing, labeling, and explaining. Controlling one's own reactions to stimulation can be learned through repetitive experiences which have been verbalized by adults and later self-verbalized.

The school-age child who is hyperactive should be monitored closely to make up for previous lack of remedial treatment. Aides could sit with such children in the classroom, repeating directions close to their ears with gentle physical pressure toward whatever should be capturing their attention. Rote learning of attention is essential at the beginning of any remedial work.

Learning to follow directions is critical for successful school learning. Remediation of hyperexcitability should ideally be initiated before the child begins school. Readiness workbooks can be used for this purpose; and the child should be required to work on a given page only up to the item where the tutor feels that the child understands the directions. Directions should be repeated for each item, and the child should verbally imitate the directions while carrying them out.

REHEARSAL This is the ability to practice input for later recall. Rehearsal is the means by which incoming information reaches the long-term memory store. Both long- and short-term memory involve the retrieval of information, whereas rehearsal involves the storage of information. Both verbal and imaginal strategies can be used to attain storage.

Verbal rehearsal can be taught remedially through giving the child an opportunity to repeat instructions aloud repeatedly until these are overlearned. There is a relatively small number of sentence patterns which, when overlearned, are triggered through a partial stimulus. The learning disabled ordinarily do not engage in overlearning. It has been noted that when these children desperately desire to engage in some motor activity (say, bike riding), they practice such an activity repeatedly. The same motivation should be activated for acquiring and using the symbol systems. Letter names, letter sequences, nouns, verbs, prepositional phrases, articles, connecting words, adjectives, adverbs, and other grammatic uses can be overlearned during the Memory Function.

Labeling objects and pictures may also be used in remediation if the child has difficulty with remembering the names of things. Such an activity, however, should not take the place of rehearsing letter and number names if the difficulty is mainly that of symbol memory.

Remediation for verbal rehearsal should include materials which provide repetitive activity such as linguistic readers. When worksheets are used, several of the same should be reproduced so that the child may work a fresh one when the previous work has been checked and corrected.

Imaginal rehearsal involves the connection of a stimulus and an internal response. It is that internal response, the image, which aids recall. Imaginative play is the way in which normal children rehearse roles and skills necessary for survival in adulthood. The learning disabled seem to have difficulty in social perception; that difficulty may have its roots in a deficit in imagery.

Remediation of imaginal rehearsal would make lavish use of nursery rhymes, finger plays, fairy tales, and songs. Opportunities for symbolic play, such as playing house and playing school, should be given. In play, children actively repeat what they have actually experienced. Through this repetition, they learn. Psychodrama is not only useful for the handicapped, but for the normal as well. It is a useful technique for helping the normal understand the handicapped. It is a useful technique for helping the handicapped understand experiences which have no meaning for them because of their handicap.

Re-Cognition Function

This function, which occurs from 8 to 12 years of age, is defined as the understanding of multiple meanings, both semantic and structural. It is the time when personal meaning is acquired. Sensory impressions are now colored by concepts, thus changing earlier cognition of the world. Children of this age engage in word play, reflecting more flexibility in thinking than during the Memory Function. This is the stage when children tell riddles and jokes, when they twist meanings of parents and teachers, and when they learn to use meaning aids such as tenses, prefixes, and suffixes. The component deficits during this function are in haptic discrimination, visualization, and figure-ground discrimination.

HAPTIC DISCRIMINATION This is the ability to note differences in the sense of touch and in muscle sensation. The learning disabled appear to have difficulty in holding a writing instrument in a somewhat relaxed manner. They grip a pencil with a great deal of tension. The kinesthetic and tactile senses help to build in recognition of meaning through body movements. As the individual develops, more senses become involved in meaning; while the auditory and visual are important during the Sensory Orientation and the Memory Functions, by age 9 or 10, arm muscle movements in writing and spelling and eye muscle movements in reading must help carry the stimulus load.

The remedial method most suitable for training kinesthetic discrimination is the Fernald method (Fernald, 1943). This method involves having the child look at a word or phrase, attempt to take a picture of it in his or her head without saying the letters, and then attempt to write it from memory while saying the word slowly. The tracing step should be avoided unless eye-hand coordination is deficient. It is important that the child pay attention to the muscle sensation while writing the word.

The word or phrase should be shown rather rapidly. If mistakes are made in reproducing it, another trial can be given. It is better to take 20 or more trials to learn something in the kinesthetic system than to try to remember it through the auditory or visual systems. The child must be encouraged to cover over the sample word while writing it from memory. A variation on this method is to have the child close his or her eyes while writing, as this enhances attention to the muscle movements. No correction or erasure of mistakes is allowed—the word or phrase must always be written as whole.

The remedial method most suitable for training tactile discrimination is to train the child to write the letters in a flowing manner, not "draw" the letters. If the child squeezes a small rubber ball in the hand opposite from the writing one, tension usually will be relieved in the hand used for writing.

Penmanship exercises are necessary to get smooth reverse movements. The learning-disabled child often has difficulty making reverse movements in writing, in reading, in thinking. It is important that the teacher show the child how to make the letter; that is, the movement of it. As the teacher makes the letter or word to be copied, the child should be watching. Meaning develops from the kinesthetic movement, not from the static form.

VISUALIZATION This is the ability to recognize wholes from sensation of the parts. It is the internal representation of overlearned symbol sequences. It is the ability to note likenesses and differences in words and things; in drawing relationships between ideas; in noting absurdities both in what is seen and heard; in understanding structural aids such as prefixes, suffixes, and root words; and in understanding words with multiple meanings, similar meanings, and opposite meanings.

Visualization requires a foundation during the Memory Function of accurate perception of all the parts within a whole context. A common problem shared by bright children and learning-disabled children is that of skipping the accurate perception of the Memory Function and operating from context clues, both in the environment and in dealing with symbols on the page. Visualization means that the context is used as much as the parts in determining meaning.

Remediation requires a careful distinction between understanding from context and perceiving parts accurately. The child must become aware of the role of tools for determining meaning from context. These tools include all previous learnings which should have occurred during the preceding age-related functions: attention which is appropriately and sequentially given to language symbols, intra- and intersensory coordination of language symbols, rehearsal of language symbols, and the ability to return to accurate examination of language symbols whenever necessary for determining meaning.

FIGURE-GROUND DISCRIMINATION This is the ability to sift the relevant from the irrelevant. The learning disabled appear to be distractible and need remedial help to focus on important features of a task. Direct connections must be made between learning a task in isolation and transferring it to new situations. For example, these children must be required to spell words correctly in text which they have learned in isolation.

Building distraction into the remedial activity is a good way to train children to concentrate on the task at hand and to ignore the distraction. This can be done by the teacher verbalizing what the child should be doing while he or she is doing it. This forces a connection between auditory feedback and action, thus closing out interfering stimuli. The child should learn to do this verbalizing for himself or herself as soon as possible.

Some examples of activities for figure-ground discrimination are "getting the main idea," "making inferences," making up titles for stories, and drawing pictures about stories.

Synthesis Function

This function, which occurs from 12 to 14 years of age, is defined as the habituation of previously learned modes of response. By this time, the senses are integrated and the acts of reading, writing, arithmetic, and spelling are fairly automatic. The system need only react when errors occur. In the learning disabled, the processes involved in the basic skills are not synthesized. Deficits are noted in monitoring and in visual-auditory-haptic coordination.

MONITORING This is the ability to note and correct errors when these occur. In this age range, correct responses may be taken for granted, but errors should arouse in the system a feeling that something is not right. Habitual accuracy and the ability to detect errors is deficient in the learning disabled.

In remediation, it is necessary to undo bad habits which the child has acquired earlier. Habits can be extinguished only when the person becomes aware of the habit and then consciously analyzes what is wrong. The focus of remediation, then, is on errors. The special teacher must detect errors, tell the child what these are, and then provide the correct response until it is overlearned. The student must consciously practice the correct responses in his or her mind.

It is best for the special teacher to ignore correct responses initially, and focus on the incorrect. After the correct response has been attained, the teacher should test only infrequently to see if the correct response has been retained. Rest periods cause the new responses to become more entrenched.

After the teacher has demonstrated catching and analyzing errors, the child should be given passages with incorrect spellings, punctuation, and tenses so that he or she may acquire a strategy for catching errors. This takes the emphasis off the child's own errors for a time.

Finally, it is expected that students will find their own errors. To do this, they must have a strategy for finding out the correct response when they do not know it. Among these strategies are asking the teacher or someone who knows, using the dictionary, thesaurus, or rulebook—whatever is most reasonable. The student should become used to checking and double-checking his or her own work. The student should constantly verbalize what he or she is doing (internally at least).

VISUAL-AUDITORY-HAPTIC COORDINATION This is the ability to associate information from all sensory modalities. Since all the senses are integrated by this age, it is not reasonable to assess individual senses for strength or weakness. Instead, it is useful to mask out those senses which appear to be overshadowing others. For example, many poor spellers cannot overcome their bad spelling because they try to remember all the letters in a word by rote. By masking out the auditory feedback of the letters, the poor speller can improve rapidly. The strategy of looking at a word fast without saying the letters and then attempting to write it from memory while slowly saying the word will serve to replace the habit of relying on auditory feedback with the habit of coordinating the feedback from seeing the word and writing the word while pronouncing the word. This strategy is what is meant by visual-auditory-haptic coordination.

Writing from dictation is an activity which forces all the senses to work together. Sounds must be blended into wholes, production of symbols must be in correct sequences, and movement must be fluid. As the student writes from dictation, the teacher must be watching for the coordination of the senses. When the pen stops, when letters or numbers are reversed, or when any other mistake is made, the teacher should model the writing, then take the model away, and have the child start again from the beginning of the word or the sentence. By beginning again each time a hesitation or mistake occurs, the student learns how to produce a coordinated whole. The material for dictation should come from the student's regular textbooks, if at all feasible. Sometimes, for remedial purposes, simpler materials could be used so long as transfer is made as soon as possible. While single words may be used, sentences are better for producing smoothness of response.

Communication Function

This last function, which begins around age 14, is defined as the process by which learned concepts and automatized modes of response are used in the service of expressing ideas to others and receiving ideas from others, both consciously and unconsciously. Synthesized skills of speaking, writing, gestures, and reading take on a personalized style, and personal responsibility is taken for the consequence of what is communicated. The learning disabled have difficulty in comprehending what they read and what others are communicating to them. This difficulty is manifested in social imperception. They also have problems expressing themselves in writing and in solving mathematical story problems. Component deficits during this function are reading comprehension, mathematical comprehension, and writing.

READING COMPREHENSION This is the ability to gain meaning from the printed page. Students with learning disability have had relatively little practice in a wide spectrum of reading experiences when they have experienced failure in the acquisition of the skill. While it is a truism to say that the more practice one gets in reading, the better one is able to read, such a statement bears repeating.

Remedial materials should be taken from textbooks used in the student's courses at school, from books written at the instructional grade level for a particular student, and from high interest books. Modeling reading with comprehension is an important place for the teacher to begin. The best means for doing this is through slow-motion choral reading. As the student reads along with the teacher, the teacher should be listening for types of mistakes, for phrasing, and for the kind of reading that connotes understanding. Occasionally, the teacher should see if the student might be able to fill in key words, phrases, and sentences without the aid of the teacher's voice.

Programmed texts are important adjuncts in remediation, but should never be used for the entire remedial curriculum. Similarly, basal readers must be used with care. They may be useful when the remedial teacher needs a refresher on the sequence and scope of abilities in reading. When basal readers are used, however, movement through the grade levels should be rapid, alternating with transferring the skills into the reading required of the student in his or her regular grade assignments. A word of caution is necessary regarding the extremely popular Richard Boning booklets (Boning, 1978). While these may be useful for giving the student the idea of comprehension, these should not be the only remedial material. Transfer from these booklets, too, should be made consistently and constantly into the student's required content textbooks.

MATHEMATICAL COMPREHENSION This is the ability to deal with quantitative concepts. Many students with learning disability have not learned arithmetic operations in an organized fashion and, thus, do not know the relationship of numbers. In order for comprehension to occur, the student must be able to work out word problems in his or her head, or at least be able to decide what arithmetic operation is needed in order to do it on paper. The basic skill needed here is to be able to hold directions in mind and visualize the operation.

Remediation should not include counting, since this is a rote activity and has probably been the student's only skill in mathematics. Sheets of paper showing the designs of numbers when these are added, subtracted, or multiplied can be drawn up by the teacher. These are not for the purpose of giving the child a ready reference to answers, but to show the "idea" of numbers.

A ritualistic dependence on each step in a sequence of solving a problem is necessary for the sequence to become automatic. Verbalizing by the teacher and the student helps to imprint the sequence. Special attention must be paid to the sign indicating the operation and the direction of working the problem. Working from the school's textbook, the teacher should help the student fill in skills which the student is lacking. Such transfer of training is essential.

Time concepts are often difficult for the learning disabled and should be included in the curriculum for teaching mathematical comprehension.

WRITING This is the ability to communicate meaning through the written word. The learning disabled often have difficulty in spelling, in syntax, and in penmanship, all mechanics of writing. They shun writing, a habit which makes the problems worse.

Copying stories, experience stories, compositions, and rewriting stories, are all necessary remedial tasks. An analysis by the special teacher should give indicators about the specific problems a student is having in expressing ideas through writing.

If penmanship is the problem, penmanship drills can be initiated. Cursive writing is important for the acquisition of smooth wholes in producing written material. If spelling is a problem, the teacher should use a modified Fernald method as described under the Re-Cognition Function. If grammatic usage is the problem, a textbook on grammar could be used, with the teacher presenting the material step by step. If punctuation is ignored, time should be spent working on that aspect of writing. Constant and consistent correction while the student is writing is important in the early stages of remediation. As students gain facility in the mechanics of writing, they will probably be more willing to write their ideas.

If ideas are sparse and deal only with concrete subject matter, the student must be given abstract material to read. He or she should then be asked to write as much as he or she can remember. Later the student can attempt to rephrase the material, using synonyms and defining concepts as he or she writes. Verbalizing what one is writing is important.

Conclusion

The philosophy of special education must be congruent with the philosophy of general education: namely, to produce responsible, useful, and self-supporting citizens. In addition, however, special education has a therapeutic mission: namely, to cure whatever is hampering an individual from attaining minimum standards for responsible, useful, and self-supporting status in society. This chapter focused on a particular view of learning disability with some remedial suggestions for critical component deficits across the age range.

Bibliography

Ayres, A. J. Sensory integrative process and neuropsychological learning disability. In J. Hellmuth (Ed.), *Learning disorders* (Vol. 3). Seattle: Special Child Publications, 1968.

Boning, R. A. *Language and reading skills series*. Baldwin, N.Y.: Barnell Loft, Ltd., 1977–1981.

Cruickshank, W. M. *The brain-injured child in home, school, and community*. Syracuse: Syracuse University Press, 1967.

Fernald, G. *Remedial techniques in basic school subjects*. New York: McGraw-Hill Book Co., 1943.

Schnorr, J. M. *Generation of psychoneurological criteria for estimating handicap in infants*. Unpublished doctoral dissertation, University of Arizona, 1976.

Strauss, A. A., & Lehtinen, L. *Psychopathology and education of the brain-injured child*. New York: Grune and Stratton, 1947.

Early Intervention with Multihandicapped Children

Carmella Ficociello Gates

Ms. Carmella Ficociello Gates defines education as a process for helping every child become as independent as possible. She sees early intervention in the education of multihandicapped children as crucial to their eventual independence, so she outlines successful intervention strategies based on a philosophy of the total child and a multidisciplinary team approach.

Education of multihandicapped children is a relatively new area in the field of special education. There is a very large number of these children who need to be served, and there is also a great need for information as how best to serve them. The establishment of the Regional Centers for the Deaf-Blind by the Bureau of Education for the Handicapped has helped to develop an awareness not only of the deaf-blind population but also of children with other multihandicapping conditions. These centers have also hastened the development of various philosophies, methodologies, and curricula to serve these children. Although these developments differ greatly in their effectiveness, one almost universal feature of them is emphasis on the need for early intervention with these children if educational programs for them are to be effective.

Two terms as they will be used in this chapter need to be defined. The first of these words is *education*. Education is operationally defined as the movement of the learner from one level of independent functioning to another level (Hammer, 1974). Thus, the traditional concept of education as the 3R's—reading, 'riting, and 'rithmetic—gives way to a new concept of education for all children: to help each child become as independent as possible. Implicit in this definition is the consideration of the individual needs of a child through the development of an individual educational plan to meet those needs. The second term is the *multihandicapped child*. For purposes of this chapter, the multihandicapped child is one with two or more physical, social, mental, or emotional problems, any combination of which may impede one or more aspects of his or her overall development.

Considering the latter definition, there are many examples of children called multihandicapped. Let's look at a few descriptions, not in an effort to label children, but rather to develop a concept of the wide scope of the term multihandicapped. The children that I am most familiar with are deaf-blind children who have some degree of sensory deficit in both vision and hearing, but who also often have other complicating problems such as congenital heart malformations, cerebral palsy, orthopedic problems as well as behavior and learning problems. Let us consider also the blind retarded or blind nonverbal child, the deaf child with perceptual problems or cerebral palsy, the genetic syndrome children, and those diagnosed as "etiology unknown."

What do these descriptions tell us about multihandicapped children?

- The descriptions make it quite obvious that all of these children may be impeded in physical, social, mental, and/or emotional development.
- It is also quite obvious that these problems do not begin when the child enters school at age five or six. It is at this age that these problems may actually become handicaps if the child has not been helped from a very early age. When problems in development are first observed, plans for early intervention must be implemented. This is not to say that early intervention will make all children "normal." However, if the intervention is begun with the child early in life, the child will attain some level of independent functioning.
- The descriptions emphasize that the population of multihandicapped children is not a homogeneous group. Each of these children has highly individual needs, and educational plans must be designed for each of the children if we are to meet these needs.

The total child approach is the major point of my paper. It is not a curriculum or a method, but rather a philosophy of looking at the individual needs of a child, emphasizing what he or she *can* do, not what he or she *cannot* do, and developing an educational plan for that child.

This approach has been found very effective with deaf-blind children, and it is quite applicable in educational programs for low-functioning multihandicapped children as well.

In order to develop such an educational plan, it is necessary to look at the *total child*. Each child exhibits several systems of behavior—physical behavior, social behavior, mental behavior, and emotional behavior. These systems can be further subdivided into visual, auditory, tactile, verbal, motor, cognitive, and so on. However, these behaviors are not separate entities occurring independently or at different intervals from each other, but rather they are integrated, often simultaneous occurrences.

Let's look at eating as an example. A child picks up a spoon, puts it in the bowl, scoops food onto the spoon, lifts the spoon to his or her mouth, puts the food in his or her mouth, chews it, and then swallows. How many systems of behavior do we see in this simple activity? First of all, there is physical behavior: vision is used to locate the spoon and, in conjunction with motor behavior, to move toward the spoon, to pick it up, to put it in the bowl, etc. There is social behavior in eating neatly, slowly, and in using a spoon. There is mental behavior in the routine and sequence of eating, in the discrimination of types of foods, and in the motor planning of eating. Maybe the emotional behavior would be the enjoyment of the food the child is eating. In this simple activity, we see the integration of many of the systems of behavior.

What does this example tell us about educating these children? First of all, it tells us that by designing separate activities to teach isolated behaviors (such as visual activities, auditory activities, tactile activities) we are only developing splintered

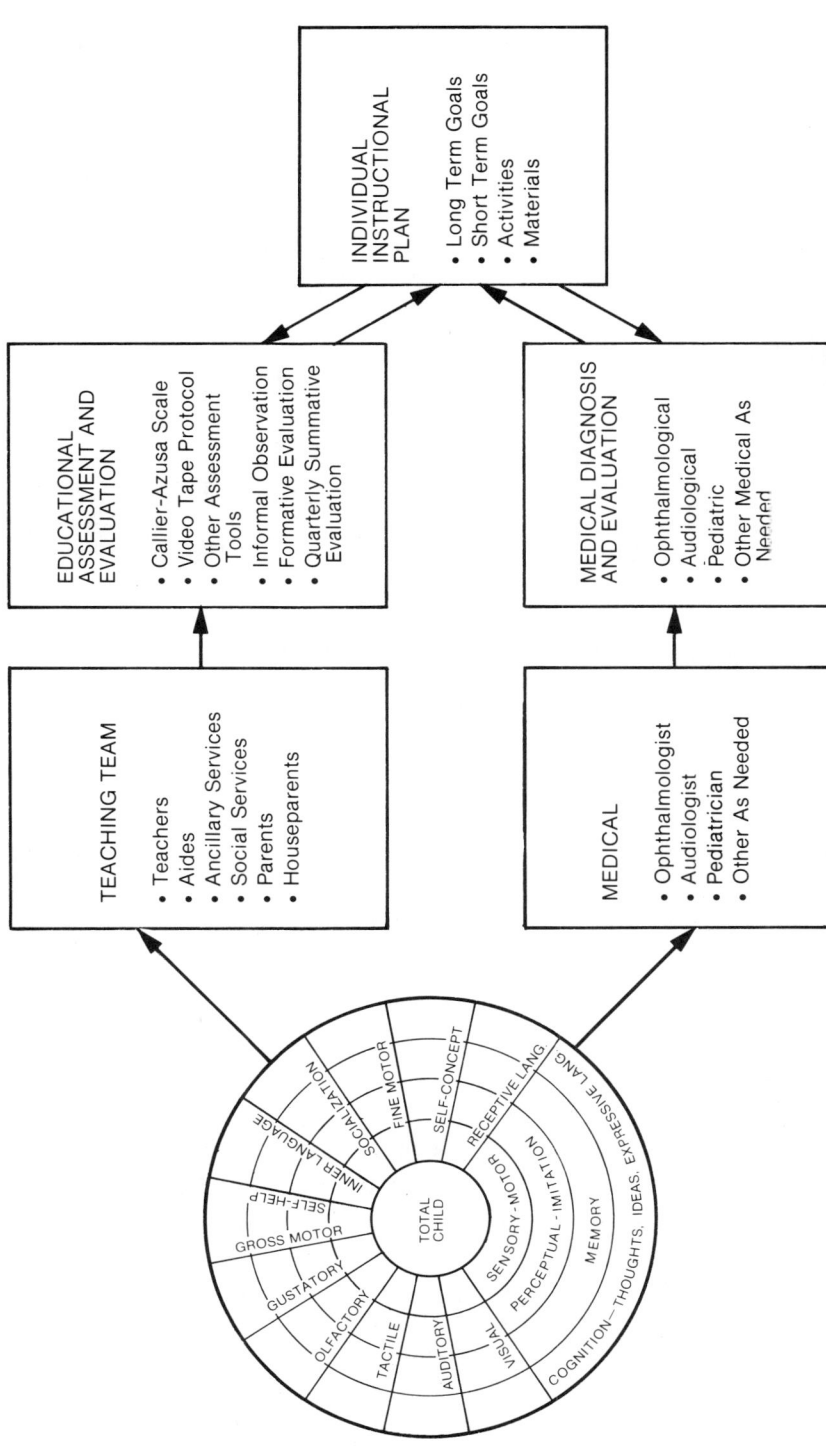

Process Teaching: Total Child Approach to Developing Child-By-Child Plans

skills which often have little or no relevance to real life situations. Secondly, it shows us the importance of designing activities which incorporate several behaviors in a realistic situation. This second point is the whole emphasis of the total child approach—designing an educational program for the *total child* by assessing each child's individual needs, by designating goals which meet these needs at his or her level of functioning in the systems of behavior, and by developing activities which integrate these behaviors in a realistic environment using realistic materials.

Thus far this paper has centered on the "why" of the total child approach. It is necessary next to discuss the "how" of developing an individual educational plan for a multihandicapped child.

Rather than one teacher to complete this task, a teaching team approach is suggested. The teaching team is similar to an interdisciplinary team in medicine. The team is comprised of *all* the people who are involved with a particular child: teachers, parents, aides, physical therapists, social workers, speech and language therapists, supervising teachers, and consultants. The use of a teaching team allows for the sharing of strategies, specializations, and methods when assessing the child's behavior and in planning and implementing an educational plan or intervention plan.

In order to incorporate the total child approach into the educational program, a format is needed. This format consists of four steps:
1. Observation
2. Planning
3. Implementation
4. Evaluation

Initially these steps occur in the progression listed above. However, what begins as a progression becomes a cyclical process, since observation, planning, implementation, and evaluation are *ongoing* in educational programs. Let us now explore each step separately.

Observation

When we observe the child, we are looking at the child's social, emotional, physical, and mental behaviors. What the child's current level of functioning is in these areas should be our primary concern. It is our starting point for the educational program. We focus on what the child *can do*, not what he or she can't do. As we have stated, planned, integrated activities develop the *total* child. In observing the child, however, it is necessary to observe these behaviors separately to assess levels of functioning and to locate problem areas. Once the child's level of functioning in each specific behavior area has been determined, this information is used to design an educational plan to meet the individual needs of the child. This information is also used to integrate behaviors in order to develop the total child.

The following is a list of specific behavior areas to serve as a guide for the observation step.

Sensory experience
    Tactile
    Olfactory
    Gustatory

Motor skills
    Gross motor skills
    Fine motor skills

Self-help
    Feeding
    Dressing
    Toileting
    Personal hygiene

Language
    Receptive skills
    Expressive skills
    Speech

Socialization
    Interpersonal skills
    Agricultural skills
    Adaptive skills
    Self-concept

Memory
    Long term
    Short term

Cognition
    Concept development
    Problem solving: relating past perceptions to experience

Tools to aid in observing these behaviors include developmental scales such as the *Callier-Azusa Scale* (1974) or the *Denver Developmental Scales* (1967). These scales give the team information about the child's level of development in each of the behavioral areas. They may also be used as a pretest and post test, as measurement of progress in the child. For example, using a developmental scale of feeding behavior, the team observing the child records that the child is able to accept soft-textured food and to finger-feed some foods; however, she is not yet able to scoop food independently. This observation gives the team information for planning a feeding program for the child in which emphasis is placed on learning to scoop food. The post test evaluation using the scale is a record of whether or not the child has made progress in this area.

Pertinent medical information should also be considered in this observation step. Information about the child's ability to develop some level of functioning in visual, auditory, and motor behavior is invaluable. Besides these formal observations of the child, each member of the team should also observe the child informally and record observations of pertinent behavior. Team members should particularly note the child's interest, attention span, self-stimulatory behavior, dependence on routine, and any problems in functioning.

Standardized tests may also be used when and if applicable, with particular stress on *when* and *if*, since experience has shown us that such tests give us more of a picture of what the child cannot do than what he or she can. Such information does not help us considerably in planning for these children.

Planning

Once all the observations have been compiled, it is then time to develop the individual educational plan for the child. We use the compiled information as baseline data. The educational plan is composed of long-term goals, short-term goals, activities, materials, and evaluation procedures.

A long-term goal is one that the child will accomplish over a period of time. The long-term goal may be for three months, six months, or a year, depending on the rate of progress of an individual child. An example of a long-term goal may be that the child sign "eat" independently in an appropriate situation, or that he or she scoop food independently.

Short-term goals are the steps leading to a long-term goal. They are sequential in nature. Short-term goals for the example of signing "eat" should be:
1. The child will give the "eat" sign when manipulated through the movement by the teacher and when food is present.
2. The child will imitate the "eat" sign after the teacher shows him or her the food and presents the sign.
3. The child will independently sign "eat" when food is presented.

Once long- and short-term goals have been developed for each behavioral area, the next step is to design activities to meet these goals. Several goals should be incorporated within each activity so that behaviors are integrated. With such integration, we thus develop the total child. (During the planning step, methods of evaluation are also designated, but these will be presented in the section on evaluation.)

An activity which would incorporate the two long-term goals of signing "eat" and scooping food would be, of course, eating. The child is seated at the table with food on the table; the teacher gives the "eat" sign; the child imitates the sign, and then the child is aided in scooping the food. The materials used in this activity are, of course, plate, spoon, cup, etc.

In planning activities and materials to use with a child, be sure not to structure the activities too much; but rather, structure the environment so that it is relevant to the child and relates to his or her needs.

What is a relevant environment for multihandicapped children? Again this relates to level of functioning. Children who are severely neurologically involved and who are barely relating to the world outside themselves need an environment that provides a great deal of sensory stimulation—visual, auditory, tactile, and motor stimulation. The materials to use with such children include things with textures, colors, lights, sounds. Therapeutic motor devices also help them develop an awareness of the world around them, provide them experiences to explore and learn about the world, and help them relate to the world and other people so they are not self-centered.

If a child is on a self-help level, a home-like environment should be provided for him or her. The classroom may resemble a home and the materials may be things found in a home. At this level, the child learns skills in dressing, eating, toileting, personal hygiene, and care of the home in a realistic setting and in the course of a *daily routine*. Daily routine is important here. The child learns to dress first thing in the morning, not in the middle of the day. He or she learns feeding skills at appropriate eating times. Developing such a routine is fairly easy in a residential program; however, with day students the teacher must work with parents to see that the child learns such things as dressing and feeding at home and carries over to the home things he or she has learned in school. Such an environment is very conducive to integrating behaviors. Vision, motor skills, and particularly language can easily be developed in the structured *environment*, as opposed to structured activities. The child will generalize "cup" much more easily when he or she is using a cup in a realistic situation of "Drink from the cup," "Wash the cup," "Put the cup away," than he or she will while sitting at a table with a cup and a shoe as the teacher says, "Show me the cup."

Implementation

The next step is implementation, actually carrying out the educational plan on a day-to-day basis. This involves setting up a daily schedule for teaching the planned goals, for engaging in activities, and for documenting or evaluating those plans.

Evaluation

Evaluation consists of both formative and summary documentation. Formative evaluation is the daily or weekly evaluation of activities and short-term goals. It may be in the form of a behavioral checklist or charts or anecdotal records. Summary evaluation occurs after a period of time. It measures all goals and activities. Summary evaluations should be completed about every three months. The information gathered from the summary evaluation is used along with continued observation of the child to develop a new or revised education plan for the child. Thus the cycle of observation, planning, implementation, and evaluation continues for the education of the multihandicapped child.

A process teaching plan is included to give a visual representation of the total child approach to the education of multihandicapped children.

In concluding, the importance of beginning these educational plans at a very early age with multihandicapped children cannot be overemphasized. Only if these children are helped when they are very young will they reap the full benefits of their education and reach some level of independent functioning.

Bibliography

Callier Center for Communication Disorders. *The Callier-Azusa Scale* (Rev. ed.). Dallas: Callier Center for Communication Disorders, September 1974.

Frankenburg, W. K., & Dodds, J. The Denver Developmental Screening Test. *Journal of Pediatrics,* 1967, *71*, 181–191.

Hammer, E. *Process teaching: A systems approach to the education of multihandicapped deaf-blind children.* Paper presented at the New Staff Orientation Workshop, Callier Center for Communication Disorders, Dallas, September 1974.

10
Working with Parents of Multihandicapped Children

Kathryn P. Meadow

Dr. Kathryn Meadow recognizes the difficulties faced by parents of multihandicapped children, and she indicates ways in which professionals can assist parents in coping with these difficulties.

There is a fine line between "too much" and "not enough" in many of the areas in which multihandicapped children and their parents need help. Much of the work that counselors do with parents consists of helping the parents to recognize that fine line and to stand both firmly and comfortably between giving too much help and too little help. The basic needs of children with multihandicaps are not very different from those of children with a single handicap; the basic needs of children with a single handicap are not very different from those of children with no handicaps. Clausen (1968) has stated that these basic needs can be met by the following activities:
1. Providing sustenance and nurturance;
2. Training and channeling of physiological needs in toilet training, weaning, sleeping;
3. Teaching the skills of locomotion, language, cognition, sociability, and self-care;
4. Orienting the child to his or her immediate world of kin, community, and society in a variety of social situations and settings;
5. Transmitting cultural goals;
6. Promoting interpersonal skills, with a concern for and responsiveness to the feelings of others;
7. Controlling the child's behavior, providing guidance and interpretations.

The nonhandicapped child, the child with a single handicap, and the child with multiple handicaps all have these needs that must be supplied by the parent or a parent-substitute. In each of the seven areas, however, it is difficult to *allow* a child with less than full potential for normal development to exercise independence in acquiring the skills that result from and contribute to his or her grasp of the world and his or her role in it. Thus, as the child grows older, it becomes progressively more difficult to determine which areas of possibly slowed development are related to his or her physical, mental, or emotional handicaps, and which are related to parental delay in the assignment of tasks that contribute to growth. Much of the important work of a teacher or counselor entails helping parents to discriminate between those tasks that are possible for the handicapped child to follow on the normal developmental time-table and those tasks which will be delayed and need special help if they are to appear.

Carol Erting offered helpful suggestions that have been incorporated into this paper.

Clausen notes the importance of opportunities for children to exercise their developing skills and abilities.

> Stimulation and the provision of models for the child is important but so is the opportunity to perform. The mother who always dresses and feeds her child does not maximize the child's ability to dress and feed himself. A good many tasks can probably be learned by children much earlier than we permit them to learn, partially because their early efforts are so ineffective that it seems simpler to give assistance or do the whole thing oneself.
>
> (Clausen, 1968, p. 142)

If parents of children without handicaps find it difficult to provide them with these self-help opportunities, it is easy to imagine that parents of handicapped children find it even more difficult. And the more handicapped the child, the more difficult it becomes. This is true for a number of reasons.

1. The handicapped child truly does exhibit some developmental lags that result in a delayed ability to perform the expected tasks of childhood. The child with cerebral palsy or with visual handicaps is delayed in the acquisition of the skills of locomotion; the child with a hearing loss is delayed in the acquisition of language skills; the child who is mentally retarded will naturally lag behind peers in some, although not necessarily all, areas.

2. It is a human tendency to extend our definition of deficit to an area that is broader than necessary. Thus, without thinking, we may assume that a lag in development of locomotion skills is linked with a lag in another area.

3. Guilt about the child's handicaps (especially if the contrast between the handicapped child and his or her parents and siblings is very great) may lead parents (and teachers) to do things for the child in an unconscious effort to expiate the guilt.

4. The usual impatience of a competent, busy, harried grown-up is to go about the business of daily life and to hurry the developing child along by doing *for* the child the things that one might *eventually* do for oneself.

The study of rubella children (many with multihandicaps) conducted by Chess and her colleagues (1971) highlights the dilemmas of parents. The authors conclude that

> If too little was expected of a child, he might be handled in such a way that he could never achieve a level of functioning close to his actual capacity. Conversely, excessive expectations could impede his adaptation by producing over-whelming stress.
>
> (Chess et al., 1971, p. 89)

These authors listed discrete self-help skills in the areas of dressing, personal hygiene, toileting, and eating. Of 153 children capable of doing at least some of the tasks listed, parents reported that youngsters actually performed only 42% of the tasks related to dressing of which they were capable and approximately half of the tasks related to personal hygiene and toileting of which they were capable. The authors saw the increased performance in the area of toileting as related to the fact that parents were unwilling to continue servicing the youngsters in this area "and worked especially hard at getting them to become self-reliant" (p. 96). The same pattern of results was found in their study of mentally retarded children also. However, level of functioning was *not* correlated with IQ test scores.

Barsch (1968) interviewed parents of children with a variety of handicaps and found that the handicapped children achieved independence at toileting later than did siblings, that the parents *expected* a delay, and that the delay was always attributed to the handicap (p. 145). In contrast, parents of children who were somewhat older reported that they expected the same help around the house with chores from the handicapped children as they did from siblings. "The legendary belief that the parents of handicapped children are remiss in imposing restrictions and making demands upon such children gained no support from these data" (p. 174). Schlesinger and Meadow (1972) reported data suggesting that parents of deaf children may scale *down* their expectations or demands on siblings in order to minimize the discrepancy between the performance of the handicapped child and the brothers and sisters.

In her interviews with parents of deaf children, Gregory (1976) noted that, while the problems these parents had were much like those of parents with normally hearing children, many parents expressed the concern of "trying to allow and compensate for the child's handicap while not spoiling him" (p. 206).

In the context of looking after deaf children, what does overprotection or rejection mean? Is it overprotective to prevent a deaf child playing in the road when one is aware that he is more in danger than his hearing siblings? Is it rejecting to send a child to boarding school when it seems (even if, in fact, it is not the case) that only such a school is in a position to provide the best learning situation for the child? . . . the balance between being fair while not spoiling or making too high a demand is difficult to establish, and parents are aware of this.
(Gregory, 1976, pp. 207–208)

It seems apparent that parents of handicapped children find it difficult to give those children the independence and the freedom of movement that contribute to optimal development. We have said, in a number of different ways, that the parents' ambivalent feelings are to some extent based on reality. In addition, they may be based on their feelings about the child's handicaps and on a common adult impatience with the slowness of the progress toward the completion of a task—an impatience sometimes increased by the nature of the handicaps.

What can parent counselors and teachers do in their work with parents? If the intervention is to be early and optimal, it will occur in infancy or soon after. Working with parents and infants during that time may make it possible to approximate the development of infants without handicaps.

For example, White (1975) believes that the period between 14 and 24 months is particularly important in the life of a child.

By two years, fundamental educational processes have developed so far that we researchers get the feeling that if we see a child for the first time at two years of age we are seeing him rather late in the game.

(White, 1975, p. 151)

The baby at this age is already engaging in exploratory and mastery activities. In order to participate in these activities, the child must have them available in the environment. The handicapped child, and particularly the multihandicapped child, may be given fewer opportunities for these kinds of activities at this age and miss an important part of this early experience. The relationship between the child and the mother, even (or perhaps, especially) at this age, is a reciprocal or interactive one. The active, demanding baby usually gets more attention and more stimulation, and therefore more opportunities for exploring and mastering the environment, than does the passive, undemanding baby. The deaf baby who does not respond to the mother's voice, the blind baby who seems not to turn toward the mother, the baby with motor problems who is slow to reach toward the mother's extended arms—all may be seen by the mother as rejecting. Thus, parents need assistance as early as possible from helping professionals.

There are four areas in which professionals might usefully intervene with parents of multihandicapped children. Not all families will need or want help in all four areas, but where the need exists, professionals should be willing and able to offer assistance.

Help with Parents' External Circumstances

Professionals working with deaf children are appreciating more and more the importance of parental involvement to the success of the child. Parental involvement, however, is possible only for those parents who are not overwhelmed by the demands of providing the necessities of life. For some families, the first step in counseling may be helping them to find an appropriate community agency to supply food, clothing, shelter, or financial assistance. This kind of help has been an important part of the New York University program for multihandicapped children and seems to be one of the major reasons for its success. (See Chapter 14, Naiman.) The counselor "provides referral services and assumes a more direct involvement if families are unable to follow through on their own" (Naiman, 1978, p.15). The importance of external influences on the developing handicapped child is pointed up by research findings indicating that the conditions of low socioeconomic status (that is, poor health care, bad diet, absent father) rather than parental *behavior,* are associated with the fact that high risk babies "apparently do better in a low risk—that is a high socioeconomic environment" (Clarke-Stewart, 1977, p. 13). For the parent whose child has multihandicaps, and who may, therefore, be overwhelmed by the multiplicity of the child's problems, other exigencies of living (such as difficulties in finding a job or adequate housing) may be even more troublesome. Energy may not be left to interact with the handicapped child, much less to contribute to the special educational and remedial activities that he or she also needs.

Help with the Parents' Internal Feelings

Parents of children with a single handicap are often beset with feelings of guilt, sorrow, anger, and deep loss. Additional handicaps may compound these feelings. Thus, a professional may need to give parents the opportunity to vent those feelings before the parents can begin to think about the child's habilitation. An emotion that tends to go unrecognized or unacknowledged in the parents of handicapped children is that of anger. It is not really acceptable for adults to know or to feel or to admit strong anger toward a child, so this emotion is often denied, hidden, or unacknowledged. Angry feelings toward a child with multihandicaps evoke even more guilt on the part of the parent. It is these angry feelings, however, that may contribute to the vacillation, to the alternate permissiveness and restrictiveness that make setting of rational, consistent limits impossible (Schlesinger & Meadow, 1976, p. 17). Naiman and Schein give some good advice to parents of deaf children.

If you are a parent who has learned recently of your child's deafness and are still filled with feelings of anguish, what can you do to help yourself get through [to] a happier more positive state? It may help to realize that there is no way to avoid going through a period of sorrow....You cannot bypass this period. You are better off if you go ahead and feel what you feel, without trying to pretend that you do not.
(Naiman & Schein, 1978, p. 7)

Professionals who work with parents need to recognize this same fact. They can be more helpful if they encourage parents to talk about their feelings than if they try to ignore them or to urge parents to "keep a stiff upper lip."

In some cases, parents who have had few experiences in discussing their feelings openly may need more help in this area. There are some instances where value systems of parents and counselors are different—where the two groups represent differing racial, language, ethnic, or socioeconomic groups. In these cases, professionals need to be particularly careful to guard against making negative value judgments about the feelings that are expressed or about parents who have particular difficulty discussing their feelings with a person who represents a different background.

Feelings will appear in some form, and the direct way is best in the long run for parents, the children, and for the professionals. This direct approach to handling parents' feelings is not something that comes easily, however. Teacher training programs need to give their trainees some experience with or some sense of how to approach this process.

Help with Information about Normal Child Development

Parents, especially those with a multihandicapped first child, may be limited in their knowledge of what to expect in child development. This can lead them to place more limitations, offer more help, and provide fewer opportunities for independence to the handicapped child than they might if they were familiar with normal stages of child development.

Help with Specialized Information Related to the Child's Handicap

It is no accident that this area of possible help to parents of multihandicapped children is last in the list of helping areas. It is my strong opinion that parents are unable to process—truly to comprehend and begin to profit from—specialized information about the handicap and how to provide habilitation for it, until they have received help in the other three areas. When too much information and too many demands are placed on parents too soon, professionals may only add to the guilt that already exists. The professionals may also make parents feel helpless and inadequate because they believe the parents are unable to attack all areas immediately.

Information about hearing aids may not be meaningful to parents who are still mourning the fact that their child is deaf. Information about mobility training may be shut out by the parent of a blind child who continues to have visions of a tin cup in the child's future. A parent who has no food in the house for tomorrow's dinner or who is worried about finding another job may never "get around to" helping the child with exercises.

The professional who feels that his or her job is to provide the specialized information and not to help parents in other areas may also be doomed to frustration, because the parents who are supposed to be learning to do the specialized tasks with the child may never get enough energy or motivation to carry through with the tasks that the professional is trying to communicate. While the professional suffers, the parent suffers more, but the child suffers most. All of these factors lead to the eventual provision (or non-provision) of an environment that contributes to the optimal development of the multihandicapped child. For parents, professionals, and children alike, the successful avoidance of hazards means walking the razor's edge.

Bibliography

Barsch, R. H. *The parent of the handicapped child: The study of child-rearing practices.* Springfield, Ill.: Charles C. Thomas, Publisher, 1968.

Chess, S., Kron, S. J., & Fernandez, P. B. *Psychiatric disorders of children with congenital rubella.* New York: Brunner/Mazel, 1971.

Clarke-Stewart, A. *Child care in the family: A review of research and some propositions for policy*. New York: Academic Press, 1977.

Clausen, J. A. Perspectives on childhood socialization. In J. A. Clausen (Ed.), *Socialization and society*. Boston: Little, Brown and Co., 1968, 130–181.

Gregory, S. *The deaf child and his family*. London: George Allen and Unwin, 1976.

Naiman, D. W. Educating severely handicapped deaf children. In *Programs for severely handicapped children and youth*. Report to Office of Education, Grants and Procurement Management Division, 1978.

Naiman, D. W., & Schein, J. D. *For parents of deaf children*. Silver Spring, Md.: National Association of the Deaf, 1978.

Schlesinger, H. S., & Meadow, K. P. *Sound and sign: Childhood deafness and mental health*. Berkeley: University of California Press, 1972.

Schlesinger, H. S., & Meadow, K. P. Emotional support parents. In D. L. Lillie & P. L. Trohanis (Eds.), *Teaching parents to teach*. New York: Walker and Company, 1976.

White, B. L. *The first three years of life*. Englewood Cliffs, N.J.: Prentice-Hall, Inc., 1975.

III

Developing the Curriculum

Assessment, Curriculum, and Intervention Strategies for Hearing-Impaired Mentally Retarded Children

Marya Mavilya

On the basis of her own work with mentally retarded hearing-impaired children, Dr. Marya Mavilya shares strategies for assessing and educating these children. She also offers an annotated list of diagnostic instruments appropriate to this population, and she recounts the successful experience of the Mailman Center in communicating through gesture with mentally retarded hearing-impaired youngsters.

Morkovin feels that a lack of purposeful and significant experience may contribute to disuse of the brain and produce a cortical inhibition which becomes irreversible. The deaf child then cannot develop an effective system by which to process information, as the normal child does. Morkovin has concluded that

Organic and inhibitory facts, which are often combined, cause educational, social and mental delay in the development of deaf children with normal brains. The main cause is that the brain is not reached in a sufficiently wide front to bring out effectively all its immense potential to compensate for these children's physical deficiencies, which often are aggravated by additional brain inhibition due to emotional stress.

(Morkovin, 1963, p. 733)

Not learning language in the early preschool years also has a deleterious effect on normal functioning. According to Penfield (1959), the capacity for learning language decreases with the pasage of time. One realizes, then, that the study of the senses is not only that of the auditory receptors but also the brain. How, then, should one look at the hearing-impaired mentally retarded child?

The difficulties of the hearing-impaired mentally retarded child assuredly are compounded by the combination of both handicaps. Whether it is the sum of the two becomes questionable when one observes this group of children. As Hardy says of deaf children, they may be deaf in different ways and in different degrees for many different reasons (Hardy, 1962), so each of these children in unique. Moreover, the same can be stated with respect to intellectual factors. Human nature is observed as a biological system, and as such has specific potential, scope, and limits (Chomsky, 1977). This is true physically, intellectually, and creatively. Moreover, Chomsky indicates that there is variability in endowment, and this variability is a source of creativity. This in turn can enrich each one of us. How can we, as educators, enrich the potential of hearing-impaired mentally retarded children and direct these children towards useful lives?

Many educators of hearing-impaired mentally retarded (HI/MR) people disclose that they are unusual as a group and quite distinct from the mentally retarded in general. Among the differences observed are that they appear happier and more popular than the mentally retarded, and they are more productive in academic work.

They also appear shy until rapport is established. Imitative behavior on the part of the HI/MR is more precise. It appears that this group is more visually oriented and so may accomplish more by observing closely. These differences are only observations and may be challenging to investigate.

Assessment

It is imperative to include a systematic study of the bio-psycho-social factors involved in the diagnoses of hearing-impaired mentally retarded children. Diagnostic studies of children's developmental stages were made by Piaget and Vygotsky in the 1920s. Present day techniques for defining deficiencies and strengths have been established by Haeussermann, Kirk, and Uzgiris and Hunt. However, there is a serious need to develop more comprehensive methods of evaluating young children who have both a hearing impairment and mental retardation. These limitations seriously impair or delay learning. The problem of communication is fundamental, for there is a basic need for self-expression and reception of thought. One must convey ideas, even if it is at such a primitive level as gesture.

Severe limitations in communication skills complicate the problem of evaluation of hearing-impaired mentally retarded children. Any assessment program should consider all factors of human life and development. It should identify conditions which interfere with effective functioning and for which remediation is available. The assessment should be repeated at regular intervals in order to monitor the progress and improve the control if necessary. The number and kinds of tests available are many, as evident in Meier's table (1978). Meier lists 58 tests covering physical, intellectual, cognitive, language, social/emotional, and comprehensive systems. All do not apply to the hearing impaired, but a composite of several are predictive.

In many educational programs for the multihandicapped, one finds that the educators have selected subtests from a number of valid tests and developed their own profile. Assessment of children with sensory deficits is difficult. Many instruments rely on highly visual and auditory systems. Tests that require language proficiency result in depressed scores of the mental capacity of children with auditory impairment. Among the tests most frequently used is the Developmental Activities Screening Inventory (DASI). The trays using wooden cubes, picture cards, beads, pegs, and cups are manipulative, so they are helpful with this population. The correlation between the DASI and standardized tests, such as the Cattell and Merrill Palmer Scale, is high thus supporting the assumption that it tests the same field.

The Callier-Azusa Scale employed with the deaf-blind is also designed to aid in assessing the mentally handicapped child's level of development and in measuring such a child's progress for program effectiveness. This test measures socialization, daily living skills, motor development, perceptual abilities, and language development. These divisions contain subscales describing developmental milestones.

This scale is based on the ongoing behaviors occurring in a classroom. It should be administered by individuals who are familiar with the child, are good observers, and have a knowledge of a child's repertoire of behavior. Several individuals, including teacher, aide, parents, and specialists, should provide a composite picture.

To make a quick assessment of measurable observable behavioral characteristics the Topeka Association for Retarded Citizens Test (TARC) may be used. The skills assessed are self-help, motor, communication, and social domain. It provides a general picture of a child's functioning based on a narrow sampling of behavior (ages 3–16). It is primarily for the mentally retarded but may be used with those diagnosed as autistic, perceptually handicapped, or learning disabled. The scoring is simple: those skills above 50 show strengths, and those below indicate weaknesses. The latter formulate the educational goals.

The Leiter International Performance Scale has been used for the hearing impaired to locate the mental age of the individual (ages 2–18). No verbal explanations are required, so that it is appropriate for the population. Such tasks as matching colors, forms, pictures; judging mass; recognizing footprints and facial expressions; classifying animals; completing forms; stating position and analogy; estimating numbers; demonstrating similarities, and other functions comprise the test.

Many programs, including the Mailman Center for Child Development in Miami, have adapted the Uzgiris-Hunt "tool of assessment which is grounded in the theory that development is an epigenic process of evolving new, more complex, hierarchical levels of organization in intellect and motivation" (Uzgiris & Hunt, 1975, p. 47). The indicators of cognitive organization are the actions of the individual himself. One can thus devise circumstances to foster the development of young children. The authors describe seven scales for assessing development: visual pursuit of objects; permanence of objects; means for obtaining desired environmental events; vocal imitation; operational causality; construction of object relations in space; and schemes for relating to objects. (Items may be selected suitable to the population intended and used for educational programming.)

Worthwhile in relation to educational planning are the Vineland Social Maturity Scale and the Arthur Point Scale of Performance Tests. The first measures the degree or level of social competence through measurement of personal social maturation (self-help, self-direction, communication, social capability, locomotion, occupational competence and promise). The Arthur Scale includes the Knox Cube Test (immediate recall), Sequin Form Board (10 shapes to be put quickly in board), Proteus Maze Test (trace shortest path), Healy Picture Completion Test, and the Arthur Stencil Design Test (reproduce complex designs by superimposing cut out stencils of various colors on a solid card). These tests are suitable for ages 5–15.

The Goodenough-Harris Drawing Test is frequently used to determine initial impression of mental ability, and it is valuable as a crude index of the mental age or development of children. It is a simple test: making three drawings, male, female, and oneself.

For the hearing-impaired population, the Hiskey Nebraska Test of Learning

Aptitude is available and provides a learning quotient (mental age and IQ) of the deaf, ages 3–16. The 12 subtests include bead patterns, memory for color, picture identification, picture association, paper folding, visual attention span, block patterns, completion of drawings, memory for digits, puzzle blocks, picture analogies, and spatial reasoning.

The Templin-Darly Tests of Articulation and the Goldman Fristoe Test of Articulation assess speech for preschool and elementary levels. The first uses 141 items grouped into 13 phoneme categories; the second is in 3 parts: sounds in words, sound in sentences, and sounds with stimulability. Both can be applied to assist in planning a remedial program.

The Boehm Test of Basic Concepts measures the child's mastery of concepts considered necessary for achievement in a school situation. It is presented orally and so may have to be adapted for some handicapped children (grades K–2). Based on the idea that each child enters school with a different background and therefore starts with a different body of knowledge and experience, the test is useful for children from varied ethnic origins and cultural backgrounds. Since the effects of deficiencies in very young children may be cumulative, attention should be directed towards early correction of initial lags in concept and language development. The test reviews reading, arithmetic, and science. The correct response is marked on a picture so that various communication systems may be used in presenting the test.

This concludes our review of formal tests presently available. For our purposes, many are not appropriate as they are written, mainly because of the communication and language delay of the hearing-impaired mentally retarded child. Some are suitable and may be used with caution to assess as accurately as possible this group of children. They may provide a guide to evolving needs in a flexible program. Educators must be aware of some assessment guidelines. The following questions may be considered when making an informal assessment, as with teacher-constructed tests or adaptations of extant tests or subtests. First, *why* are you testing, whether for broad concepts or specific information? Second, *how* do you intend to use the resulting information? Third, how much material are you trying to cover? Fourth, have you constructed a plan for your test, listing major areas and specific skills? Fifth, have you avoided ambiguities, and have you set forth clear statements? Where formal tests are a means of evaluating pupils' status and progress, teacher-made tests can be coordinated to produce an integral evaluative effort.

In conclusion, diagnostic assessment of the HI/MR child should be comprehensive: a medical assessment including history and examination; communication assessment, incorporating audiometric measure, language, and speech evaluation; educational/psychological assessment, covering cognitive development, sensorimotor skills, and academic achievement; social assessment, incorporating social, family, and cultural background; and adaptive behavior assessment and level of functioning (Healey, 1975). In order to assist in the development of prescriptive individual programs, these assessments should disclose causes and effects of the combined problem. At this point in time, the challenge is to provide a repertoire of tests, formal and informal, to furnish a composite picture of the strengths and weaknesses of the hearing-impaired mentally retarded child.

Curriculum

Without curriculum to implement an evaluation, an assessment remains a blank sheet of paper. Once hearing impairment and problems in intellectual functioning or adaptive behavior have been confirmed by comprehensive interdisciplinary assessment, program planning begins. Such planning must guide comprehensive services to ensure individual achievement. These services include an educational plan, periodic educational reassessment, periodic psychological reassessment, special education, and vocational education. The curriculum must be varied, broad, and flexible enough to provide for efficient learning. Assessments are only words which are used hundreds of times in numerous reports for many years; they must be backed by solid planning.

A good curriculum has goals, such as unlocking potential abilities in each handicapped person and developing maximum independence to function in an open or sheltered society. Whatever the setting—full-time special classroom, resource room, regular classroom with supportive services, home/hospital services, or residential placement—comprehensive skills must be developed. Among these might be listed self-care activities, basic skills, communication skills, occupational skills, and recreational skills. Goals in these areas should be commensurate with the potential of each person.

Within each skill, we can catalogue the following objectives. Self-care activities entail:
1. Cleanliness: washing, drying, bathing; care of hair, teeth, and nose;
2. Eating: managing solid food; drinking liquids; using utensils; observing table manners; using vending machines;
3. Safety: coping with weather; travelling safely in vehicles; crossing streets safely; becoming aware of potential danger;
4. Dressing and undressing;
5. Toileting and health: maintaining posture; recognizing sickness; obtaining first aid; grooming;
6. Personal development: gaining self-knowledge; utilizing personal information (name, age, etc.);
7. Social interaction: attending and relating to others; behaving appropriately sexually; becoming independent; caring for property;
8. Social amenities: physical; verbal;
9. Leisure: using media; playing or listening to music; dancing; participating in table games.

Basic skills encompass:
1. Sensorimotor skills: tactile, gustatory, olfactory;

2. Position in space: developing body image; learning body parts; understanding directionality;
3. Motor coordination: stationary movements (bending, reaching, kneeling); locomotion (walking, running); object movement (rolling, pushing);
4. Coordinated exercise; and
5. Visual-motor coordination: acquiring rhythm; maintaining balance.

The goals in communication skills of the HI/MR population must be a function of the capabilities of each person. These individual capabilities affect the selection of the most appropriate method of communication. Those who have severe learning problems frequently use a combination of oral and manual communication. Some may adapt the McGinnis method. Those with moderate to mild learning dysfunctions may be capable of learning limited oral skills of communication and may be educated in a resource room with supportive services.

Whatever mode of communication is used, the training of prelinguistic behavior is paramount in language development. One must inculcate eye contact and attention in order to initiate the development of meaning. The perceptual attributes (shape, movement, and size) play a distinctive role in building meaning. To develop meaning further, a child must have an experiential base, and in the early years the most suitable base is meaningful play. The child can learn through symbolic play to communicate wants, needs, and ideas. During play, appropriate responses may be established, for the element of imitation, particularly motor imitation, is strong.

One employs the child's natural environment as a tool in language training. Strategies that may be used are motor imitation, then sound imitation, and later play imitation. Of course, such imitation must be related to meaningful situations. For example, the parent or educator may use the child's favorite toy for this activity: "Push the car up the hill. The car goes zzzz." The parent or teacher uses action words first, such as "push," "throw," and "move." The parent or teacher may have the child imitate the action, and then ask what the child did. As soon as the child can imitate, the adult can use the action and the words in social interaction. As soon as verbal production is developed from imitation, the child can learn the value of communication. Repetition is important at this stage for cognition to take place. The parent or teacher has to teach the child to use contextual clues when learning to decipher the relation of words and the environment.

One of the crucial aspects in learning language is the development of memory. To develop memory, one must repeat information, organize units by spacing or exaggerating, and learn to use visual clues. When rehearsed sufficiently, generalization may occur. The parent or teacher should capitalize on such strategies as breaking down concepts into basic ideas or breaking down activities into basic acts. Those simple steps can be arranged sequentially so that their effect can be cumulative. Such sequencing and accumulation are fundamental techniques in developing memory, which is so crucial to learning language.

As part of language development, receptive vocabulary must be cultivated, too. The receptive vocabulary will concern concepts of self, food, clothing, shelter, everyday activities, family, friends, and physical environment. To the degree that the person is able, he or she will learn written language: reading, copying, and writing. Prereading skills include visual discrimination, visual memory, identification of letters, naming sight words (safety words, public signs). Prenumber skills entail identification of numerals; understanding concepts of "more," "dozen," etc. More complex number skills make possible handling money, making change, shopping, and counting. Other complex number skills are measuring, using a calendar, telling time, and telling temperature. Other numerical operations are simple addition and subtraction.

A number of current curriculum guides (such as *A Catalog of Instructional Objectives for Trainable Mentally Retarded Students,* 1974; *Home Teaching Activities Center for Early Development,* 1973; *Developing a Child's Potential,* 1972; *Joy of Learning,* 1976; and the *Readiness Curriculum, Reading Curriculum, and Math Curriculum for Deaf Multi-Handicapped Unit of California School for the Deaf,* 1974), include materials designed to reinforce concepts and skills taught by the teachers. Some include patterns and suggestions in the appendices. Others develop individual learning centers helpful in establishing independent work habits and in fostering a sense of responsibility. These abilities help reduce frustration and anxiety as well as help in building skills needed in occupations later in life.

Concepts in the *Joy of Learning* are broken down into their component parts. As the child succeeds with those small steps, they are combined to build a foundation for more advanced academic skills. This strategy is one that has been employed for many years with the slow deaf child and one that can be pursued with HI/MR children, too. It is necessary both to seek the basics of a task and to present concepts of the task in many different ways since each child is unique in his or her mode of learning.

Individualization is the focus of education today, and it is only through personalization that the child can learn at his or her own rate. In developing materials a teacher should keep in mind a child's specific interest. Materials should be varied, as nearly indestructible as possible, clearly made, attractive, yet not over stimulating. The Oregon program, for example, uses independent work areas and learning stations where a child works in a one-to-one relationship with a teacher. There are two teachers to eight pupils.

Individualization involves making appropriate learning materials and keeping records on what the child is doing. When good records are kept, the teacher has a file on each child that indicates the results of pretests and post tests and lists objectives. This file becomes an account of the child's own achievement without comparison to others. This is one way that a hearing-impaired mentally retarded child can become self-confident and be motivated to learn new tasks.

Programs and projects developing the hearing-impaired mentally retarded citizen have direct implications for vocational adjustment and community living. One must develop general work skills (such as sorting and assembling), work habits (such as attending, following rules, cooperating), and work concepts (such as independence and productivity). Skills necessary to maintain a position—whether it be domestic service, shop service, or speciality jobs—often extend into the community, so counselling and referral agencies may have to provide support services for the most severely impaired. Practical experiences, such as training for independent living and trial job placements, should be offered when possible. Often the involvement of a family is imperative to serve as an inspiration.

Intervention Strategies

It is interesting that a natural gesture system was initiated with a number of children in order to develop a communication system (Mavilya, 1978). In 1977, the Mailman Center for Child Development conducted a study to assist in developing a system of communication for multihandicapped hearing-impaired infants and toddlers. The study involved six multihandicapped children between the ages of 2½ and 5 years. They were taught by graduate students during this period. These children had a combination of disabilities that rendered them severely handicapped. They were both hearing-impaired and had one or more disabilities, such as cerebral palsy, mental retardation, perceptual problems, and emotional disturbances. The Natural Gesture Language System was employed to initiate communication between educator and child. The children were assisted in acquiring strategies to deal with daily familiar situations. The children's interaction with the models provided discovery and practice in communication. Imitation may be a crucial learning strategy in a child's acquisition of nonverbal communication.

The original study focused on gestures characterized by an essential physical movement. The gestures utilized are easily recognized by an untrained observer. Most of the gestures collected are complexes of motion, and they may be analogous to sentences. For example, to shrug the shoulders and then extend the arms would indicate, "I don't know where it is." We have excluded any specialized gesture system, such as ritual gestures found in secret organizations, American Sign Language, or game gestures. The collection gathered is by no means complete, for an infinite number of gestures is used almost unconsciously by most people.

These familiar body and facial gestures incorporate feelings, wants, and emotions. The descriptions cannot be complete in all instances since the context in which gestures are made lends more information. The semantic labels range from the very general "Where?" to the specific "Me." Simple illustrations can capture the essence of the movements for easy recognition and reproduction.

When gestures are used with a hearing-impaired mentally retarded population, they must be accompanied by verbal utterances at all times since they are known as words in the context of the situation. A smile along with a clapping of the hands and accompanied by the word "Good" is obvious in meaning. We use gestures in conjunction with the verbal message, including intonation and appropriate stress, in order to maintain normal communication and engender, if possible, any auditory response that may be present. The visual reinforcement in speechreading may prove to be a clue for understanding the message. The multihandicapped child does require more dynamic or dramatic movement and special consideration. If the child is unable to lipread or read signs, the natural gesture system can be used as an entity in itself or as a supplement to oral language.

It has been documented that nonverbal communication predominates during the first year of life of a child (Vetter, 1969). At this age a child speaks with the whole body at first. It seems plausible, and it became evident in the study with the multihandicapped infants and toddlers, that they could learn to communicate using this mode of communication, a natural gesture language. It is conceivable that this technique could establish a communication mode until a child could learn to read lips or to develop standard sign language. This proved to be true of an 11-year-old child and others in several classes for the multihandicapped deaf in the primary grades.

In those primary classes, educational intervention with the children consisted of daily one-half hour language lessons incorporating action-bound gestures. The intent of the program was to employ natural gestures in a language-oriented activity, anticipating that the child would receive and express these gestures. Various concepts were used such as "up" (climbing *up,* lifting oneself *up,* moving objects *up,* and stretching arms *up*). By working individually, the teacher was able to assess the needs and progress of the child. The language lessons resulted in both receptive and expressive communication.

There is limited knowledge about the benefits of gesticulation with severely handicapped children. This investigation and a few results reported by teachers in this group assisted in establishing communication and proved to be provocative. The children responded to the gestures and initiated some of the language expressively. Some incorporated vocalization in conjunction with the gestures. Those children with physical involvements adapted and modified the gestures in ways which proved to be recognizable and valid. These results can be regarded as a stimulus to further investigation, for it would be of inestimable value to know the extent to which this mode of communication, a natural gesture language, can be used to establish communication among the hearing-impaired mentally retarded.

Conclusion

Perhaps one may view some of the suggestions offered in this chapter as unconventional. In the domain of assessment, we consider informal teacher-made adaptations; in curriculum, we offer many teacher-made materials, all helpful in building skills needed by this very special group of children; among educational strategies, we recommend devising a simple, natural gesture system as a communication mode. All of these ideas serve as catalysts to propel the education of the hearing-impaired mentally retarded. No one technique is perfect, but we cannot always be prudent or wait forever for *the* solution. We may stumble over the solution. Perhaps the only way to succeed is by really trying.

Bibliography

A catalog of instructional objectives for trainable mentally retarded students (Funded under Title VI-B Grant awarded Duval County School Board). Tallahassee, Fla.: Department of Education, 1974.

Chomsky, N. Current perspectives in acquisition and use of language. Luncheon speech at ASHA Conference. Chicago, November 4, 1977.

Davis, E. *Curriculum activities guide for severely retarded deaf students.* Indianapolis, Ind.: Marion County Association for Retarded Citizens, 1973.

Debbie School Programs, Mailman Center for Child Development. *Child progress monitoring system.* Miami, Fla.: University of Miami, July 1977.

Eaton, P., & Eiring, L. *Joy of learning.* Beaverton, Oreg.: Dormac, Inc., 1976.

Gearhart, B., & Willenberg, E. *Application of pupil assessment information for the special education teacher.* Denver: Love Publications, Inc., 1974.

Haeussermann, E. *Developmental potential of preschool children.* New York: Grune and Stratton, Inc., 1958.

Hardy, W. C. Human communication: Ordered and disordered. *Volta Review,* 1962, *64*(7), 354–362.

Healey, W. C. *The hearing-impaired mentally retarded: Recommendations for action* (Document funded by Department of HEW, Social and Rehabilitation Service). Rehabilitation Services Administration, 1975.

Home teaching activities (Supported by Grant S F 500. Center for Early Development and Education. University of Arkansas). Office of Child Development, Department of HEW, 1973.

Hyde, S., & Engel, D. *Potomac Program: A curriculum for the severely handicapped deaf.* Beaverton, Oreg.: Dormac, Inc., 1977.

Jordan, E. S. *Developing a child's potential* (Funded under Title III). Boise, Idaho: State Department of Education, 1972.

Luria, A. R. *The mentally retarded child.* Washington, D.C.: Office of Technical Service, U.S. Department of Commerce, 1962.

Mavilya, M. *Natural gesture language and spoken words: Mode of communication for the multiply handicapped hearing-impaired infants and toddlers.* Paper presented at CEC Convention. Kansas City, Mo., May 1978.

Meier, J. Dimensions of early detection of developmental disabilities. In *Themes and Issues.* Chapel Hill, N.C.: 1978.

Morkovin, B. V. Organic and inhibitory factors of speech perception and speech production disturbances in children with hearing disorders. *Proceedings of the International Congress of the Deaf.* Washington, D.C.: Gallaudet College, 1963, 726–734.

Penfield, W., & Roberts, L. *Speech and brain mechanisms.* Princeton: Princeton University Press, 1959.

Peterson, B., & Schoenmann, S. *Building blocks for developing basic language.* Beaverton, Oreg.: Dormac, Inc., 1977.

Power, D. J., & Quigley, S. P. *Problems and programs in the education of multiply disabled children.* Champaign, Ill.: University of Illinois Press, 1971.

Readiness curriculum, reading curriculum, and math curriculum for the Deaf Multihandicapped Unit (Funded under ESEA. Title I). Riverside: California School for the Deaf, June 1974.

Uzgiris, I., & Hunt, J. McV. *Assessment in infancy.* Chicago: University of Illinois Press, 1975.

Vetter, H. J. *Language behavior and communication.* Itasca, Ill.: F. E. Peacock Publishers Inc., 1969.

Developing the Curriculum for Severely Disturbed Hearing-Impaired Students

Larry G. Stewart

Emotional disturbance affects a significant proportion of the hearing-impaired student population. Dr. Larry Stewart estimates as much as 25% of a typical class of deaf children may suffer emotional disturbance. In response to this problem, he sets forth a curriculum designed to eliminate patterns of inappropriate coping behavior and to teach adaptive coping to these youngsters.

The needs associated with emotional disturbance among hearing-impaired students have generally been overlooked by educators. In addition, few specialists are trained to work with this group of children. As a result, we do not have a great deal of knowledge to draw from as we attempt to design educationally oriented treatment strategies. Therefore, I will draw primarily from my own experience over the years in working with students and teachers as a psychologist.

Definitions and Limitations

Permit me at the beginning to define some of my terms and outline several limits to keep in mind as we consider the topic of planning educational programs for emotionally disturbed hearing-impaired children.

DEFINITIONS In order to insure clarity and mutual understanding, I offer these definitions of terms as I use them in this chapter.

Hearing-Impaired Children For my purposes, this term will refer to children who have a significant hearing loss which necessitates special efforts from helping persons in the area of one-to-one communication. These special efforts will usually involve the use of sign language, carefully enunciated speech, or both.

Severely Disturbed This term refers to children whose overt behavior is such that they experience interpersonal conflict with other students and teachers, and this conflict interferes significantly with classroom learning and everyday coping. It is assumed here that psychotic conditions are not present in the child, or, in other words, the child's thought processes are basically intact.

Curriculum This term is used here to refer to educationally oriented classroom activities. Implicit in this definition is the concept that schools are not hospitals; schools are not mental health institutions; schools are not mental health treatment clinics; and school personnel are not specialists in psychotherapy. Regardless of what schools could be, regardless of however much one might wish schools could be everything to everyone, the fact is that schools are oriented toward educating children. Because of the nature of the educational process in America, it would be best if we were to keep in mind that there are very real limitations as to what the typical school can do for an emotionally disturbed child, deaf or hearing, Public Law 94-142 or no Public Law 94-142.

Do not misunderstand me. Someday public schools and schools for the deaf can and will be doing a very great deal more than they are now doing for disturbed children. However, for now, the reality is that many disturbed children are being further disturbed by the very fact of their being in regular educational settings. Treatment personnel and support systems simply do not exist for these children in most schools. Accordingly, my discussion will not get into what can be done for those children who should not be in school because of the severity of their disturbance, any more than should a child with a temperature of 105° or acute influenza.

LIMITATIONS My remarks are intended for classroom teachers, not for mental health specialists. It is assumed that teachers have access to a competent psychologist and/or a capable psychiatrist who can provide qualified diagnostic services for the child and consultation for the staff in designing and implementing an effective treatment program for the individual child. When a teacher does not have access to a psychologist or psychiatrist, the danger of educational malpractice exists. I think that too often educators tend to underestimate the seriousness of some emotional disorders or behaviors suggestive of disturbance. In my experience, children with behavior problems are overlooked until the problems involved can no longer be tolerated. Then, when it is recognized that there is a *big* problem, it is often too late to take effective corrective measures. Thus, it is my hope that teachers will *insist* on professional diagnostic assistance with any child whose behavior is suggestive of emotional disturbance. Teachers should also demand from administrators the provision of guidance from a mental health specialist when they attempt to plan an educationally oriented treatment program. Tender, loving care is indispensable to all children, and especially so to disturbed children. A good teacher can and must offer TLC. However, TLC is not enough. Expertise in treatment is mandatory.

The Population

Before getting into curriculum, I would like to emphasize the size of the task insofar as disturbed hearing-impaired children are concerned. Qualitative considerations aside for a moment, there is conflicting information on the probable size of the population of hearing-impaired emotionally disturbed children. For example:
- Schlesinger and Meadow (1972) have estimated that possibly as many as 17% of the children in schools and classes for the deaf have a significant emotional disturbance.
- Of the 44,949 hearing-impaired children reportedly enrolled in October 1976, in schools and classes for the deaf in the United States, 1,253 (2%) were reported to have a social/emotional disturbance.

- A Presidential Commission on Child Mental Health in 1971 reported that one out of every ten persons in the United States can be expected to spend some time in a mental health institution. This represents 10% of the population.

My own estimation is that as many as 25% of a typical school or class of deaf children may have emotional disturbance of such a nature that special educational assistance is needed. However, validation of these estimates must await a concentrated attempt to identify this population on a national basis.

Curriculum Planning

The essential difference between the deaf child with significant emotional disturbance and the deaf child without significant emotional disturbance is found in the area of coping skills. The disturbed child has significantly diminished ability to cope with the demands of his or her environment and typically responds to these demands by either withdrawal behavior or acting out behavior. The former results in failure to respond, the latter in behavior that disrupts the learning process both for oneself and for others. Moreover, this behavior is characterized as a pattern, a continuing response, rather than a temporary or transitory response to adverse circumstances. Everyone can and does become "disturbed" under severe stress, but emotional disturbance, as we define it, exists when there is a continuity of disturbed behavior under ordinary stresses.

Curriculum planning thus must aim to break up this patterned, non-coping behavior and to provide the child with behavioral responses that permit adaptive, coping behavior. In order for this process of change to occur, the following logical steps are required:
1. Identify the behavior and behavioral patterns that are preventing the child from coping adequately.
2. Identify the reinforcers that are maintaining the child's maladaptive behavior.
3. Identify potential reinforcers of adaptive, coping behavior.
4. Plan and implement a program of activities whereby reinforcers of maladaptive behavior are eliminated or at least minimized, and reinforcers of coping, adaptive behaviors are substituted or maximized.
5. Monitor behavioral progress and evaluate outcomes on a systematic basis, providing feedback to the child and persons involved in educational programming.

IDENTIFICATION OF PROBLEMS The first step in this five-stage process of curriculum development for the hearing-impaired child is crucial. It permits identification of both the problem behaviors of the child and, equally important, the settings where these behaviors occur.

The steps of identification should be:
1. Referral for assistance, usually to the principal or psychologist.

2. Provision of a psychological evaluation to determine the child's abilities, interests, and behavior characteristics.
3. Examinations by specialists (vision, physical, neurological) when indicated.
4. Acquisition of prior and current reports from teachers and parents concerning the child's behavior. For residential school children, dormitory reports are vital.

PROGRAM PLANNING Once identification information has been acquired, it should be organized and presented to concerned staff members. A staff meeting of involved teachers, dormitory personnel, and others is required for this purpose. The objectives of this staff meeting, led by the mental health specialists, should be to plan treatment with a prescriptive approach.
1. Identify problem behaviors.
2. Identify length and duration of behavior patterns.
3. Identify reinforcers of problem behaviors.
4. Identify student assets and their reinforcers along with other potential reinforcers of coping behavior.
5. Set goals for eliminating problem behaviors and replacing them with coping behaviors.
6. Set specific objectives for attainment of goals.
7. Determine objective-oriented activities. Identify what will be attempted by whom and how, and according to what timeline. Select one person to act as coordinator of efforts on behalf of the child to insure accountability.
8. Determine method of progress monitoring and outcome evaluation.

MONITORING ACTIVITIES Curriculum activities must be monitored very closely. Otherwise, staff efforts will most likely become weakened and disorganized. Monitoring is facilitated by the use of reporting forms used by staff members to provide feedback to the activities coordinator. The coordinator, in turn, synthesizes these reports and provides an evaluation or progress report to all involved staff members. Meetings of the staff may be held to share information and to modify treatment approaches.

To clarify this identification and prescription process, one case will be presented as an example.

Richard: A Case Study

BACKGROUND Richard was a 17-year-old deaf student attending the school for the deaf. He was husky and muscular and was on the varsity football and wrestling teams. A quiet young man, he was known to have occasional explosive outbursts of temper and to engage in physical assaults on other students who had disagreements with him. There were no other recorded overt signs of emotional disturbance aside from a tendency to keep to himself and stubbornness. Referral was initiated by the

Dean of Students following a fight in which Richard battered a peer so badly the latter was in the hospital for two days.

PSYCHOLOGICAL EVALUATION A psychological evaluation reported a Wechsler Adult Intelligence Scale (WAIS) Performance Scale I.Q. with even subtest scatter. Bender-Gestalt Test results were borderline, suggestive of a minor degree of visual-motor impairment but without strong signs of neurological malfunction. Stanford Achievement Test (SAT) scores were more or less typical, with reading comprehension at slightly below fourth grade and a similar Word Meaning grade level score. Arithmetic computation was at sixth grade level. Personality assessment revealed an immature level of personality development, with evidence of poor impulse control and underlying aggressive/hostility trends. Self-concept measures suggested a poor self-concept and resentment against his parents. No thought disorder was present.

MEDICAL CONSIDERATIONS Medical examination revealed no physical problems other than deafness. Richard was in excellent health. An EEG exam performed the year before at the request of the parents was normal.

PRIOR REPORTS An examination of Richard's school records and other records on file showed him to be a mediocre student, having obtained primarily C grades and a few Ds and Fs. Dormitory reports referred consistently to aggressive, acting out behavior as well as periodic episodes of resistance to authority. Other comments referred to tardiness, a couple of instances of going to town without permission, and two instances of drinking wine with other students on campus. It was clear that Richard had had behavior problems throughout the time he was enrolled in school, but none of these problems were considered important enough to raise a red flag with school officials until the most recent fight.

Records revealed that the parents were separated, with the father living in another state. The parents were well-off financially, and the mother, socially prominent in her hometown, was active in club affairs. She appeared to be at a loss in helping Richard; she deferred discipline to the father's infrequent visits to the home. When the parents visited the school, the mother would be reticent, deferring to her husband in decision making with respect to Richard. Neither parent could use sign language, and Richard, being congenitally deaf and with no usable speech, did not seem to relate to the parents when the three were observed together.

Richard had a history of participation in school athletics, being especially effective in football and wrestling. In the latter sport, he was champion of his weight class for two straight years. He was clean and neat in his dress and personal hygiene, and he had good work habits as observed in the dormitory and in vocational training classes. He had two close friends but did not seem to enjoy social activities.

Richard's teachers reported that he seemed to have only minimal interest in school. When he became bored, which was often, he would retreat into himself and appear to be daydreaming. When asked to return to his work, he would seem irritated and at times would say crossly, "Leave me alone" or, if angered, make an obscene gesture to his teacher or stalk out of the room until he had calmed down. His teachers were reluctant to crack down on him too closely because of his temper. The teachers were especially wary of Richard fighting with other students, since this had happened often enough in the past.

Richard has been receiving counseling from a school counselor for several months, specifically for helping him with his temper outbursts.

Richard's primary area of interest was motorcycles, which he enjoyed riding and reading about.

PROGRAM PLANNING The information gained in the identification process was compiled by the psychologist during the initial case study. A staff meeting was then called by the principal, and attended by the following:
1. Principal
2. Counselor
3. Richard's classroom teachers
4. Richard's dormitory counselors (Houseparents)
5. Psychological consultant
6. School Nurse

Case findings were reviewed, with comments from staff, if present. At the completion of this review the following specific findings were noted:
1. *Problem Behaviors*
   a. Temper outbursts
   b. Physical aggression
   c. Irritability toward others
   d. Disrespect toward teachers and dormitory counselors
   e. Disregard for expected standards of behavior in the classroom
   f. Lack of interest in school
2. *Length and Duration of Problem Behavior*
   a. Records revealed Richard's behavior patterns had existed since childhood, with an increase in intensity during the past year.
3. *Reinforcers of Problem Behaviors*
   Records and staff review suggested the following reinforcers:
   a. Parental conflict
   b. Ambivalence in handling discipline in the home
   c. Communication frustrations in the home
   d. Richard's need for recognition in view of his poor self-concept
   e. Lack of meaningful involvement in day-to-day school activities
   f. Lack of future direction
   g. Teacher reluctance to be firm with Richard
   h. Lack of consequences for past aggressive behavior

i. Language frustrations
4. *Student Assets, Positive Reinforcers*
   a. Physical strength and peer respect
   b. Personal attractiveness and good hygiene
   c. Achievement in athletics and peer respect
   d. Interest in motorcycles
   e. Ability to get along with others when no pressures were present
   f. High level of intelligence
   g. Home values (cleanliness, care for personal affairs, achievement orientation)
   h. Potential for academic success and some interest in attending junior college
5. *Objective Setting*

   As a result of this meeting and the identification of Richard's problem behaviors, problem reinforcers, and positive reinforcers, the staff established the following objectives:
   a. To help Richard learn to cope with his aggressive behavior tendencies and improve control of his feelings
   b. To help Richard develop new areas of interest, both socially and personally
   c. To help Richard's parents to become more effective in their relations with Richard
   d. To assist teachers and dorm counselors to be more effective in their work with Richard
6. *Objective-Oriented Activities*

   To achieve these objectives, the following activities were decided upon:
   a. The psychological consultant would develop a list of problem behaviors and positive behaviors and assign weighted scores to each. This list would be distributed to all staff members coming into contact with Richard on a regular basis. The completed forms would be returned to the counselor, as mental health coordinator, each week. The psychological consultant would review the results with Richard each Friday afternoon.
   b. The psychological consultant and counselor would meet with Richard, review with him identified problems and staff concerns and plans, and seek his full participation in treatment plans.
   c. Richard's parents would be called upon to share in the staff findings and would be requested to (1) cooperate in treatment plans, (2) seek guidance regarding their relations with Richard, and (3) take manual communication classes.
   d. Since Richard's father had planned to buy him a motorcycle in June (it was February), it was decided to use the motorcycle as a primary reinforcer. The cost of the motorcycle was set, and the amount Richard would have to earn each month in order to have the required amount by June was set ($450.00 divided by 4 = $112.50 per month or $28.12 per week). A value was set, using money values, for each type of negative or problem behavior and each

type of positive or coping behavior. Serious behaviors were assigned a high value ($15.00 for pushing someone, $25.00 for hitting) and less serious behavior a lower value ($1.00 for making unpleasant faces). Conversely, positive behaviors were assigned similar value, with normal behavior assigned a low value and especially helpful behavior a high value.

Thus, Richard was faced with direct reinforcers for both positive and negative behavior. Observations by teachers and other staff would lead to ratings, which, in turn, would lead or not lead to a motorcycle.

Importantly, each Friday Richard's tabulations were added up and his earnings discussed. He then took the ratings to the business office, where his father had deposited $450.00, and the clerk would transfer the earned amount to Richard's own account.

e. The counselor would meet with Richard each week to discuss his progress, review his problems, and consider outlets for his frustrations.

7. *Progress Monitoring and Outcome Evaluation*

Every two weeks the psychological consultant would summarize Richard's progress and report, via memo, to participating staff members. This would permit staff feedback and progress evaluation.

This was the plan that was followed over a four-month period with Richard. A copy of the teacher rating scale is in Form 1. A copy of the progress summary form is in Form 2.

I am pleased to report that this plan was highly successful. Initially, Richard had difficulty with many of the behaviors so firmly entrenched within him, but as the weeks went by, he gradually eliminated his problem behaviors and started to accumulate coping behaviors in impressive style. At the end of the year, he had few overt behavioral problems and no major acting out difficulties. He earned the money he needed to buy his motorcycle, and in the process developed a new repertoire of coping behaviors.

Not all curriculum planning has such pleasant outcomes, but as one can see, the job can be done with careful planning and monitoring. The identification and prescription model presented here can be replicated with many problem areas.

Support Systems

Obviously, the task of meeting the needs of disturbed deaf youth is a complex one. The model presented will not always work. However, given basic support systems, this model and others have an excellent chance of being effective.

What are support systems? Basically, they are positive reinforcers that are readily available to a teacher and to the child. Some of these systems are:
- Qualified diagnostic personnel
- A capable staff with positive attitudes
- A meaningful overall school curriculum

FORM I
STAFF RATING FORM FOR RICHARD*

Staff Member _____

Week of _____

	Frequency					
	Monday	Tuesday	Wednesday	Thursday	Friday	Saturday

Behavior Problem

1. *Physical Aggression*
    a. Verbal
    b. Physical
       1) Mild
       2) Moderate
       3) Serious

2. *Anger*
    a. Verbal
    b. Gestural

3. *Disrespect*
    a. Verbal
    b. Gestural

4. *Disinterest*
    a. Mild
    b. Moderate
    c. Serious

Coping Behavior

1. Classroom
2. Dormitory
3. Athletics
4. Dining Room
5. Other (specify:)

   _____

   _____

Comments: _____

*Use one checkmark per incident.
**Use one checkmark for exemplary behavior.

FORM II
PROGRESS SUMMARY FORM FOR RICHARD

For 2 week period from _____ to _____ .

	2 Week Total Incidents	Cumulative Total

Behavior Problems

1. *Physical Aggression*
   a. Verbal
   b. Physical
      1) Mild
      2) Moderate
      3) Serious

2. *Anger*
   a. Verbal
   b. Gestural

3. *Disrespect*
   a. Verbal
   b. Gestural

4. *Disinterest*
   a. Mild
   b. Moderate
   c. Serious

Coping Behavior

1. Classroom
2. Dormitory
3. Athletics
4. Dining Room
5. Other (specify:)
   _____

   _____

Totals

- A meaningful after school activity
- An effective parent education program
- Community interaction
- Counseling and guidance activities
- Access to community mental health resources
- Models (e.g., qualified deaf professionals) for deaf youths.

These amount to resources for both treatment *and* preventive mental health. The old adage, "An ounce of prevention is worth a pound of cure," is no more true than with mental health. Experience has shown that with the appropriate support systems, mental health problems need never occur, or, at least, can be minimized. Considering the complexity of treating disturbed youth, and the dearth of trained therapy personnel, preventive mental health must necessarily be "the treatment of choice." If a school lacks the support systems it needs for this approach, then change is in order. Meanwhile, we now have a model for treating the disturbed deaf child that has been shown effective with a fairly large number of deaf children.

In closing, let me emphasize once again that treating disturbed deaf children requires a professional, individualized approach, but professional diagnosticians and treatment specialists are also indispensable members of the team. With this interdisciplinary team and emphasis on early diagnosis and treatment, the rate of success will be pleasantly high.

Bibliography

Schlesinger, H. S., & Meadow, K. P. *Sound and sign: Childhood deafness and mental health.* Berkeley: University of California Press, 1972.

Assessing and Remedying Perceptual Problems in Hearing-Impaired Children

Charlotte Shroyer

Noting that the term "learning disability" has been used imprecisely, Dr. Charlotte Shroyer favors the term "learning problem" in her paper. She defines such phenomena as perception, visual discrimination, and figure-ground discrimination. She tells how these skills can be assessed in hearing-impaired students with learning problems, and she describes remedies for deficits in these areas.

By definition, the field of learning disabilities has excluded learning problems primarily attributable to sensory handicaps, to physical handicaps, or to cultural disadvantage. This point is illustrated in the definition evolved by the National Advisory Committee on Handicapped Children (1968):

Children with special learning disabilities exhibit a disorder in one or more of the basic psychological processes involved in understanding or using spoken or written languages. These may be manifested in disorders of listening, thinking, talking, reading, writing, spelling, or arithmetic. They include conditions which have been referred to as perceptual handicaps, brain injury, minimal brain dysfunction, dyslexia, developmental aphasia, etc. They do not include learning problems which are due primarily to visual, hearing, or motor handicaps, to mental retardation, to emotional disturbance, or to environmental disadvantage.

(p. 4)

This position of exclusion has been justified by a pragmatic need for allocation of funds for the education of a group of children previously excluded from special education services, namely, those children manifesting learning problems.

Although the definition itself has been exclusive, the field of learning disabilities has become multidisciplinary, resulting in an accumulation of knowledge from professionals within other disciplines such as psychology, linguistics, and special education services for other exceptionalities. The field of education of the deaf has been excluded by definition, but professionals within the field of education of the deaf have shown an interest in identifying learning disabilities as secondary handicaps accompanying the primary handicap of deafness.

References to learning disabilities within the deaf population are apparent in the literature. Jensema (1975) analyzed the results of administration of the Stanford Achievement Test Battery to a sample of 16,882 deaf students. Of that total, 4,031 were reported to have at least one handicapping condition in addition to deafness. Four hundred twenty-seven were identified as having learning disabilities. When compared to other subsets of secondary handicaps, such as emotional disturbance, epilepsy, severe visual impairment, orthopedic disabilities, to mention only a few, the category of learning disabilities ranked third. When perceptual-motor disabilities, often considered a subset of the more general category of learning disabilities, were included within the learning disabilities category, the total of 833 students ranked second only to emotional problems with a total of 885. In a similar report, Jensema and Mullins (1974) found that 1,262 students of a total sample of 23,704 students were exhibiting behaviors associated with perceptual-motor dysfunction in addition to the major handicap of deafness. In addition to references in the literature, subjective observation has revealed that teachers of the deaf report existence of what they perceive to be learning disabilities in a segment of the population of deaf children with whom they work on a day-to-day basis.

It remains to be seen whether the so-called learning disabilities currently reported in deaf children are observable and measurable behaviors which can indeed be attributed to specific learning disabilities, or whether they are an apparition explained to some extent by societal emphasis on learning disabilities.

Despite references in the literature to learning disabilities in deaf children, and despite current interest in the matter, there has been little attempt to clarify the use of the term as it applies in this context. Does the term connote some demonstrable dysfunction in learning? Is it pertinent to some deaf children who are exhibiting learning patterns deviant from the learning patterns of most deaf children? Does it refer only to perceptual-motor difficulties? Is it another label for distractable behavior? The definition of learning disabilities as it pertains to the deaf child is ambiguous.

This paper is not intended as an argument against the existence of learning disabilities in a deaf population. On the contrary, there are many indicators which point to an inferential relationship between the two. Johnson and Myklebust (1967) define a learning disability as psychoneurological in nature, meaning "that the behavior has been disturbed as [the] result of a dysfunction in the brain and that the problem is one of altered processes, not of a generalized incapacity to learn" (p. 8). Implicit in the term is an assumption that a dysfunction in processing, probably neurological in nature, exists. If we accept that definition, it seems logical to suppose that sensorineural hearing loss may affect other processing areas of the brain, thus resulting in a learning dysfunction in addition to the hearing loss. However, this relationship, although logically clear is at best inferential.

For all of these reasons, the term learning disabilities will not be used in this paper. Instead, the more generic term "learning problem" will be incorporated to apply to the deaf child who does not appear to be learning in a manner similar to that of his or her deaf peers. Because the deaf child is more dependent on visual processing for information about the environment than are hearing peers, this chapter focuses on visual-perceptual problems in a deaf population as they affect learning.

What Is Perception?

Perception is the "process by which we gain first-hand information about the world around us" (Gibson, 1969). The child does not come into the world with his or her perceptions predetermined. Although some types of perception, such as depth perception, are apparent as early as one month of age with some indication that the ability may be functional from birth (Stone, Smith, & Murphy, 1973), adult perception of the world must be learned.

Perception is an active process which occurs in the brain. Because it does occur in the brain, and because it is basically an "internal cognitive process" (Ross, 1976, p. 32), the intactness of its functioning is difficult to assess. One can only infer its functioning on the basis of observable responses which may involve skills other than perception. Even the use of sophisticated mechanical devices, such as the electroencephalogram (EEG), does not reliably explain or represent what is occurring in the brain (Satterfield, 1973).

Perception is a selective process. The visual stimuli bombarding each individual are too numerous to mention. As part of the learning process, the individual learns how to extract the necessary information from those stimuli within the environment. This process appears to be developmental in nature (Crane & Ross, 1967; Stevenson, 1972).

Although the process is learned, much of what is learned is learned in a developmental manner through the interaction of the child with the environment and those within his or her environment. If, for some reason, this process is not proceeding in the normal developmental fashion, the child will be handicapped in learning how to deal with the world. This handicap may be reflected in different behavior at various chronological levels and in varying degrees of severity. The fifth grade child who has difficulty discriminating between b and d; the child who can't understand Mother's facial expression when he laughs at being punished; the child who has not learned how to match the cylinder with the round hole in the wooden toy—all have problems which may not be due in toto to perceptual problems, but which may be attributable in some degree to perceptual deficits.

Assessment of Visual Perception

The assessment of visual perception is not an easy matter. The nature of the process itself may be responsible, at least in part, for this difficulty. Because perception is a process which occurs within the brain, any quantification related to the intactness of the process must be based on some kind of observable response occurring externally in the environment. Even then one can only infer the efficiency and the effectiveness of the process.

The Developmental Test of Visual Perception (Frostig, Maslow, Lefever, & Whittlesey, 1964) represents one of the attempts to measure visual perception through inference on the basis of demonstrated, observable responses such as drawing, copying, and making appropriate shapes on five subtests: Eye-Hand Coordination, Figure-Ground Perception, Form Constancy, Position in Space, and Spatial Relations. Scoring on at least three of these subtests depends heavily on the accuracy of the motor responses by the child (Hammill, 1975). Tasks which rely heavily on accuracy of motor response by the child may be considered to assess visual-motor processes, not visual-perceptual processes.

Tasks which require the child either to point or to indicate "yes" or "no" in either a verbal or nonverbal fashion may be considered more appropriate measures of visual perception. Although the response is still a motor response, the motor component has been minimized. The Motor-Free Test of Visual Perception (Colarusso & Hammill, 1972) is representative of such a format. Items are multiple choice; the child looks at visual forms (nonsense, common objects, and letter forms) and points to the response of his or her choosing.

Assuming that motor response is intact (as determined by observation) and assuming that visual-motor integration difficulties are suspected, the teacher might wish to administer both the Frostig Developmental Test of Visual Perception and the Motor-Free Test of Visual Perception. Although Colarusso and Hammill (1972) found a correlation of .73 between the two tests, it must be noted that statistical procedures indicate that these two tests may "measure some unique abilities" (Colarusso & Hammill, 1972, p. 17). Judgments based on such results must be considered tentative.

For the deaf child suspected of having minimal visual-perceptual and/or perceptual-motor difficulties, these two tests may be used with their limitations kept in mind. There is one additional limitation: the lack of any standardization on a deaf population. Although the Frostig test does include directions (available upon request) for administration to deaf youngsters, there are no norms for deaf youngsters in the manual. Likewise, the Motor-Free Test of Visual Perception has no available data on standardization with the deaf.

For the deaf child suspected of or manifesting more severe visual-perceptual problems, however, neither the Frostig nor the Motor-Free Test will provide a reliable valid assessment of visual-perceptual or visual-motor skills. Much of the assessment information obtained must be acquired on an informal basis. For the child who is most likely limited in his or her language ability, this necessitates a professional who is extremely skilled in the observation of children and who is familiar with developmental norms. Of course, the interpretation of such data acquired from informal observation is at best tentative, and this fact must be kept in mind.

A four-year-old deaf child, on one of many occasions, was observed during a free play period as he assembled a truck into its corresponding template. Instead of completing the task in the usual manner by placing the bed and body of the truck within the template and then sequentially placing six colored blocks representing the load carried by the truck, he did the manipulation in reversed order. First, he placed the six blocks carefully in their correct spatial position within the template. This was followed by the correct placement of a rectangle representing the window and a circle representing the headlight of the truck. The final manipulation involved the placement of the bed and body of the truck in their correct positions. Without his performance on any standardization test, this observation and subsequent observations in free play revealed data essential to an informal assessment of perceptual functioning. The child had given some indications that he remembered where the respective parts of the truck were to be placed (visual spatial memory) and that he discriminated among the component parts of the truck (visual discrimination).

It is apparent that judgments related to the intactness of perceptual functioning on the basis of one anecdotal incident can only be considered extremely unreliable. However, "a series of valid anecdotal records systematically collected over a period of time, once obtained, can be analyzed for emerging patterns and needs . . . " (Zigmond, 1976, p. 2.14). It is important to remember that any anecdotal observation should be *descriptive* and *objective*. It is only after descriptive information has been collected that the interpretive process can begin.

The remainder of this paper deals with some general approaches to the assessment and remediation of visual-perceptual difficulties in the deaf child. The term "general" is emphasized because it must be realized that each child, whether multihandicapped or not, is an individual with his or her own unique learning style. The types of assessment utilized will depend to some extent on the nature of the presenting behaviors. Remediation will be prescribed not only on the basis of the strengths and weaknesses which the child exhibits, but also on the basis of the child's affective behaviors. The prescription also depends on his or her behavioral responses to variables of the environment, including response to spatial environment and the effectiveness of group versus individual instruction, to mention only two. In other words, the remediation should be tailored to the child's unique learning style. Once aware of certain educational principles and developmental concepts, the teacher can create a series of tasks specific to the child's profile.

What Is Visual Discrimination?

Visual discrimination may be defined as "the ability to differentiate one object from another" (Lerner, 1976, p. 175). According to Gibson (1969), the development of perceptual skills in children, among them the skill of visual discrimination, can be explained by a theory of differentiation in which the child learns to make perceptual judgments on the basis of distinctive features. "*Distinctive features* are characteristics that identify a stimulus and make it distinct from other stimuli" (Blake, 1976, p. 320). For example, the feature distinguishing the R from the P is the diagonal line attached to the R. The discrimination of the letter R when presented with the letter K, however, is based on the recognition of a different distinctive feature, namely, the circular portion above the diagonal.

Objects within the child's world are rarely simple. Many of those objects contain visible features in addition to the distinctive feature but which do not provide any information necessary to the discrimination. These irrelevant features may only serve to make the discrimination task more difficult for the child (Blake, 1976).

Informal Assessment of Visual Discrimination

There are a number of ways in which a teacher may assess a child's skills in visual discrimination. The following informal activities can give a teacher working knowledge of a student's strengths and problem areas.

MATCHING OF THREE-DIMENSIONAL FORMS Place a familiar object in front of the child. Give the child two additional familiar objects from which to choose. One of these objects should be identical in every detail to the initial object placed in front of the child. Indicate through demonstration and gesture that the child is to match objects. If this task is too difficult or if you suspect that the child does not understand the requirements of the task, give the child only one alternate object to match. Demonstrate what he or she is to do. If the child still does not perform correctly, the teacher should place a hand over the child's hand and physically manipulate it through the task.

MATCHING OF TWO-DIMENSIONAL FORMS Show the child pictures of concrete objects, abstract geometric forms, and/or letter forms. From a selection of two, three, or four cards with pictures of similar forms, the child selects the appropriate matching form.

MATCHING OF A THREE-DIMENSIONAL OBJECT WITH A TWO-DIMENSIONAL OBJECT Ask the child to match familiar three-dimensional objects within the environment with pictures of the object. Objects such as keys, a comb, a paper clip, etc., which can be placed directly on the picture make good selections.

DISCRIMINATION OF ABSTRACT TWO-DIMENSIONAL SYMBOLS For the deaf child with learning problems who is ready for academic learning, the teacher may want to include a survey of his or her ability to discriminate letter forms. Many of the readiness tests on the market provide good models to follow when devising informal measures to assess the child's ability with this task (e.g., Letter Recognition subtest of the Metropolitan Readiness Test by Nurss & McGauvran, 1976).

Remediation of Visual Discrimination Deficits

Although most children learn the discrimination of objects by an almost incidental process, many exceptional children, including the deaf child with perceptual problems, may not. For these children, the teacher must define those distinctive features in a structured, sequential fashion. The following are offered as general guidelines for the teacher as he or she designs this instructional sequence:
1. Identify the distinctive feature which distinguishes one object from another.
2. Start with discriminations which can be made on the basis of only one distinctive feature.

3. Reduce irrelevant features within the task. As the child achieves success with these tasks, the irrelevant features may gradually be added to the form.
4. Emphasize the distinctive feature itself. The highlighting of the distinctive feature enables the child to focus on or attend to the important component of the task. The use of color, added texture, exaggeration of distinctive features, and the presentation of the distinctive features in isolation are only a few of the techniques which can be used for emphasis.

COLOR In using color to emphasize distinctive features, the teacher must keep certain principles in mind. Color can be used as a highlight, but it should not be used in a manner which requires the child to make an additional association. For example, writing a P in blue and an R in red does not serve to emphasize distinctive features. It may only serve to confuse the child because now he or she is required not only to discriminate P from R but also to discriminate blue from red and associate a color with the appropriate form. Color information used in this fashion would be irrelevant and redundant. A more viable alternative would be to write only the diagonal downstroke of the letter R in a color to draw the child's attention to the distinctive feature.

TEXTURE The teacher can use Elmer's glue to outline the distinctive features of forms. Then the child traces around the shape with his or her finger or hand.

PRESENTATION OF DISTINCTIVE FEATURES IN ISOLATION Schreibman (1975) employed a fading technique by which she taught autistic children to discriminate between comparable visual forms. An adaptation of her technique may be of value to the deaf child with perceptual learning problems. The distinctive feature is presented in isolation with exaggeration of size and position until the child responds consistently. Upon initiation of the sequence, the teacher should select one of the two stimuli to which she or he wants the child to respond. Upon presentation of that stimulus, the child puts a button in a box, places the card in a pile, or responds in any other observable manner decided upon. Irrelevant features are gradually added to the task.

What Is Figure-Ground Discrimination?

Figure-ground discrimination is the "ability to distinguish an object from the background surrounding it" (Lerner, 1976, p. 176). The child's inability to focus on relevant features of a stimulus interferes with the correct interpretation of the stimulus. This reaction to both the important (figure) and the unimportant (ground) features of the stimulus with little differentiation in behavior may result in distractible behavior on the part of the child. This list suggests behaviors which may be exhibited by the child with figure-ground discrimination difficulties. This list is not intended as a checklist to be used in the diagnostic assessment of the multihandicapped deaf child, but it can assist a teacher in identifying a child's difficulties and in making appropriate referrals for formal testing.

The student may:
1. Have difficulty differentiating an object from its background.
2. Have difficulty differentiating part from whole.
3. Experience difficulty in completing work on a "busy" or crowded worksheet.
4. Omit parts of worksheets, tests, etc.
5. Have difficulty keeping his or her place while reading printed material.
6. Have difficulty attending to the task or staying on task.
7. Be easily distracted by visual stimuli within the classroom.
8. Have difficulty locating a reading word on a page when presented with a model.
9. Have difficulty copying written material from a book or the chalkboard.
10. Have difficulty locating an object from among an array of objects.

The role of contrast as a factor affecting the efficiency of figure-ground discrimination in the learning disabled child has not been fully explored. However, Werner and Strauss (1941) noted that brain-injured children walked with a more nearly normal gait when their shoes had been painted white. In a more recent study, May (1978) found that the drawing performance of cerebral palsied children improved when the children were asked to draw on black paper with white pencil in comparison to their performance when drawing with black pencils on white paper.

The perception of the contrast within a stimulus may depend not only on the illumination of the room in relationship to the object but also on the amount of light reflected by the stimulus itself. "The reflection of a surface is the ratio of the amount of light reflected to the amount of light that strikes the surface" (May, 1978, p. 258). White has a reflecting index of 85% in comparison to a reflecting index of 14% for black (Forgus, 1966).

Assessment of Figure-Ground Discrimination

For the academically oriented student, a standardized test such as the Motor-Free Test of Visual Perception (Colarusso & Hammill, 1972) may be administered. The same cautions about the Motor-Free Test and its limitations in assessing visual perception apply when the test is used to determine figure-ground difficulties, especially with deaf children.

For the more severely affected deaf child, the teacher may want to assess his or her figure-ground discrimination abilities in an informal setting by a task which requires the child to discriminate among objects in the environment. The teacher shows the child a comb. Then the teacher places a second comb similar in every detail in a box or on a table with other objects. The teacher demonstrates that the child is to find that comb. Additional variations of the task include location of a specific button among other buttons, location of an object among nuts and bolts, location of a can of vegetables from among a display of canned goods.

The teacher should observe the child's responses when complexity of the task is varied (e.g., a comb placed on one object versus a comb among several objects).

Remediation of Figure-Ground Deficits

Two principles related to the manipulation of the figure-ground contrast and to the degree of complexity within the stimulus may provide the teacher with added direction for the creation of remedial techniques.

COMPLEXITY OF STIMULUS For the child operating at a picture level, the use of transparent overlays may prove effective. The task starts with one pictured object (e.g., ball) on an overlay; the teacher adds a second overlay, which includes grass; then he or she adds a third, which includes a tree. At each stage the child is asked to locate the ball. The reverse of this technique may also be utilized.

For the child who is reading, the teacher may cut out an oak tag window which the child can move as needed.

CONTRAST Although more research is needed in this area, the notion of contrasting figure and ground through the use of color appears to show promise in the remediation of figure-ground deficits. Placing white or light stimuli on dark backgrounds may prove useful.

What Are Spatial Relations?

Spatial relation refers to ". . . perception of the position of objects in space. This dimension of visual functioning implies the perception of the placement of an object or a symbol (pictures, letters, numbers) and the spatial relation of that entity to others surrounding it." (Lerner, 1976, p. 175) Not only must the child learn the relationship of objects within space to himself as a nonstatic and static object in that environment, he must also learn the relationship of one object to another object within that environment. The relationship of object to object and individual to object may change with the individual's movement and change of position in space. "The cat is *beside* the table" when viewed by the viewer from one vantage point in the environment; but "the cat is in *front* of the table" when viewed from a different vantage point.

The acquisition of spatial concepts may be impeded by the complexity involved in making the transfer from three-dimensional tasks to two-dimensional tasks. "Around the table" implies a different visual orientation in three-dimensional space than does "around the table" in two-dimensional space. Predicting the location of objects when they move is easy for 3½-year-old to 6½-year-old children, but when the move is symbolically represented (as in a picture), it becomes a more difficult task (Schantz & Watson, 1968–71). The normal child handles this differentiation with time; however, some children do not.

There is little evidence that there is one-to-one correlation between the ability to perceive spatial relationships and the ability to reproduce in drawing the same spatial relationships (Piaget & Inhelder, 1967). This discrepancy between perception and reconstruction may be illustrated by the example of the child who can identify faces with the features in their respective position, but who cannot draw the features in the appropriate places. The reconstruction of objects appears to depend upon a process by which the child coordinates his or her motor activities and mental representation of space.

Assessment of Spatial Relations

The observation that a discrepancy may exist between the perception of objects and the reproduction of objects has direct implications for assessment of spatial relations. Many of the formal tests on the market (e.g., The Developmental Test of Visual Perception) require the child to draw forms with the underlying assumption being that there is some correlation between the two processes. Friedland and Meisels (1975) dispute this assumption on the basis that spatial development in the child may at first be topological in nature and then Euclidean, as described by Piaget (1953).

For the preacademic or academic deaf child suspected of difficulties with spatial relations, a test, such as the Motor-Free Test of Visual Perception, which does not require the child to draw figures, is recommended.

Also, the teacher may design a series of tasks similar to those utilized in the Motor-Free Test. For example, the teacher may direct the child to find the one which is not the same among figures such as these:

Additionally, the teacher should observe how the child moves through space. A series of anecdotal observations may be of value for analysis and for later reference.

Remediation of Spatial Deficits

USE OF THREE-DIMENSIONAL AND TWO-DIMENSIONAL OBJECTS The teacher can plan an instructional sequence to help the child make the transition from three-dimensional space to two-dimensional space.

The teacher may stack blocks. The child then selects a card which represents three-dimensional relationships in a two-dimensional format. The child can reproduce the relationship two-dimensionally by placing felt blocks in the same relationship on a felt board.

USE OF VISUAL CUES TO HELP THE CHILD ORGANIZE WRITTEN WORK Graph paper provides both vertical and horizontal cues for vertical alignment of numbers. This is a great help for column addition.

A color, a number, a dot, an arrow (or any other cue meaningful to the child) can provide an external cue to remind the student where to start on a written task.

A transparency with quadrants placed over a picture can help the child scan the material in an organized, sequential manner.

SPATIAL MANIPULATION OF LETTER FORMS Nonverbal forms may be confused because of their similarity. Spatial discrimination of these nonverbal forms can be facilitated by either vertical or horizontal alignment of these objects, depending on the characteristics of the objects themselves (Sekuler & Rosenblith, 1964; Huttenlocher, 1967). Hallahan and Kauffman (1976) extended this finding to include letters which are often reversed. A vertical presentation of b and d (e.g., $\genfrac{}{}{0pt}{}{d}{b}$) results in fewer discrimination errors than a horizontal presentation. However, the vertical presentation of b and p (e.g., $\genfrac{}{}{0pt}{}{p}{b}$) results in more errors when compared with the horizontal presentation (e.g., $\genfrac{}{}{0pt}{}{b}{p}$). Hallahan and Kauffman (1976) suggest that the teacher utilize this information in instruction by initially presenting the child who is experiencing difficulty with left-right reversals with a teacher-made task in which the b and d are vertical on a card. In successive tasks, the teacher gradually aligns the letters closer to the horizontal plane.

$$\genfrac{}{}{0pt}{}{b}{d} \qquad \genfrac{}{}{0pt}{}{b}{d} \qquad b_d \qquad bd$$

Conclusion

In closing, it must be noted that there is negligible evidence of any significant relationship between visual perception and academic performance (Larsen & Hammill, 1975). Furthermore, any enhancement of reading skills as a result of perceptual-motor training has not been demonstrated. For the deaf child who is experiencing visual-perceptual difficulties but who is reading, it is advisable to incorporate the remedial techniques into the task. For example, as an activity for facilitation of figure-ground discrimination, show the child a word on a card and ask him or her to locate it in a story.

On the other hand, many deaf multihandicapped children will exhibit visual-perceptual problems but will not be ready for academic tasks. For these children, many of the tasks dealing with objects and manipulation of objects in the environment may be appropriate.

Bibliography

Blake, K. A. *The mentally retarded: An educational psychology.* Englewood Cliffs, N.J.: Prentice-Hall, 1976.

Colarusso, R. P., & Hammill, D. D. *Motor-Free Visual Perception Test.* San Rafael, Calif., 1972.

Crane, N. L., & Ross, L. E. A developmental study of attention to cue redundancy introduced following discrimination learning. *Journal of Experimental Child Psychology,* 1967, *5,* 1–5.

Forgus, R. H. *Perception: The basic process in cognitive development.* New York: McGraw-Hill, 1966.

Friedland, S. J., & Meisels, S. J. An application of the Piagetian model to perceptual handicaps. *Journal of Learning Disabilities,* 1975, *8,* 20–24.

Frostig, M., Maslow, P., Lefever, W., & Whittlesey, J. R. B. *Marianne Frostig Developmental Test of Visual Perception.* Palo Alto, Calif.: Consulting Psychologists, 1964.

Gibson, E. J. *Principles of perceptual learning and development.* Englewood Cliffs, N.J.: Prentice-Hall, 1969.

Hallahan, D. F., & Kauffman, J. M. *Introduction to learning disabilities: A psycho-behavioral approach.* Englewood Cliffs, N.J.: Prentice-Hall, 1976.

Hammill, D. D. Assessing and training perceptual-motor processes. In D. D. Hammill & N. R. Bartel (Eds.), *Teaching children with learning and behavior problems.* Boston: Allyn and Bacon, Inc., 1978.

Huttenlocher, J. Discrimination of figure orientation: Effects of relative position. *Journal of Comparative and Physiological Psychology,* 1967, *63,* 359–361.

Jensema, C. J. A note on the achievement test scores of multiply handicapped hearing-impaired children. *American Annals of the Deaf,* 1975, *120,* 37–39.

Jensema, C., & Mullins, J. Onset, cause, and additional handicaps in hearing-impaired children. *American Annals of the Deaf,* 1974, *119,* 701–705.

Johnson, D. J., & Myklebust, H. R. *Learning disabilities: Educational principles and practices.* New York: Grune and Stratton, 1967.

Larsen, S., & Hammill, D. The relationship of selected visual-perceptual abilities to school learning. *The Journal of Special Education,* 1975, *9,* 281–291.

Lerner, J. W. *Children with learning disabilities.* Boston: Houghton Mifflin Co., 1976.

May, D. C. Effects of color reversal of figure and ground drawing materials on drawing performance. *Exceptional Children,* 1978, *44,* 254–260.

National Advisory Committee on Handicapped Children. Special education for handicapped children. First Annual Report. Washington, D.C.: U.S. Department of Health, Education, and Welfare, 1968.

Nurss, J. R., & McGauvran, M. E. *Metropolitan Readiness Test.* New York: Harcourt Brace Jovanovich, 1976.

Piaget, J. How children form mathematical concepts. *Scientific American,* 1953, *189,* 74–79.

Piaget, J., & Inhelder, B. *The child's concept of space.* London: Routledge and Kegan Paul, 1967.

Ross, A. O. *Psychological aspects of learning disabilities and reading disorders.* New York: McGraw-Hill, Inc., 1976.

Satterfield, J. H. EEG issues in children with minimal brain dysfunction. In S. Walzer & P. H. Wolff (Eds.), *Minimal cerebral dysfunction in children.* New York: Grune and Stratton, 1973.

Schreibman, L. Effects of within-stimulus and extra-stimulus prompting on discrimination learning in autistic children. *Journal of Applied Behavior Analysis,* 1975, *8,* 91–112.

Sekuler, R. W., & Rosenbluth, J. F. Discrimination of direction of line and the effect of stimulus alignment. *Psychonomic Science,* 1964, *1,* 143–144.

Shantz, C., & Watson, J. Relation of spatial egocentrism and spatial abilities of the young child. *Merrill-Palmer Institute Report #7,* 1968.

Shantz, C., & Watson, J. Spatial abilities and egocentrism in the young child. *Child Development,* 1971, *42,* 171–181.

Stevenson, H. W. *Children's learning.* New York: Appleton-Century-Crofts, 1972.

Stone, L. J., Smith, H. T., & Murphy, L. B. (Eds.). *The competent infant: Research and commentary.* New York: Basic Books, 1973.

Werner, H., & Strauss, A. A. Pathology of figure-background relation in the child. *Journal of Abnormal Social Psychology,* 1941, *36,* 236–248.

Zigmond, N. K. *Teaching children with special needs.* Dubuque, Iowa: Gorsuch Scarisbrick Publishers, 1976.

Educational Programming for Hearing-Impaired Mentally Retarded Adolescents

Doris Naiman

Dr. Doris Naiman describes a demonstration program for mentally retarded hearing-impaired adolescents. This day program serves youngsters living with their own families, those in sheltered foster care, and those in residential institutions. Consequently, the demonstration program has devised curricula for the education of the students as well as strategies for engaging parents, foster parents, and residential staff in the progress of the students. Another salient feature of the program is its emphasis on broadening the students' experience of their own community and preparing them for eventual work and independence.

This chapter describes a demonstration program that has been effective in educating severely mentally retarded deaf adolescents. With the support of the United States Office of Education, Bureau of Education for the Handicapped, we have established special classes and developed curriculum, procedures, and materials to use with the students, their parents, and staff members. About half of the students have been living in institutions where these developments can be used.

Our results, in terms of measurable progress made by each student, have been positive enough to show that even severely retarded students can be helped to learn. The project was planned with the goal of making it as easy as possible to replicate in other settings and with a range of individuals. Hence, the basic considerations and approaches used in the program should be useful and adaptable when planning for less severely retarded hearing-impaired students as well as those functioning on a very low level.

Included in this chapter are some considerations for planning the placement and overall programming of mentally retarded deaf students. The chapter also offers an overview of the program in action, the assessment process, the curriculum, the program for parents and institutions, and the results. Figure 1 depicts the components of our demonstration program and indicates relations among them.

Placement

In planning educational programs for hearing-impaired mentally retarded students, it is essential to keep in mind that the individuals are very different from each other and that no one setting and no one curriculum within a setting could possibly meet all needs. It is important not to lump together all retarded deaf students and not to allow any student to be stuck in a special placement that becomes a holding operation. A range of educational placements should be provided, and flexibility within and between various settings should be allowed as far as possible.

The major components of the demonstration program have been based in a local day school for deaf children. From the outset, provisions have been made for the students to attend the school from home or from custodial institutions, and to "graduate" from the school into integrated programs with hearing children. The system is dynamic and provides for children to move back and forth to more appropriate educational settings instead of remaining fixed in one placement.

The students are not labeled, and those who at first receive instruction at home do so always with the expectation that they will go to the school as soon as possible, perhaps part-time at first. Similarly, students who at first receive instruction in custodial facilities are transferred to their families and small special classes in the day school as soon as their self-help skills and social behavior improve sufficiently. As severely retarded students in special classes make progress, they are moved along to classes with students fuctioning on a higher level. Some may be able to learn satisfactorily in regular classes for deaf children, if they have the support of part-time resource room teachers and if regular classroom teachers are given assistance in handling them. A few may be able to learn in an integrated program with hearing children with the help of an itinerant or resource room teacher.

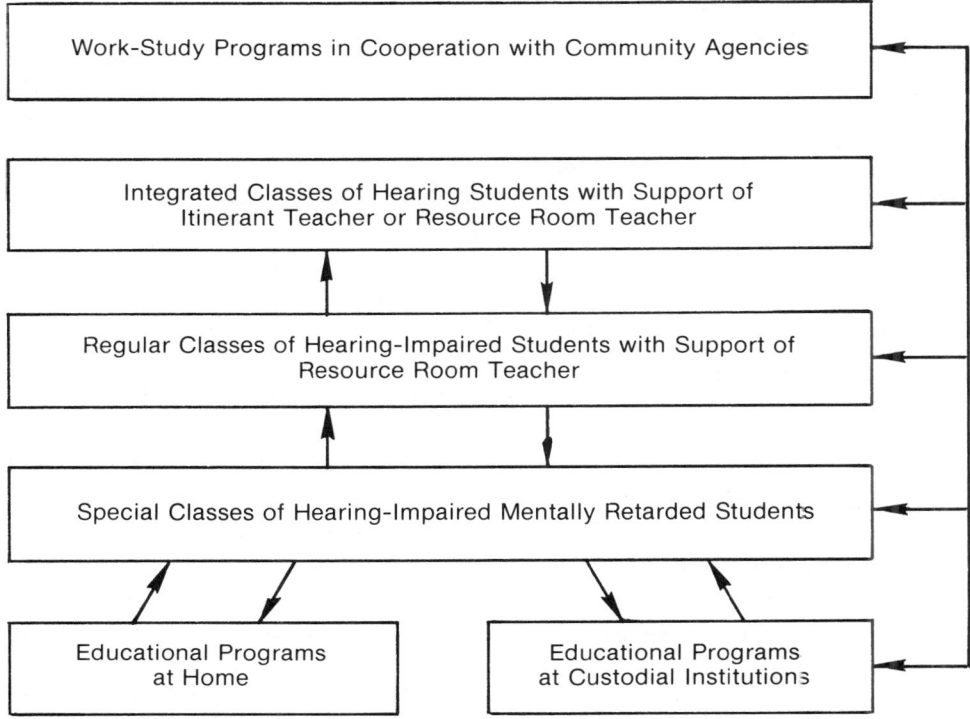

Figure 1
Programming for the Education of Hearing-Impaired Mentally Retarded Adolescents

Contact with the Larger World

For many students a realistic goal is to develop self-care and communication skills sufficient to function in a sheltered workshop. But it is important to build into the system educational options that allow for an increasingly normal setting and that encourage (rather than limit) expectations on the part of the child, the parents, the teachers, and the professional team involved in diagnosis and prescription of education plans.

The rationale for the hierarchy of educational treatments in the demonstration program is based on the philosophy that hearing-impaired mentally retarded adolescents need an educational environment as nearly normal as possible. Clearly, very specialized education and training are required to help this group develop to their fullest potential. But, as far as possible, the education should be provided in a setting that enables them to be in contact with the larger world and the mainstream of education. Even for the severely retarded students who may continue to need highly specialized placement, there is the major advantage to the students of being in contact with normal deaf and hearing students, both so that they can interact part of the time and so that they will have role models to help them develop appropriate social behavior.

The students live at home with their own families and in their own community whenever possible. Intensive assistance is given to families to help them manage their children at home. The program also provides them with effective help at home to reinforce the help they are receiving at school. This plan provides an opportunity for even severely mentally retarded hearing-impaired students to develop independence and social learning skills in a realistic home setting. Where there is no family able to care for the child, foster home placement is sought.

The Program in Action

We have chosen to develop the program in a facility which must cope with real-life problems instead of in a specially devised laboratory school. Because we want our results to be as generalizable and useful as possible, we have wanted to demonstrate what can be accomplished in an existing setting where there are no special facilities for accommodating these students, where the teachers have had no previous training to prepare them for work with these children, and where it is necessary to deal with typical local problems. Hence, our program is centered around a public day school for deaf children, Junior High School 47. It is located in the heart of New York City and must deal with the problems of an inner city population and manage with limited resources.

Commitment by administration is important in order to achieve the long-term special programming required by hearing-impaired mentally retarded students. The principal of the school has been involved in the implementation of the program from the beginning, and an assistant principal serves as school coordinator.

Five classroom teachers participate in the project, and each manages a class of six children. Each teacher is assisted by a graduate student in the New York University Program for Teachers of Deaf Children. Because progress depends on a great deal of systematic one-to-one instruction, it is necessary to have at least two adults in the classroom. This additional person may be a teacher's aide, a parent, or a volunteer working under the teacher's supervision. Other staff members are a curriculum specialist, an educational psychologist, and a parent counselor. Also available are part-time supportive staff members from the school, including a physical therapist, a speech therapist, and a coordinator of medical services. Peer tutors, who have been selected from higher functioning classes, assist in the classrooms twice a week.

Thirty hearing-impaired students functioning at a profoundly retarded level have been placed in the five classrooms. Two-thirds of the students are adolescents between 12 and 18 years old. Students are placed in classes on the basis of age, developmental level, and general overall functioning.

When they entered the program, many of the students could not feed or dress themselves. They had no means of communication other than by gross physical actions. Some were totally withdrawn and did not interact with anyone. Others displayed violently disruptive behavior and were difficult to control. Most had never been in any kind of educational program suited to their needs.

Assessment Procedures

Our goal in the assessment process is to identify a student's level of functioning in a way that has direct implications for prescribing institutional strategies. Since a prescriptive approach is used with each child, the process of assessment, prescription, and reassessment is basic to the demonstration program. Each child's curriculum is shaped according to the specific needs determined by the ongoing assessment.

In addition to an initial assessment, we evaluate daily the effect of our program on child performance. We need to know whether our instruction is having the desired effect in terms of regular progress by the student, and if not to make changes at once. In order to interweave assessment even more closely with instruction, in the second year of the project we have devised a new assessment instrument related directly to the curriculum that provides the core of our daily instruction program. This means that the assessment instrument itself lays out the sequence of developmental steps, indicates the precise point along that sequence where the child is functioning, and then indicates what the next step in the development of the terminal skill would be. The daily assessment form provides a simple way for the teacher to assess pupil performance on the tasks being taught and to evaluate the effects of each lesson as soon as it is taught. This ongoing information allows us to identify weaknesses quickly in the program for individual students and to identify elements which might be revised to meet the student's needs better.

Besides the measures which are directly related to instructional goals, we continue to use other instruments for initial assessment and again at the end of each year to provide a broad-based evaluation. The comprehensive assessment is used to monitor the student's overall development in all general areas of the curriculum, whether those areas are currently targeted for instruction or not. It serves to insure that all areas of the student's development are considered on a regular basis and that if lags continue in some areas, there is a restructuring of the child's program.

The Behavioral Characteristics Progression (BCP) has been especially useful for initial assessment and for obtaining data on each child's progress. The BCP is an assessment, instructional, and communication tool which provides a comprehensive chart of pupil behaviors. The chart assists in identifying those behavioral characteristics which a child does or does not display. All labels for ages and handicaps are eliminated.

The classroom teacher, an administrator, a parent, and other relevant people study the assessment data and determine a series of instructional objectives for each child. In setting priorities for instruction, the team considers the areas in which the child is most deficient relative to peers and the deficiencies which cause the most difficulties for him or her and the people with whom the child lives. Priority is given to establishing behaviors that are important for safety and to developing skills that contribute to future learning and adjustment. The focus is on positive behavior to be developed, but the group also identifies negative behavior that needs to be eliminated in order for learning to take place.

Students sometimes have difficulty in performing daily living tasks, such as brushing teeth and eating with a fork, because they have not yet developed the prerequisite perceptual-motor skills that are needed for accomplishing the tasks. Hence, though it is important to provide daily opportunities for practicing these activities in a natural setting, this provision is not sufficient. It is necessary to prescribe a systematic structured curriculum that, step by step, helps the child to develop the basic perceptual-motor skills necessary to perform the daily living tasks.

It is important that assessment procedures take as little time as possible. In the first year of the project, teachers and their assistants found that testing interfered with teaching. Since it is essential that assessment procedures not consume a great deal of the teacher's time, we subsequently have concentrated on devising assessment procedures that are easy to follow and clearly useful in setting specific behavioral goals, planning daily instruction, and monitoring a child's program.

The Curriculum

Programming has been complicated because of the varying kinds of experience that had to be provided. Students need (1) structured daily individual lessons in prescribed areas and (2) group experience in a natural context. It would have been simpler to manage if we had focused only on scheduling the individual sequential lessons. But we also wanted to provide many opportunities for the children to learn to interact with each other and to take part in group activities. With careful planning and structuring of the daily schedule, the teachers have been able to achieve this. A group breakfast in the cafeteria with other children in the school is the first activity of the day. After this, most of the structured individual lessons take place in the mornings, and most of the other kinds of experiences in the afternoon.

Our goal has been to make each child as socially competent as possible. The emphasis is on the development of skills and habits needed for independent living and social interaction. For some children, this means an educational and training program that, in the beginning, helps them learn basic self-care skills such as dressing and washing themselves. For other children, the focus is on achieving self-control of intemperate behavior or on learning to interact with other children.

We have adapted the Social Learning Curriculum (SLC) developed by the Curriculum Research and Development Center in Mental Retardation of New York University. The SLC is structured so that a sequential variety of activities can be used daily to facilitate the students' social functioning and independent living skills. Activities include many types of teacher-student interaction, such as role playing, motor involvement, art, and games. Lessons are presented in developmental sequence, and the activities are designed to have relevance to the students' immediate environment and, at the same time, to be a foundation for learning in the future.

The curriculum has as its core the common personal and social skills all people need to learn. These skills include drinking, eating, dressing, undressing, toileting, basic grooming, preparing for and cleaning up after meals. The curriculum consists of three components: Perceptual-Motor, Concept Formation, and Social Learning.

The Perceptual-Motor component is concerned with the motor skills needed to perform a personal or social skill. It breaks the movements down into small tasks, teaches the student how to perform each task, and finally shows how to put them together to perform the total skill. Each student has at least one practice session daily, usually individually, although the teacher sometimes works with two students on the same level. The teacher begins by giving the student simple verbal and sign directions. Most students also need to see a demonstration of what is wanted, and the teacher then models the task. If the student still needs help, the teacher uses a manipulation procedure of taking the student's hand and physically guiding him or her through the entire task two or three times. This gives the child an understanding of what is to be done and also provides the positive experience of having done it. Finally, in order to help the student learn to do the task independently, the teacher uses a backward chaining technique and provides physical manipulation with diminishing assistance.

The Concept Formation component of the curriculum introduces students to basic concepts which are prerequisite to more difficult concepts and skills. The concepts are presented in the form of experiences and are chosen because of their relation to the phase being worked on.

The Social Learning component provides the opportunity to interact with others while participating in one of the skill areas. The social learning experiences are taught to the total group in natural settings and situations, as far as possible. All students, regardless of their perceptual-motor ability, are included in the activities. Since there is little correlation between motor skill and social skill, students can benefit from social training, even if they have not mastered the perceptual-motor skills and may need the assistance of aides in order to take part in the activity.

Broadening the Range of Experiences

Hearing-impaired students frequently have an experiential deprivation related to a restricted environment and to the communication difficulties that sharply decrease outside input and limit opportunities for interaction. For students who are also mentally retarded, the experiential deficit is even more marked. Some of the severely retarded students have been out of their homes, custodial institutions, or contained classrooms only rarely. Hence, they never have had any of the common, everyday experiences that most people take for granted, such as walking around the neighborhood, going to the grocery store, or mailing a letter.

Normal life experiences need to be built into the daily routine of these students. Teachers need to plan for them in a systematic way in addition to taking advantage of informal opportunities both to enlarge the range of the students' experiences and also to increase the amount of active participation.

The teachers have started by broadening experiences within their own classrooms. They have encouraged visitors, such as the school nurse, the principal, the custodian, and the cook, to come into the room. They have introduced the guests to the students and have seen to it that the students do not sit and watch passively. The students are shown ways of acknowledging the guests by shaking hands, signing or speaking, or interacting in some other way.

In building new experiences for the severely retarded students, the teachers have not been limited by the four walls of their own classrooms. They have found other areas in the school to which the class could venture out, look around, and see what the possibilities are. They have used a kitchen, where the students have prepared meals and eaten together family style in the dining area. They have participated in the school workshops and interacted with different teachers in different settings. These students need to experience different settings and see things happening in context. Transfer of training is difficult for the severely retarded students. If the students cook in the kitchen, rather than on a hot plate in a corner of their classroom as often happens, they are more likely to learn what people do in kitchens. If they actually cook on a stove, they will know what to do with a stove when they see one at home or in another place.

It is better if the students do not do everything in a group. Some students may have a special strength or a special need that requires more individualized planning; others may be ready to go out on their own and join another class for an activity.

We have found ways to structure informal interaction between the retarded students and the other students in the school. The students eat lunch together in the cafeteria and ride the same school buses. The severely retarded students often do not have access to the playground and other public areas of a school; when they do, it is often at a time when they are segregated from the rest of the school population. By making sure that these students have common experiences with peers from other classes, it is possible to build in more opportunities for role modeling. Holidays and other special occasions provide an opportunity for social interaction between classes during a party. One special class hosted a Valentine's Day party and invited another class to share the celebration. The students from both classes ended up dancing and playing games together. The level of interaction was greater than could have been achieved without the participation of the visiting students.

In selecting sites for excursions outside the school, we concentrated on the ordinary experiences that are routine for most of us. Something as simple as a walk outside the school has been a new experience for many of the students. We have made a list of common experiences and places accessible to our school, and we have regularly arranged for our students to be outside in the neighborhood.

Just being out and seeing the world is worthwhile for these students, but in order to make the trips as meaningful as possible, the teachers have prepared the students ahead of time. They have planned the route and taken pictures beforehand of the places to visit. Then with the aid of the pictures, they have role played the situations the children are likely to encounter. For example, the teachers have shown students how to walk on the sidewalk and attend to the traffic light when crossing streets. Teachers have helped students understand "stop" and "go" and other concepts they must know for safe travel outside the school. Role playing also has included appropriate behavior in a store, a restaurant, or on a public bus, such as how to pay for items at the counter or how to put a token in the machine. Because many of the students have not had these everyday experiences, preparation with pictures and role playing has helped them to understand what is happening.

Trips have been made to the neighborhood playground, the ice cream store, McDonald's, and the 5¢ and 10¢ store. In each case, the teachers have anticipated the specific experiences and the special problems which might occur. A child going to the 5¢ and 10¢ store has to learn about making choices, and the choices probably have to be limited. He or she must learn that everything cannot be touched. Then there is the experience of waiting in line to pay for purchases; it may be the first time the student has ever paid for anything in a store. What happens if there is change to be received? What do we do with money when we are leaving a store and must go out onto the street? These are some of the more obvious new experiences, and there are others, many more subtle. The teachers have been alert to find ways to help students understand and know how to live in the world.

Trips to the laundromat have been an experience new to most of the students. Everyone must know about washing clothes, and these students cannot be an exception if they are to become more independent. They need to see how people wash clothes and learn how to use the machines properly, and they need to try it for themselves. The students took towels and clothes from the classroom, and they were prepared with soap and change for the machines. It took some practice for the students to learn to measure the right amount of soap and to fit the right coins into the slots, but the students learned by doing the real thing, and they were able to do better the next time.

We have taken along a Polaroid camera on the trips. We then could discuss what happened on the spot, and later we used the pictures to review the trip and the entire learning experience.

Prevocational Training Program

The entire curriculum contributes to the long-range goal of making the students as independent and self-supporting as possible. For some students, the beginning is developing skills in self-care, emotional control, and basic communication. Learning social skills and having the opportunity to be in contact with the community helps prepare students for possible functioning in the world of work.

We have developed a prevocational workshop where work samples simulate sheltered workshop tasks. Appropriate work behavior is emphasized, and a token economy is used to reinforce appropriate behavior.

Work samples for the severely retarded population have consisted of packaging, sorting, collating, and assembling. These are tasks which are most commonly found in workshops. We have used task analysis to break down tasks into the smallest elements necessary for completion and to teach each element successively. Reward and reinforcement follows each successful learning step.

We have used techniques of cue removal in skill training. We have also found that use of a cue (color coding) in training an assembly task is an efficient learning procedure, especially when the teacher has many students with whom to work.

It has been useful in teaching to have students match completed work items to a picture of the completed item at the work site. For example, the student will keep working until all pictures are covered with one completed work unit. This has helped to increase independence and to provide a measure of achievement which students can identify.

For higher level students, we have presented tasks by providing a model of finished work and trays containing component parts. Instructions to students are to make one like it. This allows for individual achievement, trial and error. We have begun with a few component parts in order for the students to experience success regularly. For many students this will not be realistic, but teachers should always remain alert for those who gain by it.

Developing Communication

A major goal is to help students develop a way to communicate. All methods of communication are used where feasible. For students with severely limited communication, experience has shown that teaching manual communication in a meaningful context of daily life situations is an effective way to develop communication ability. In fact, our focus has been on developing a meaningful context of daily life situations as an effective way to develop communication. The emphasis has been on communication that involves visible action and results. The general principle in developing communication skills is the same as in developing other kinds of behavior. In order to shape the desired behavior, any response approximating it is rewarded. With a noncommunicating student, the first objective is to get an approximately appropriate response.

Our experience in helping the students develop language indicates that the students have more success when language development activities are in the context of meaningful communication and interpersonal interaction rather than in formal drill. Important considerations are that there should be a large amount of language input and that it be complete, unamibiguous, and understandable to the student. Our experience is consistent with recent research in the language development of both hearing and deaf students.

Inservice Training

Our emphasis has been on instruction in specific methodologies effective with hearing-impaired students. Special skills included:
1. Methods of teaching communication skills and functional language; the importance of building a mode of communication by using all methods, including pantomime and gesture; special problems of amplification for hyperactive students.
2. Application of behavior modification principles to teaching daily living and independence skills; improving skills in interpersonal relations and social adaptation; using the Social Learning Curriculum.
3. Strategies and techniques for remediating handicapping conditions associated with various types of disabilities.
4. Special instructional materials: sources, selection, adaptation.
5. Developing and implementing plans for individual students; working with the psychoeducational team to provide an appropriate sequence of goals, activities, and consequences for each student.
6. Classroom management and handling of individual behavior problems.
7. Assessment of student's progress.
8. Special approaches to working with adolescents: work-study programs, prevocational training.
9. Vocational possibilities and special services available.

Inservice training has continued through the year. Manual communication instruction has been provided for project staff, and seminars were provided on specific subjects such as adaptation of the Social Learning Curriculum, class management, and problems in providing one-to-one individualized instruction. It has been our experience that individual conferences with classroom teachers and assistants are an especially effective form of inservice training. Hence, we have had weekly individual conferences with each of the classroom teachers and graduate assistants.

Parents and Residential Staff

An important part of the project has been a program that has assisted families and foster families in contributing effectively to the social and academic growth of the students. The program has included child-care workers and other staff members in the residential institutions and group homes in which some of the students live.

The program with parents and residential institutions has included the following activities:

FAMILY INVOLVEMENT IN INDIVIDUAL PRESCRIPTIVE PLANS The project staff and the parents have worked together to develop and implement the individual prescriptive plans. The staff and parents have cooperated to assist the students in achieving the behavior goals set for them in the home situation.

FAMILY COUNSELING ACCORDING TO NEEDS Having a hearing-impaired retarded child frequently causes the parents to have feelings of guilt, anger, disappointment, and frustration. Parents have been encouraged to talk about these feelings and handle them in a way which contributes to a satisfying relationship with their child.

PROVISIONS OF SOCIAL SERVICES AND ADAPTATIONS FOR SPANISH-SPEAKING FAMILIES To assist with financial, housing, medical, and general social service needs, project staff have provided referral services and assumed a more direct involvement if families were unable to follow through on their own. In many families, the parents spoke only Spanish and in others, English was spoken as the second language. Spanish interpreters have been involved in all contacts with these families, both in home visits and group programs.

ASSISTANCE IN LANGUAGE AND SOCIAL DEVELOPMENT In addition to the student's prescriptive program, parents have been given information and explanations about hearing loss, cause of deafness, the use and care of hearing aids, speechreading, and the effect of deafness and retardation on language development. Parents discovered ways of developing a rich language environment at home and of counteracting the isolation of the child by special efforts to involve him or her in the family and neighborhood. Project staff members have increased parents' awareness of the child's need to engage in social activities outside of the school environment and have provided information about recreational and entertainment facilities in the community.

Parents have been helped to assist their teenager in developing the daily living skills needed to enable him or her to function more independently. They were shown the importance of teaching responsibility and of giving the teenager the opportunity to make decisions. Discussions in home visits and group meetings have centered on how the parent and the family could help in the development of adaptive social behavior.

ASSISTANCE IN MANAGING HOME BEHAVIOR Basic principles of behavior modification have been explained, and parents have received guidance and support in implementing these techniques. Parents have learned how to shape behavior by setting small initial goals for their child, by using rewards along with social praise for appropriate behavior, and by ignoring inappropriate behavior. Parents have been encouraged to establish rules for the home and to be consistent in rewarding their child for following them. Staff has helped parents understand the need to build their child's self-confidence by having him or her experience success regularly. As far as possible, the focus has been on building positive behavior rather than punishing negative behavior.

Because the development of improved communication skills directly affected the parents' ability to manage their child's behavior, phrases useful in managing behavior have been discussed and learned. Increases in communication and the concomitant increase in mutual understanding have reduced frustration.

CONTACT WITH DEAF ADULTS Because many of the families never had been with deaf adults, deaf staff members and graduate students have participated regularly in home visits and group activities as discussion leaders, teachers, and counselors. The opportunity to interact with deaf adults was an important factor in improving parents' understanding and acceptance of deafness.

Results

The most important single fact about the project is that every student has made measurable progress that is clearly discernible in each of the curriculum areas. Assessment instruments and instructional sequences divided into small incremental steps have made it possible to observe gradual, cumulative building of skills. This kind of clear evidence of progress is important for teachers, parents, and children. It gives a needed sense of success and accomplishment and offers encouragement to others who are concerned with providing appropriate education for profoundly handicapped hearing-impaired students.

Some of the students have made enough progress to warrant new class placement and a new focus in curriculum. Six students have been moved to a class designated as a transition class with the goal of providing more academic work. Eight students have moved from institutions for the mentally retarded and are now able to manage satisfactorily in foster or group homes.

Significant progress has been made in the aspects of development that are emphasized in the curriculum. These results are similar to those reported by other researchers who indicate that severely handicapped students learn and make regular gains in those areas in which instruction is presented consistently and daily in a systematic way.

Suggested Readings

Behavioral characteristics progression. Palo Alto, Calif.: Vort Corporation, 1973.

Donlon, E. J., & Burton, L. J. *The severely and profoundly handicapped: A practical approach to teaching.* New York: Grune and Stratton, 1976.

Fredericks, H. D., et al. *A data-based classroom for the moderately and severely handicapped.* Monmouth, Oreg.: Instructional Development Corporation, 1975.

Goldstein, H. *Social Learning Curriculum.* New York: Curriculum Research and Development Center in Mental Retardation, New York University (mimeo).

Haring, N. G. (Ed.). *Developing effective individualized educational programs for severely handicapped children and youth.* Washington, D.C.: U.S. Department of Education, Bureau of Education for the Handicapped, 1977.

Haring, N. G., & Brown, L. J. (Eds.). *Teaching the severely handicapped.* New York: Grune and Stratton, 1976.

Healey, W. C. *The hearing-impaired mentally retarded.* Washington, D.C.: American Speech and Hearing Association, 1975.

Meier, J. H. Screening, assessment, and intervention for young children at developmental risk. In B. Z. Fridlander, G. M. Sterritt, & J. E. Kirk (Eds.), *The exceptional infant* (Vol. 3). New York: Brunner/Mazel, 1975, 605-650.

Naiman, D. W., Schein, J., & Stewart, L. New vistas for emotionally disturbed deaf children. *American Annals of the Deaf,* 1973, *118,* 480-487.

Naiman, D. W. Preface. Seminar on behavior modification methods for psychologists working with deaf children. *American Annals of the Deaf,* 1970, *115,* 458.

Naiman, D. W. Picture perfect: Photography aids deaf children in developing language skills. *Teaching Exceptional Children,* 1977, *9,* 36–38.

Naiman, D. W. *Needs of emotionally disturbed hearing-impaired children.* New York: Deafness Research and Training Center, New York University, 1975.

Naiman, D. W., Turney, G., & Muller, R. Parents of multiply handicapped deaf children. *Proceedings of the Forty-seventh Meeting of the Convention of American Instructors of the Deaf.* Washington, D.C.: U. S. Government Printing Office, 1976.

Naiman, D. W. Education of severely multiply handicapped deaf children. *Proceedings of the Forty-eighth Meeting of the Convention of American Instructors of the Deaf*. Washington, D.C.: U.S. Government Printing Office, in press.

Naiman, D. W. Proposed model for preparation of personnel. In J. D. Schein (Ed.), *Education and rehabilitation of deaf persons with other disabilities*. New York: Deafness Research and Training Center, New York University, 1974.

Naiman, D. W. *Inservice training for after class staff in residential schools*. New York: Deafness Research and Training Center, New York University, 1972.

Schein, J. D. *Education and rehabilitation of deaf persons with other disabilities*. New York: Deafness Research and Training Center, New York University, 1974.

Somer, R. Toward a psychology of natural behavior. *APO Monitor,* 1977, *8,* 1-7.

Sontag, E., Burke, P. J., & York, R. Considerations for serving the severely handicapped in the public schools. *Education and Training of Mentally Retarded,* April 1973, *8,* 20-26.

Webster, E. J. *Professional approaches with parents of handicapped children*. Springfield, Ill.: Charles C. Thomas, Publisher, 1976.

Wehman, P., & Bates, P. Education curriculum for severely and profoundly handicapped persons: A review. *Rehabilitation Literature,* 1978, *39,* 2-14.

A Curriculum Development Project for the Multihandicapped Hearing-Impaired Child Ten Years Later

Lillian C. R. Restaino

Dr. Lillian Restaino, principal investigator for the Cooperative Research Endeavors in the Education of the Deaf (CREED), reports on ten years of research and applications among multihandicapped hearing-impaired children. She highlights progress in task analysis for teaching attention, memory, understanding, and problem solving.

I became aware of the problem of multihandicapped hearing-impaired children 11 years ago, after a pilot survey of children in schools for the deaf in the state of New York indicated that a majority of the children were defined as having varying degrees of learning disorders. The 12 administrators whose schools participated in the survey were alarmed by the findings and decided to use discretionary state funds to determine the nature of the children's learning problems beyond those expected as a consequence of their hearing impairment. Subsequently, the administrators supported the development of a special program for multihandicapped hearing-impaired children.

Cooperative Research Endeavors in Education of the Deaf (CREED) was established as a project of the consortium. As principal investigator of the project from 1968 through 1973, my task was to mobilize a staff to develop for young deaf children a battery of tests appropriate for educational diagnosis; to test all children ages three through eight years in all the schools for the deaf in New York State; and to develop a curriculum—all formidable tasks. The relative success of our endeavors is a testimony to the dedication and talent of the staff, to the concern and cooperation of the teachers, and to the interest and support of the administrators. All of us wanted to learn more about the multihandicapped hearing-impaired child whose needs and problems we had been overlooking until that point in time. The body of work that came out of the projects was an important beginning for the schools for the deaf in New York; it generated an atmosphere in which many exciting programs for the multihandicapped hearing-impaired child were developed. These programs range from cognitive instruction with the three-year-old to career development with the sixteen-year-old.

But what were the factors of immediate significance that the CREED projects contributed to the education of the multihandicapped hearing impaired? I believe it was the redirection of attention to educational diagnosis—first, as analysis of the *learner's abilities* in terms of what it is that he or she will need in order to succeed with the educational task and second, as analysis of that *task* into all of its component parts.

The CREED project's diagnostic battery was strongly influenced by the work of Piaget, who helped us to understand what we could expect of any child at a given level, and by newly emerging information processing theorists, whose work helped us determine the complex operations required of the child in perception and memory.

Our analyses of educational tasks were based on the task analysis procedures of Robert Gagne. We integrated Gagne's procedures with those of the other theorists in our design of the CREED Five Curriculum.

But, we conceived the structure of these projects more than ten years ago, and we began applying our ideas well over seven years ago. We have since become more sophisticated in our research, theory, and educational practice, and some dramatic changes have occurred in all three. It is those changes that I should like to report in this chapter.

Some Unchanging Basics

Before we report the current status of diagnosis and instruction of the multihandicapped hearing-impaired child as presented in CREED Projects Three through Five, we should note several elements of the tests and curriculum for which our endorsement has remained constant and unchanged.

First, and perhaps foremost, is the extensive involvement of the teacher in the development and implementation of both the tests and the curriculum. Teachers were viewed not only as resources in the problem areas which the CREED staff would address in tests and program development but, in addition, they (rather than "experts") administered the tests and evaluated the curriculum at every step of its design. Their systematic input was obtained from the construction of behavioral objectives to the piloting of methods and materials to help the child master those behavioral objectives. We were convinced at the outset of the CREED projects that teachers had to be intensively involved with and responsible for both tests and program development. These convictions, judged by the results, were well founded.

A second element of the CREED projects is the behavioral objective as the defining unit for instructional development. Many educators look with disfavor upon attempts to translate curricula into specific objectives; others argue that the more significant aims in education are too global or affective to be transformed into specific objectives. I disagree with both positions. Significant aims are fulfilled by our children through small, accumulated experiences—experiences that teachers have a responsibility to communicate. In defining specific objectives for children to master, we hold ourselves as responsible as the children for their fulfillment.

Finally, and of greatest inportance, is the CREED premise that teaching can be successful only when there has been systematic analysis of the subcomponents of the educational task, as well as analysis of the learner's characteristics directly related to the mastery of those subcomponents.

While in CREED Five, tasks were analyzed in terms of hierarchies of skills, these sub-skills are more likely to comprise some hypothesized sequence rather than a hierarchy; nevertheless, no matter how the order of difficulty is arranged, sub-skill analysis is absolutely essential to the education of all children.

These three principles were the foundation for all the CREED projects. They were perhaps most clearly defined in the General Assumptions section of the CREED Five Curriculum. (See Appendix A.)

The Multihandicapped Hearing-Impaired Learner Today

Initially in developing a test battery that would provide teachers with the information that they needed, we limited ourselves to four domains: attention, memory, visual analysis, and conceptualization. The major theories in each of the four domains were delineated to help the teacher with diagnosis and instruction. Today, these four are subsumed under the general label of cognition or information processing.

When we interviewed teachers of multihandicapped hearing-impaired children, they urged that our work in diagnosis and instructional programming be directed toward skills and abilities defined as attention, memory, visual perception, and concept development. In operating upon their suggestions, we defined these areas according to research and theory then available; and, as there have been dramatic redefinitions in the research and theory in these areas, so must there be change in our transformation of that research and theory for the educational practitioner.

Table 1 is an attempt to transform current theories and research in the four domains into lists of processes that *all* learners need to master. Educational tasks range from the simplest to the most complex. These lists appear to be different from the four domains in the CREED Five Curriculum. But they are not so much changed as they are expanded, and with that expansion comes increasing opportunities for teachers to find alternatives and to develop new hypotheses to help their children to learn. What are these changes and how can the teacher of the multihandicapped hearing-impaired child capitalize upon them? I shall cover each of the four areas about which the original CREED project teachers voiced concern, elaborate upon our current knowledge of their functioning, and indicate what teachers can do with this knowledge.

I shall cover some of the new and significant findings in cognitive theory; I shall describe how they are involved in the learning processes of children and how this information can be used to help MHHI children.

ATTENTION In the CREED Three Test Battery and in the CREED Five Curriculum, we combined attention and memory in one section and concentrated on isolated tasks for evaluation and training in these areas. The more sophisticated status of our current knowledge is nowhere better represented than in our redefinition of the processes of attention and memory. As Table 1 clearly indicates, very specific processes

Table 1
The Strategies and Processes Used by Successful Learners and Thinkers

Strategies for the Central Processing System	General Store of Information and Strategies		
	For Visual Analysis	For Understanding	For Problem Solving
1. General strategies for automatic attention.	1. Rules for pattern recognition.	1. Rules for concepts, categories, and classes.	1. General rules for problem solving.
2. General strategies for selective attention.	2. Feature categories and hierarchies of feature categories.	2. Rules for dimensional orderings.	2. Creative rules for problem solving.
3. General strategies for searching long-term memory.	3. Rules for images.	3. Rules for relating concepts to episodes.	
4. General strategies for using expectancies for the target item and context.	4. Rules for relating patterns to contexts.	4. Specific strategies for automatic attention.	
5. General strategies for constructing meaning in short-term memory.	5. Specific strategies for automatic attention.	5. Specific strategies for selective attention.	
	6. Specific strategies for selective attention.	6. Specific strategies for searching long-term memory.	
	7. Specific strategies for searching long-term memory.	7. Specific strategies for using expectancies.	
	8. Specific strategies for using expectancies.	8. Specific strategies for processing, organizing, and holding information in short-term memory.	
	9. Specific strategies for processing, organizing, and holding information in short-term memory.	9. Specific strategies for entering information in long-term memory.	
	10. Specific strategies for entering information in long-term memory.		

of attention are required for visual analysis and conceptualization, or understanding and problem solving, as we now define it.

We know now that when successful learners encounter a new object or event or symbol, not only do they visually discriminate it and form a concept about it, but also they figure out strategies for scanning it and focusing upon it so that they can identify it more quickly and accurately the next time they meet it. Some of these strategies are general rules for looking, but there are also ways of scanning and focusing that are very specific to objects in the environment, for example, as compared with symbols for numbers and letters.

Further, we now know that successful learners do not attend to every part of what they are identifying; they use repeated experiences with objects, events, symbols, language, and text to build rules for very educated guesses. They use what we call expectancies, so that they do not need to put forth the great effort demanded of conscious attention processes for every aspect of a task.

Finally, successful learners know how to identify objects or events at some level below conscious awareness without directing their overburdened conscious attention processes to them, thus freeing these conscious, selective attention mechanisms to focus upon the more complicated levels of the task before them. Psychologists label this level of recognition "automaticity"; this is, however, a very special use of the word. It means that we have learned to do some part of a task so thoroughly that we can respond to it directly through the long-term memory; we do not need to tax our conscious attention. Really successful learners of any task—ranging from reading to driving—always direct some parts of a task to an automatic level to free them for the really complex aspects of the task. The skilled reader relegates letter, word, even phrase recognition to automatic levels—freeing the reader to concentrate on the complex points being made in the text. The driver relegates steering corrections to automatic levels, to free him or her to watch for the unpredictable perils of the road.

Unfortunately, all these attentional strategies are seriously undermined by the tendency of what we call "task specificity" or "context specificity." Task specificity defines our inability to use what we have learned about past experiences in understanding new experiences. For example, when the child learns the concept of five with marbles, he or she is not immediately or automatically able to develop expectancies for the rule of five with people or cars or fingers. Such task specificity is not an obstacle restricted to young learners, however; the sophisticated learner is equally hindered by changes of context. Only when the learner sees the applicability of the same rule over many contexts can he or she use it to predict or fill in what is in a given task; only then can he or she use expectancies.

How would these new descriptions of the mechanisms of attention be interpreted with respect to the multihandicapped hearing-impaired child? Table 2 compares unsuccessful and successful learners in terms of the attention processes they can marshal. My experience indicates that when children are having serious problems (as described in the column headed unsuccessful learner), they need help in building systematic ways for scanning and focusing; they need very deliberate help in learning some tangible rule for recognizing the elements of a task that they have repeated experiences with; and they need very special help in recognizing these elements when the tasks differ slightly from time to time, i.e., from context to context.

Teachers of the multihandicapped hearing-impaired child need to help their children very deliberately to build the kinds of conscious and automatic attentional processes that successful learners have constructed on their own. Teachers need to engage in the following actions:

Whenever the child is learning a new task, very deliberately direct him or her to the elements that differentiate the task from other tasks. Help the child each time to find the cues that will be most likely to occur again whenever it is presented. If the child is left to figure out what to look for, he or she may well fix on salient but irrelevant components. Unfortunately, most of the materials we use to "teach" concepts really "test" those concepts without directing the child to what he or she is supposed to be looking for.

Help the child to use the differentiating cues to build expectancies, that is, rules to use it to identify an object or event or symbol without having to investigate its every part. Teachers should make an important part of their program the encouragement of thoughtful anticipation, guessing, and filling in. They should help the

Table 2
Attention Processes

The Processes	The Unsuccessful Learner	The Successful Learner
1. It requires effort and skill to decide where to focus attention, where to look, what to ignore, what will pay off.	1. Has not yet learned most efficient ways to allocate focused attention (as in reading print and performing other academic tasks).	1. Has learned strategies for attending on his or her own, as a consequence of pay-off.
2. These decisions are based on familiarity from past experiences, which generate expectations, cutting work load.	2. Is beginning to organize structures from past experiences to generate expectations.	2. Can generate expectations based upon his or her more extensive experiences.
3. New contexts and task specificity work against habituation and familiarity.	3. Finds new context too confusing to utilize strategies.	3. Is less confused by context specificity.
4. One must learn to attend automatically to much information in an event, to concentrate effort on complicated parts.	4. Requires more focused attention for lower level tasks; hasn't yet directed these tasks to automatic levels, freeing him or her for working out more complex levels.	4. Can attack more complex levels as he or she directs over-learned, organized aspects to automatic attention.

child construct responses based upon incomplete information with thoughtful guessing. The child must become aware that such thoughtful anticipation is not only acceptable, it is rewarded. In encouraging such behavior, the teacher must differentiate between errors that are the result of a *real* attempt to work at the task and impulsive guessing. One can encourage the use of expectancies through directing the child to focus upon the elements that are likely to lead to the right answer, and such direction can be used with the simplest or most complex tasks.

VISUAL ANALYSIS In CREED Three and Five, our definition of visual analysis was heavily based upon a theory of distinctive features; we concentrated our efforts on the invariant component of a pattern—be it an object, symbol, letter, or number. We sought to order the tasks in terms of increasing difficulty. Nevertheless, theorists were only beginning to determine the high level thought processes required for visual discrimination, so even our careful efforts fell short of current theories.

Our current descriptions of visual analysis have been greatly elaborated, as in Table 3. The words most conspicuous in these new descriptions are *rules* and *categories*. Today, we have revised our earlier global definition of visual analysis as "discriminating distinctive and invariant features." We know now that the discrimination of invariant and distinctive features is the end product of complicated categorization processes. Visual discrimination is rule-governed behavior. We build categories for symbols and patterns, based upon a set of attributes, and our recognition of these patterns is a consequence of these rules. The letter "a" can be seen in many different perspectives, sizes, even shapes. In order to determine that what we are looking at is an "a," it must consist of some of the attributes of the category "a," included in the rule for "a" that we have constructed over time.

Further, researchers have determined that we force children to discover on their own what the complicated rules of the discriminating game are. That is, they must learn, by trial and tribulation, what we expect them to call "different" and what we will accept as "the same." And, what is more, adults change the rules with the task; where shape may be an important feature for differentiating a circle from a square, the shape of the "a" must be ignored in making a decision about "same" or "different."

Finally, we now know that, while multisensory input does indeed facilitate learning, merely exposing the learner to such input is not sufficient. The learner must be very deliberately helped to see where the visual features overlap with the tactile, and how the visual features coincide with their linguistic analogies if these multisource inputs are going to increase the retrievability and availability of the object for future use.

What do these changes say to the teacher of the multihandicapped hearing-impaired child? In Table 3, under Visual Analysis, we see the emphasis upon visual analysis as rule-building. Clearly, when the child does not discriminate between patterns, it is because he or she has not developed the systematic recurring rule for

Table 3
Visual Analysis

The Processes	The Unsuccessful Learner	The Successful Learner
1. Categories and rules must be constructed in order to discriminate symbols, patterns, objects, events in the world; without the rules or maps for seeing, we do not discriminate and organize, either now or in the future.	1. Needs to build rules for pattern relationships from simple patterns (shapes) to complex (letters, words, etc.).	1. Has stable and usable rules and strategies for analyzing text, patterns, events, and continues to add to them.
2. The rules for visual analysis are complex and hierarchical. They relate patterns to their contexts.	2. Must learn strategies for scanning to help in visual analysis; must learn how to use information in the periphery of his or her vision.	2. Knows how to use peripheral information to tell where to look next; has constructed "visual maps" for analysis from similar past experiences; knows how and when to use them.
3. We use a variety of strategies for scanning exhaustively and efficiently.	3. Has to learn the adult rules for calling objects, symbols, text, events the "same"; must learn how rules change (the context problem again).	3. Has learned many of "the rules of the game" and how to "ask the right questions" in order to distinguish the differences being asked of him or her.
4. Visual imagery can be supported by language and vice-versa, but the relationships *have to be deliberately constructed*.	4. Does not use language effectively to organize visual experience.	4. Uses language to help him or her perceive and organize images and vice-versa; understands these as useful aids to learning.

finding the features that make Pattern A different from Pattern B, but the same as Pattern A₁. The child has not figured out what it is that we will accept as the same, or what we will accept as different. Traditionally, we have left these very complicated deliberations to the child's reasoning abilities—without even the simplest direction. Look at the workbooks or games we give to children to "teach" them to discriminate; they present the problem as a *fait accompli*. We ask the child to "find the one that is different" or "find the one that is the same"—with little or no direction on what he or she is to look for or at. The child is expected to construct the most complicated rules for discriminating between the patterns, and—what is worse—the patterns and the rules change rapidly and without warning.

How can teachers of the multihandicapped hearing-impaired child use current research and theory to help their children in the visual analysis of tasks?

Teachers must be very clear about the dimensions of difference and sameness on the tasks children are working with. Teachers must provide directions for their children so that the students know what they are supposed to be doing. When they are correct, they must be asked or told why; when they are in error, they must be helped to see why.

Because we consider the discriminating features of any pattern to be attributes of a category, the teacher must determine what the attributes are and then articulate the rule for using these attributes to identify the symbol or letter, and so forth. While teachers traditionally do this for simple forms (for example, the line and crossbar for "t"), they tend to expect that the older children can do it on their own when encountering far more complex and detailed forms. This tendency is particularly unfortunate because more complex forms, such as words and maps, require hierarchies of categories for discrimination. Thus, the teacher should not abandon the older children to their own devices in building and using rules for the more demanding discriminations they must make.

UNDERSTANDING AND PROBLEM SOLVING Perhaps the most dramatic changes within the 10-year period have occurred in research and theory in the area of understanding and problem solving. While the CREED Three and Five Projects focused upon Piaget's theory, today the higher reasoning processes have been the subject of intensive reexamination. As a matter of fact, theory and research in both Piaget's theory and in information processing have undergone a number of changes. Nevertheless, the overriding focus of both is *organization*. The emphasis is upon the description of ways that we organize the events of our lives in a sensible, useful way.

One of the most significant contributions in information processing theory has been the principle of the *schema,* or framework, as the organizing structure for all our concepts and classifications, all the ongoing events of our lives. What these theorists are telling us is that we do not organize our experiences in neat little categories of objects, people, places, and so forth. We do, of course, build such categories, but more important, these categories themselves play a role in and are defined by larger, more meaningful frameworks of experience. In other words, we do not build concepts in isolation; we build them embedded in the contexts of many different events, and the events become the basis for a framework of similar concepts. Concepts that have to do with school are given added meaning through being a part of a school *schema,* or framework. The concept of *teacher* is related to that of *student* in the framework. This schematic grouping of concepts is not just an interesting theory; it provides all educators, and most especially educators of deaf children, with a powerful instrument for helping the child to build meaning. Bob Pehrson, coordinator of language instruction at the Lexington School for the Deaf, has constructed an exciting new program based upon this theory of *schema.*

Piaget's theory has always been based upon the processes of organization and adaptation. The principles of organization have been most familiar to us in terms of his stages of thinking. However, the adaptation processes in his theory are of singular importance; more specifically, equilibration, as accomplished through assimilation and accommodation. An important change in emphasis has occurred in writings based on Piaget's work; while the process of equilibration was defined as one of the four factors upon which intellectual development depends (the others being maturation, experience, and social transmission), equilibration has been more precisely defined and well elaborated. Equilibration is the feeling of dissonance or conflict, the thrust to know, when one perceives some event in the environment that does not fit the current state of one's knowledge. The feeling of conflict, along with the other three factors, generates the intellectual activity that Piaget characterized as stages of logical development.

What are the implications of these theoretical principles for teachers of multihandicapped hearing-impaired children? In Table 4, we see that unsuccessful learners have very limited frameworks for building and giving deeper meaning to new concepts. They not only need to build classifications, concepts, and hierarchies of classes and concepts, but they also need to build more elaborate and extensive frameworks to provide relationships between these concepts and classes, and thus make them more meaningful.

How should we expect to see the multihandicapped hearing-impaired child function in terms of Piaget's logical operations? What level of conflict will he or she experience in the intellectual tasks in the environment? As important to Piaget's theory of information processing is the issue of task specificity. The child may well be able to classify material he or she has had much experience with (may, for example, be capable of seeing the need to call dogs both dogs and animals) but, when asked to do the same class inclusion task with other materials, he or she fails. Thus, the teacher should not expect a child to function with the organizing processes of classification and seriation by seeing disequilibrium in tasks and attempting to solve them, unless the child has had much former experience with the materials involved in that task. The child should not be expected to activate higher level reasoning on items he or she must first learn to discriminate and identify.

How can the teacher help children develop these higher level reasoning and understanding processes? We can suggest at least three ways. First, as we discussed "sameness" and "difference" in visual analysis, we indicated it is essential that teachers analyze the concepts that they expect their students to learn. Before teachers can expect their students to build concepts, they must have a very clear picture of the dimensions of a concept, its attributes, and the combining rules for those attributes.

Secondly, the framework for concepts is the instrument for building meaning through the relationships among concepts. Teachers should never build concepts in isolation; they must always build them in a structure that provides meaning through reciprocal relationships. Pehrson's language program does just that; the child is helped to build a framework of associated concepts for any new concept. Such activity provides a familiar structure for the new concept; the new concept enriches the framework and is enriched by it. The concept in a framework is more easily retrieved when necessary and so is more readily available for future tasks.

Table 4
Understanding and Problem Solving

The Processes	The Unsuccessful Learner	The Successful Learner
1. Rule construction is the basis for all thinking. It helps to make sense of the world through organizing, classifying, problem solving. Piaget tells us that our life's work is discovering and using the logical rules for organizing the world through classifying and ordering.	1. Develops concepts and rules, but cannot deal with complex and hierarchical concepts. Problem solving is restricted to narrow methods.	1. Shows superiority over the unsuccessful learner because of more experiences to increase the breadth of frameworks and contexts and because of increasing knowledge and use of higher level rules.
2. We organize according to the larger context of our experiences. We organize and think in terms of analogies between our experiences. We build frameworks to include similar experiences.	2. Has frameworks for experiences and their concepts, but they are similarly restricted; has difficulty going beyond specific contexts, and has not developed rules for high level classification.	2. Has organized more experiences and used more rules for such organizing and so has more information available and can use more strategies for working over that information.
3. Building isolated concepts from personal experiences is difficult. We must isolate the concept from the total context.	3. Needs to have direction for building relationships and rules.	3. Is extending concrete operations and is on the way to the highest levels of thought—formal operations.
4. Piaget says: (a) We need disequilibrium to build concepts. When we can see the question and engage it through systematic ways of solution, we increase our intelligence. (b) We need physical experience, social interaction, and maturity to move from one level of thinking to the next, and we need cognitive conflict to integrate the other three factors. (c) The younger child doesn't see the conflict the older child sees. He or she thinks differently. The adolescent thinks differently from the older child. All use the prerequisites of later stages of thinking.	4. Can use rules for first level concepts and for learning about higher level rules and organizations.	4. Is becoming a very efficient understander and problem solver, but always in spite of the problem of context specificity.

Thirdly, multihandicapped hearing-impaired children of the same age differ in their level of logical operations just as do other children. Kevin Keane, at St. Joseph's School for the Deaf in New York, has designed an ingenious modification of Piaget's classic concrete operations tasks for administration to multihandicapped hearing-impaired children. I watched his tapes and observed that the differences in the level and types of responses were astonishing. Such individual differences provide teachers with exciting possibilities of using more advanced children as resources for challenging their peers. Piaget tells us that social interaction, where a more advanced child poses questions, points to the errors of thought, and shows another the reality of a situation, is a powerful means for activating higher levels of thinking in less advanced children.

Teachers, too, can challenge the child, even when they do not expect the child to function at that level. Children do not advance in logical operations without challenge. The essential principle to remember is that any thoughtful response is the result of the child's hypotheses. The child is not in error; he or she needs further questioning and time to think about the questions. However, Kevin Keane cautions teachers that, because there is necessarily heavy emphasis upon language in education of the deaf, frequently the child may give an acceptable answer without mastery. Keane's work suggests that supportive, nonjudgmental probing questions, in the traditional clinical method of Piaget, should provide the teacher with an incredible wealth of information about the ways of the child's thoughts.

SHORT- AND LONG-TERM MEMORY   The coverage of short- and long-term memory in the CREED Five Curriculum, while basically correct, is now superseded by ten explosive years of research and theory. Once again, our early definitions have been not so much changed as expanded and elaborated, providing exciting direction for educators.

In the expansion and elaboration of the descriptions of short- and long-term memory, the major overriding principle is *organization:* initial and ongoing organization of information in the short-term memory so that we can work to understand that information; organization of information in long-term memory so that we can make it available for use. We now know that, when information is well organized in the long-term memory, we can use that organization to hold it in short-term memory when working on it in a new situation. Today, researchers and theorists describe understanding and retrieving information as different phases of the same process. As the learner seeks to understand a new situation, he or she tries to find ways in which the new situation is similar to concepts and frameworks already organized in the long-term memory. We understand new events by searching our long-term memory for analogous events.

Finally, perhaps the most exciting new direction is that labeled somewhat pretentiously "metamemory," or more recently "metacognition." Both these terms describe the learner's level of awareness of the strategies he or she is using to learn, to organize, to understand, to remember, and to retrieve information. Researchers and theorists assert that successful learners have a much greater awareness of what it takes to succeed on tasks; they are aware of what they are doing that increases their level of success. Even young children tell them, "I repeated it in my head," or "I looked for all the red ones first." The culmination of such awareness of strategies is found, of course, in the successful problem solvers, who have defined for

Table 5
Short- and Long-Term Memory

The Processes	The Unsuccessful Learner	The Successful Learner
1. Everything we attend to, perceive, understand, and solve, and the strategies we use to do so, are organized in our long-term memory and must be retrieved to be known and used.	1. Is still building rules for organizing; rules for retrieving are not systematic and task specific.	1. Is becoming more sophisticated in the use of the same rules used to classify, order, or find analogies between similar experiences; can use them to help retrieve past information and to help understand current situations.
2. We think through our short-term memory processes. They are of limited capacity and time; we must develop ways to overcome these limitations, or we limit our thinking.	2. Has inefficient short-term memory processing; has not developed specific strategies for organizing or holding information in short-term memory, so loses information if it is beyond short-term memory capacity at any one time.	2. Uses those rules, plus specific strategies for rehearsing or "chunking" information to hold it in short-term memory as he or she works it out.
3. All of the rules for organizing information and for using that information are used to retrieve old information to understand new experience.	3. Lacks experience; lacks efficient organization of such experience as he or she has had; lacks retrieval strategies; consequently, retrieval of old experience to clarify new experience is limited.	3. Is becoming aware of the strategies that assist in thinking and those that don't; is building a repertoire of the successful ones.
4. The efficient thinker, organizer, and retriever is aware of what it means to think, organize, and retrieve. He or she deliberately develops ways of doing all of these.	4. Has not yet become fully aware of the existence or the role of efficient strategies for organizing, thinking, and retrieving information.	4. Is beginning to think about his or her thinking.

themselves the complex sequence of steps required to generate the information they do not have from the information they do have.

How can teachers of the multihandicapped hearing-impaired child take advantage of these new ideas? First of all, once again, I urge teachers to analyze the instructional tasks they are providing for their children. In this case, teachers must determine the best way to organize the material for processing by both short- and long-term memory. Teachers must examine tasks in terms of the specific components to be learned, the distracting components of the different contexts in which the task is presented in repetition, the number of components to be handled at any one time, and the order in which these components must be worked upon. Such analyses should provide the basis for task presentation for organization in short-term memory and in long-term memory. For short-term memory, the teacher should analyze tasks into small groupings of information, with opportunities for repetition in recognition of time and space limitations; for long-term memory, the teacher must analyze tasks in terms of past frameworks, signal words, and ideas to aid retrieval and to utilize strategies for remembering. Such analysis sounds complex, burdensome, and difficult for any one teacher, and so it may be; but groups of teachers and their curriculum advisors can and should perform these analyses. To fail to do them is to doom the child to failure.

Secondly, the children must be helped to increase their awareness of the activities they engage in to learn. Teachers cannot leave the means for mastery of instructional tasks—no matter how well analyzed and how often repeated—to the trial and error strategies of the learners. Teachers must begin to focus upon what successful learners actually do to organize, to understand, to retain, to retrieve, and to use information. Then teachers must help less successful learners not only to use these strategies but also to be aware of how, why, when, and where to use them. Successful learners know what they are doing to be successful; we must let all learners in on these secrets.

Summary

While I have been able to provide only a very brief abstract of new research, current theory, and educational implications, there is much here of value to educators.

In summary, I would like to share with you a comment that David Klahr made in 1976. He thought the results of our research were intriguing, but he was far more interested in what the individual children who succeeded did, and what the individual children who failed did; he was particularly interested in the individual differences that all of the children manifested in their actions on the task, rather than the end product of their performance scores. How did they succeed? How did they fail?

He congratulated us on defining the nature of the task, but he urged that we view these components in their relationship to the different ways learners work upon them. He was talking as a researcher to us, as researchers, but his comments affected us profoundly as educators.

Determining the unique learning abilities of our children in relationship to their performance on task components is, however, easier to recommend than to do, because it requires task and learner analysis more complex than that practiced in other fields. Task analysis requires that the teacher:
1. Determine the rules that must be mastered, whether the task emphasizes perception, concepts, classification, or language.
2. Determine how these rules are best organized for learning, retention, and retrieval.

Learner analysis requires that the teacher:
1. Truly determine the child's "strengths." Educators of exceptional children always teach "to their strengths," but we must expand our description of these

strengths. In defining strengths, we must ask questions such as: What rules for discriminating letters does he or she have? How does he or she use them? What frameworks for our concepts does he or she have? How rich are these frameworks? How does he or she use them?

2. Carefully diagnose the child's abilities. Teachers can find out such information about their children who are both deaf and learning disabled only through diagnostic procedures far more thorough than current commercially available tests. They must know a great deal more than they do now about what a learner needs to know and to do in order to master a task, if they are to determine what a particular child does or does not know and can or cannot do.

Such intensive procedures of task and learner analysis are already being used at all levels of education, including the education of the multihandicapped hearing impaired. The analysis that Bob Pehrson has made of the frameworks for concepts of the deaf children he works with is exactly the type of analysis I am describing. With his sophisticated knowledge of the structure of concepts themselves and the frameworks or schema that a child already has, he determines the needs of the child. He has designed exciting procedures for developing the schema necessary for the meaning of the concepts being taught. It can be done. All it takes is a group of educators in tune with the newest, most creative principles of cognitive psychology, who, with the support of enlightened administrators, can transform these principles into the analysis of their instructional tasks and into instruments for determining the level of needed skills for these tasks in their children. As I mentioned earlier, the single most significant principle of all the CREED projects I directed is that the *teacher* must have primary responsibility for the educational diagnosis and instruction of the multihandicapped hearing-impaired child. Consequently, we need to provide training and support for our teachers to enable them to engage in the learner and task analyses I have described.

I have always been convinced that the teachers of the multihandicapped hearing-impaired children with whom I have worked in the CREED projects have the motivation for a complex undertaking. With the appropriate support and training, perhaps ten years hence, we shall be discussing their new and exciting innovations in diagnosis and instruction.

Bibliography

Anderson, R. C., Spiro, R. J., & Montague, W. E. (Eds.). *Schooling and the acquisition of knowledge*. Hillsdale, N.J.: Lawrence Erlbaum Associates, 1977.

Appel, M. H., & Goldberg, L. S. (Eds.). *Topics in cognitive development* (Vol. 1). New York: Plenum Press, 1977.

Bates, E. *Language and context: The acquisition of pragmatics*. New York: Academic Press, 1976.

Bjork, R. A. Short-term storage: The ordered output of a central processor. In F. Restle, R. M. Shiffrin, N. J. Castellan, H. R. Lindman, & D. B. Pisoni (Eds.),

Cognitive theory (Vol. 1). Hillsdale, N.J.: Lawrence Erlbaum Associates, 1975.

Bobrow, D. G., & Norman, D. A. Some principles of memory schemata. In D. G. Bobrow & A. M. Collins (Eds.), *Representation and understanding: Studies in cognitive science*. New York: Academic Press, 1975.

Bourne, L. E., Jr. An inference model for conceptual rule learning. In R. L. Solso (Ed.), *Theories in cognitive psychology: The Loyola Symposium*. Hillsdale, N.J.: Lawrence Erlbaum Associates, 1974.

Brannan, A. C., et al. *The hearing impaired/mentally retarded: A survey of state institutions for the retarded*. Lubbock, Tex.: Research and Training Center in Mental Retardation, Texas Technological University, 1975.

Brown, A. L. The development of memory: Knowing, knowing about knowing, and knowing how to know. In H. W. Reese (Ed.), *Advances in child development and behavior* (Vol. 10). New York: Academic Press, 1975.

Combs, A. W. *Educational accountability: Beyond behavioral objectives*. Washington, D.C.: Association for Supervision and Curriculum Development, 1972.

Craik, F. I. M., & Jacoby, L. L. A process view of short-term retention. In F. Restle, R. M. Shiffrin, N. J. Castellan, H. R. Lindman, & D. B. Pisoni (Eds.), *Cognitive theory* (Vol. 1). Hillsdale, N.J.: Lawrence Erlbaum Associates, 1975.

Craik, F. I. M., & Levy, B. A. The concept of primary memory. In W. K. Estes (Ed.), *Handbook of learning and cognitive processes: Attention and memory* (Vol. 4). Hillsdale, N.J.: Lawrence Erlbaum Associates, 1976.

Cronin, F., & Restaino, L. C. R. *Curriculum development for young multihandicapped children: One approach*. Monograph of the Bureau for Physically Handicapped Children. Albany, N.Y.: State Education Department, 1973.

Day, M. C. Developmental trends in visual scanning. In H. W. Reese (Ed.), *Advances in child development and behavior* (Vol. 10). New York: Academic Press, 1975.

Estes, W. K. Memory, perception, and decision in letter identification. In R. L. Solso (Ed.), *Information processing and cognition: The Loyola Symposium*. Hillsdale, N.J.: Lawrence Erlbaum Associates, 1975.

Flavell, J. H., & Wellman, H. M. Metamemory. In R. V. Kail, Jr. & J. W. Hagen (Eds.), *Perspectives on the development of memory and cognition*. Hillsdale, N.J.: Lawrence Erlbaum Associates, 1977.

Gallagher, J. M., & Easley, J. A., Jr. *Knowledge and development: Piaget and education* (Vol. 2). New York: Plenum Press, 1978.

Gibson, J. J. The theory of affordances. In R. Shaw, & J. Bransford (Eds.), *Perceiving, acting, and knowing: Toward an ecological psychology*. Hillsdale, N.J.: Lawrence Erlbaum Associates, 1977.

Greeno, J. G. The structure of memory and the process of solving problems. In R. L. Solso (Ed.), *Contemporary issues in cognitive psychology: The Loyola Symposium*. Washington, D.C.: V. H. Winston & Sons, 1973.

Hagen, J. W., Jonglward, R. H., Jr., & Kail, R. V., Jr. Cognitive perspectives on the development of memory. In H. W. Reese (Ed.), *Advances in child development and behavior* (Vol. 10). New York: Academic Press, 1975.

Healey, W. C., et al. *The hearing impaired mentally retarded: Recommendations for action.* Department of Health, Education, and Welfare, Social and Rehabilitation Service, Rehabilitation Services Administration, Division of Developmental Disabilities, 1975.

Inhelder, B., Sinclair, H., & Bovet, M. *Learning and the development of cognition.* Cambridge, Mass.: Harvard University Press, 1974.

Just, M. A., & Carpenter, P. A. *Cognitive processes in comprehension.* Hillsdale, N.J.: Lawrence Erlbaum Associates, 1977.

Kaufman, R. A. *Educational system planning.* Englewood Cliffs, N.J.: Prentice-Hall, 1972.

Kintsch, W. *The representation of meaning in memory.* New York: John Wiley and Sons, 1974.

Klahr, D. (Ed.). *Cognition and instruction.* Hillsdale, N.J.: Lawrence Erlbaum Associates, 1976.

Kreutzer, M. A., Leonard, C., & Flavell, J. H. *An interview of children's knowledge about memory.* Monographs of the Society for Research in Child Development. (Vol. 40). 1975.

La Berge, D. Perceptual learning and attention. In W. K. Estes (Ed.), *Handbook of learning and cognitive processes: Attention and memory* (Vol. 4). Hillsdale, N.J.: Lawrence Erlbaum Associates, 1976.

La Berge, D., & Samuels, S. J. Toward a theory of automatic information processing in reading. *Cognitive Psychology,* 1974, *6,* 293–323.

Lindsay, P. H., & Norman, D. A. *Human information processing* (2nd ed.). New York: Academic Press, 1977.

Norman, D. A. *Memory and attention: An introduction to human information processing.* New York: John Wiley and Sons, 1969.

Paivio, A. Imagery and long-term memory. In A. Kennedy & A. Wilkes (Eds.), *Studies in long-term memory.* New York: John Wiley and Sons, 1975.

Paivio, A. *Imagery and verbal processes.* New York: Holt, Rinehart and Winston, 1971.

Piaget, J. *The development of thought: The equilibration of cognitive structures.* New York: Viking Press, 1977.

Presseisen, B., Goldstein, D., & Appel, M. H. (Eds.). *Topics in cognitive development: Language and operational thought* (Vol. 2). New York: Plenum Press, 1978.

Relihan, J., & Restaino, L. C. R. *Effects of training in organizing upon the solving of class inclusion problems in young children.* Paper presented at A.E.R.A. Conference, San Francisco, April 1976.

Restaino, L. C. R. *Individual differences in logical operations: An information processing analysis*. Monograph of the Seventh Interdisciplinary Conference on Piagetian Theory and Its Implication for the Helping Professions (Vol. 2). Los Angeles: University of Southern California, 1979.

Restaino, L. C. R., et al. *Curriculum for young deaf children*. Project CREED Five (Cooperative Research Endeavors in Education of the Deaf—PL 89-313). Albany: New York Division for Handicapped Children, State Education Department, 1972.

Restaino, L. C. R., & Socher, P. A. *Psycho-educational assessment of young deaf children*. Project CREED Three (Cooperative Research Endeavors in Education of the Deaf—PL 89-313). Albany: New York Division for Handicapped Children, State Education Department, 1969.

Restaino, L. C. R., & Socher, P. A. *Curriculum development for young deaf children with specific learning disabilities*. Project CREED Four (Cooperative Research Endeavor in Education of the Deaf—PL 89-313). Albany: The State Education Department, 1970.

Scardamalia, M. Information processing capacity and the problem of horizontal decolage: A demonstration using combinatorial reasoning tests. *Child Development*, 1977, *48*, 28–37.

Shaw, R., & Bransford, J. Introduction: Psychological approaches to the problem of knowledge. In R. Shaw & J. Bransford (Eds.), *Perceiving, acting, and knowing: Toward an ecological psychology*. Hillsdale, N.J.: Lawrence Erlbaum Associates, 1977.

Shiffrin, R. M. Short-term store: The basis for a memory system. In F. Restle, R. M. Shiffrin, N. J. Castellan, H. R. Lindman, & D. B. Pisoni (Eds.), *Cognitive theory* (Vol. 1). Hillsdale, N.J.: Lawrence Erlbaum Associates, 1975.

Shiffrin, R. M. Capacity limitations in information processing, attention and memory. In W. K. Estes (Ed.), *Handbook of learning and cognition: Attention and memory* (Vol. 4). Hillsdale, N.J.: Lawrence Erlbaum Associates, 1976.

Stewart, L. G. *Serving hearing-impaired developmentally disabled persons*. Tucson: The Rehabilitation Center, College of Education, The University of Arizona, 1977.

Unruh, G. G. *Responsive curriculum development*. Berkeley, Calif.: McCutchan Publishing Corporation, 1975.

Wright, J. C., & Vlietsra, A. G. The development of selective attention: From perceptual exploration to logical search. In H. W. Reese (Ed.), *Advances in child development and behavior* (Vol. 10). New York: Academic Press, 1975.

Young, F., & Lindsley, D. (Eds.). *Early experience and visual information processing in perceptual and reading disorders*. Washington, D.C.: National Academy of Sciences, 1970.

Appendix A
General Assumptions and Objectives
of the CREED Five Curriculum

The CREED curriculum was designed for the teacher of the young deaf child with special learning disabilities. The CREED curriculum provides the teacher with a description of developmental objectives, and methods for fulfilling these objectives, in the areas of gross motor development, sensorimotor integration, visual analysis, attention and memory, and conceptualization. These objectives and procedures were based upon several very important assumptions about the children for whom they were developed. These assumptions are the product of the interaction of the CREED staff with classroom teachers and supervisors, as well as consideration of current research and thought in psychology and education.

In proposing the assumptions we recognize that the teacher must be provided with special resources to help the special deaf child's performance on motor, perceptual, and conceptual tasks. Of equal importance to us, however, is providing the teacher with special resources to help the child's affective development.

The success that the child achieves in the five motor-perceptual-conceptual areas is inextricably related to the motivation, ego-strength, and positive expectation the child brings to these tasks. We believe that it is essential that these factors be considered by each school and each teacher in implementing the objectives and procedures of the CREED Five Curriculum.

The CREED staff expects the teacher to view these objectives and activities as *specific content* which may fit into varied instructional modes. In other words, the objectives and activities are designed for use in many educational structures; they are not an educational structure in and of themselves.

The general assumptions are those that we strongly believe each school and each classroom teacher must consider in the development of all instructional activities that involve the deaf child with special learning disabilities.

ASSUMPTION 1 Deaf children with special learning disabilities move through the stages of development in the same sequence as other children. As in all children, the many skills they need to function in school may develop at different rates. The CREED Three Project indicated that the performance of most special deaf children does not reflect bizarre behavior patterns; rather, they may be at very early developmental levels in one skill area and at higher levels in others. They should, however, move through these developmental stages as any other child would, and they must be provided with the opportunities to do so.

ASSUMPTION 2 The deaf child with special learning disabilities is seriously hindered in meeting the demands of classroom learning without prerequisite skills. The demands of classroom learning in subject areas are such that subordinate skills must be mastered before we can expect any child to succeed in them. Many children acquire these subordinate skills without the direct aid of the teacher. The teacher of the special deaf child, however, must give careful consideration to the structure of these skills and to the environment in which they can be mastered. The subordinate skills must be analyzed and specifically described, and the environment must be carefully prepared for the child if he or she is to progress through it toward readiness for instruction in subject areas.

ASSUMPTION 3 Because the child's limited experience with elements in the environment leads to greater rigidity of behavior than that of other children, the structuring of the environment by the teacher to insure progress in motor, perceptual, and conceptual skills may further encourage such rigidity. As we stated in Assumption 2, we must structure the environment for the child when introducing new learning to help the child master it, but we must also recognize that such deliberate structuring may provide little opportunity for the child to adapt even to small changes confronting him or her.

It is essential that we systematically provide for the development within the child of the ability to react without confusion when presented with several alternatives and to make decisions based upon such alternatives. Because our goal is to lead the child to the highest level of functioning of which he or she is capable within the environment, we must systematically provide opportunities for the child to develop strategies to meet changes in this environment.

Because the special deaf child depends on adults to make decisions for him or her to a greater extent than do most children, we must also systematically train the child to assume an increasing responsibility for, and a larger role in, aspects of his or her own development.

Such training, in the case of independent behavior and problem solving strategies, can be provided using elements of the CREED Five Curriculum after careful consideration of each child's cognitive and affective level of development.

ASSUMPTION 4 The classroom experiences of the special deaf child constitute a greater proportion of his or her opportunities for learning than for other children; therefore, the interaction between the special deaf child and the teacher is more critical to that child's education than it may be for other children. Other children are better able to select from and integrate the varied, unstructured sources of experience outside the classroom; the special deaf child is far more dependent upon the classroom structuring of experience for building a framework for knowledge. Thus, the teacher's role in the child's development becomes far more critical than for other children. Because the teacher is so important to the child's progress as a thinking and feeling human being, the nature of interaction the teacher has with the child becomes as important as the content of instruction.

ASSUMPTION 5 The deaf child with special learning disabilities has experienced failure to a greater degree than other children. Therefore, our attention must be directed not only to progress in motor, perceptual and conceptual skills, but also to the enhancement of the child's ego-strength, expectation for success, and pleasure in trying. We must analyze skills to their fundamental levels and develop activities with small levels of increasing difficulty not only to provide the opportunity eventually to master skills at their highest levels, but also to provide the opportunity to succeed at some level. The teacher must provide continuous opportunities for successful performance in order to help develop a positive feeling in the child about his or her ability to do something well. Such positive feeling is an important source of motivation, and it is absolutely essential if the teacher expects the child to persist at tasks he or she finds more difficult.

ASSUMPTION 6 There is, within the group of deaf children with special learning disabilities, as wide a range of individual differences as in the group of typically deaf children. These differences are found in their affective behavior as well as in their cognitive behavior. We have urged that teachers and supervisors observe individual children intensively in order to diagnose abilities and disabilities in perceptual-motor-cognitive areas; it is also essential that they study children's behavior for cues to the kinds of communication and interaction patterns that seem to be productive or obstructive to their learning.

IV

Developing Language and Communication Strategies

Structuring the Communication Program for the Needs of Multihandicapped Hearing-Impaired Children

David Tweedie

Recognizing seven functions of communication, Dr. David Tweedie reviews the work of Jan Van Dijk with deaf-blind children. Tweedie indicates how Van Dijk's methods develop those functions of communication with deaf-blind children. From there, Tweedie considers the options of teachers developing communication skills among deaf-blind children. He suggests that such teachers may view their options as occurring along a sign language continuum. Their task, then, becomes one of selecting the optimal point of the continuum for a unique and particular child.

Communication is a process basic to all human beings. Each way we move our bodies, or more importantly, specific parts of our bodies, provides a "bit" of information for the receiver of our communication. Even that lack of movement is a form of communication that can be interpreted by the receiver. The way we position our bodies and the way those positions have been perceived by others have led to the study of "body language." The way facial expressions are consistently paired with feelings and emotions illustrates an additional form of movement language.

Each of our senses provides us with information concerning our environment or communication from the environment. If our senses provide us with information about our environment and its effect on us, then our conscious reaction to that stimulation through expression, movement, or some other appropriate action is a communicative response to our environment. Normal hearing children develop their language and communication system through the variations in sensory input and the consistency of sensory input. Halliday (1975) discussed the communication functions of normal children and categorized their explorations of development from 9 months to 18 months of age. His discussion of this development identified seven discrete communication functions:

1. Instrumental—to satisfy the child's own bodily needs;
2. Regulatory—to exert control over the behavior of others;
3. Interactional—to establish and maintain a communication contact with those in the child's environment that had significance to him or her;
4. Personal—to express his or her own individuality and development of self-awareness;
5. Heuristic—to explore the objective environment;
6. Imaginative—to create an environment of one's own;
7. Informative—to convey information.

Through these communication functions the child attempts to learn about the environment and to interact with that environment.

Through these communication functions, the infant begins to be less at the total mercy of the environment and acts upon it, as it acts upon him or her. The beginning of awareness of this concept is the basis for language development in the infant. Through the "constants" communicated by the environment to the child, he or she learns the language of the society in which he or she resides. By pairing individuals, movements, and objects to the sensory stimulus they provide, the child builds a repertoire of linguistic concepts representing the actual experience.

In the deaf-blind multihandicapped child, however, this patterning or pairing is interrupted or not consistently provided because of the sensory impairments. It has often been said that deaf-blind multihandicapped children live "within themselves." Therefore, they have not been able to learn about their environment or to progress through the stages of communication discussed by Halliday. The communication patterns developed by normal hearing children within their environment, which provide them with information about their environment and their role in it, are severely impaired in deaf-blind multihandicapped children. This sensory isolation prevents them from learning about their environment through exploration and communication. Because of this lack of normal movement experiences in the severely multihandicapped children's world, their experiences in the main are those which act upon them without permitting them to react with their environment. Therefore, their behavior and communication is directed inward and, typically, becomes egocentric.

The severely impaired communication system of the deaf-blind multihandicapped child was observed by Jan Van Dijk (1965) and led him to develop his theory which encouraged the development of language in this population through movement. Van Dijk recognized that developmental or motor activity was one of the early ways a child learns about the world and about his or her own body. He believed that the basis for our concept development lay in the motor patterns we receive by working with objects in our environment. This movement within our environment instructs us in our *relationship* to our environment. In Van Dijk's approach, the body is the basis for learning language, and movement is the medium to experience the world and the body as a unit. The Van Dijk approach builds awareness of the body and teaches how to move the body in space.

The Van Dijk approach is not a technique or method but a philosophy, a way of looking at a total child within a flexible, theoretical framework. Van Dijk has commented that educators of the deaf-blind have, over the years, tended to overemphasize gestural and oral communication with a disregard for the many and various levels of communication functioning as prerequistes to a readiness for a gestural, sign, or oral communication system.

Van Dijk's outline of progress in language development for deaf-blind children is provided by Dr. Hammer in Chapter 17. In the beginning of the Van Dijk program, efforts are directed to the removal of the child from the ego-consciousness state in which he or she has been functioning. This communication towards the self must be directed outward before any higher functioning in communication can be developed. Activities suggested by Van Dijk develop the "me-not me" concept of the world and the child's place in it. Training in this area exploits the stimulus hunger of the deaf-blind multihandicapped child. This training also attempts to build through reinforcement a set of behaviors that may be observable. Most language development programs for deaf-blind children rely on a systematic reinforcement program to increase responses. A token system of reinforcement is used at the beginning of training; however, a deferred gratification or total praise reinforcement system is striven for as soon as possible.

The next stage of instruction and monitoring is the building of motor patterns for experiences. Here the attempt is made to increase further the movement experience of deaf-blind children. In this stage children are provided experiences moving their bodies in space through walking, running, jumping, and moving over, under, upon, above, through various planes, textures, and objects. Here also movement is experienced in various "atmospheres" to help the children experience differences in sensation on their bodies. Movement through water, sand, styrofoam pellets, or other media provide the children differentiation in environmental influences. Through these states the concepts of out, in, under, and through may be developed. They can be reinforced in the swimming pool. Without a symbol system at this point, the children are building sensory concepts of what these experiences mean. Later experiences with a symbol system hopefully will be paired with the experience-building from this stage.

Perhaps the most important stage of development in preparation for a formal communication system within the Van Dijk approach is level III, the Development of Body Schema or Body Image and its movement towards level IV, Natural Gesture. During these stages, the transition from cohesive through coactive to imitative behavior attempts to continue the movement experience of the child through space as well as to initiate communication to other human beings.

It is at this point in training that an interpersonal dialogue should develop between the teacher and student through movement. Here also a beginning gesture system is initiated from the behaviors typically exhibited by the deaf-blind youngster. Through the close body contact between teacher and student during the cohesive stage, the teacher permits the student to initiate the communication most important to him or her. For example, during the rocking behavior of a severely involved deaf-blind student, a pushing or shoving motion directed towards the teacher to secure permission to continue with "rocking behavior" is an integral part of the deaf-blind youngster's repertoire at this point in development. This close interpersonal contact between teacher and student would also identify other gesture needs of the child. In initiating a communication gesture system in this manner, the child for the first time in his or her existence is able to communicate his or her wants to the outside world. The movement of his or her body upon another's (the teacher's) would bring the child into the *regulatory stage*, as described by Halliday in his seven discrete communication functions. This seemingly minor sequence of events, if appropriately undertaken, is the basis for gesture and eventually sign communication for severely and multihandicapped deaf-blind individuals.

The coactive stage as well as its growth into the imitative stage provides a series of events that develop the child's memory and anticipation skills. These skills are all important to true language development in severely handicapped individuals. The sequencing of movements plus changes from one movement to another builds confidence in the child. It also challenges the child while becoming more and more complex. As sequenced activities become more complex, they also assist in developing attention span.

When the imitation level is reached, a major objective of the imitating of gross body movements, body positions, and limb movements will be transferred into smaller, more complex, symbolic hand movements as signs and possibly even fingerspelling. (See also the discussion by Stremel-Campbell, Chapter 19.) Care must be taken in the program not to move too rapidly into a sign system without proper regard for prerequisite behaviors. At this point the teacher more and more directs the activities of the student by determining the "natural gesture" most appropriate to the activity in question. For example, gestures involving objects are not introduced prior to their natural facilitation with that particular object. If the child is bouncing a ball, the gesture for the ball would be movement of the hand in an up and down fashion to denote the "bouncing of the ball." Other objects familiar to the child would also have a gesture to denote their presence when they are not within the immediate environment of the student.

In the progress towards a sign system these activities or gesture-like activities would be paired to transfer their meaning to a formal sign. Once again, it must be pointed out that extreme caution should be exercised and care taken not to move too quickly through these all important stages of transference. It is at this critical time that many teachers incorrectly interpret a student's mastery of some signs as an indication that the student is ready for more complex linguistic involvement. Here linguistic splinter skills would develop, and the student could become "programmed" for providing answers to questions through sign without the proper understanding of the meaning or use and transference of the sign symbol.

As the student gains vocabulary enrichment through this stage, decisions must be made about the sign system to be used throughout the next stages of instruction. To the novice attempting to understand the various sign language systems, selecting the most appropriate system for these children may prove to be very complex and extremely confusing. Table 1 illustrates the so-called sign language continuum. This continuum could be thought of as being consistent with the Van Dijk approach: it provides for transition from a nonverbal communication system (using mainly pantomime, gesture, and facial expressions) as the important prerequisite for language development through body movement on to an English representation of language through fingerspelling. The overwhelming majority of deaf-blind multihandicapped students, however, need some combination of "sign language systems." The decisions regarding pure use of any system will need careful study and will succeed only if basic prerequisites for language development were adequately covered in the prior stages of the training program.

Table 1
Sign Language Continuum

	Characteristics	Relation to English	Examples
Nonverbal Communication	Pantomime, natural gestures, facial expressions, body movement	No representation of English elements	
In-group Signs			
American Sign Language (ASL)	Standard signs, fingerspelling, elements of pantomime; has syntax of its own; is ideographic, idiomatic One sign—one concept	Some representation of English elements	American Sign Language (ASL), also known as Ameslan
Signed English	Standard signs, fingerspelling, a lot of English syntax One sign—one concept	A great many English elements	Sign English Signed English Manual English
Manual English	Some standard signs, supplemented with invented signs to represent visually the syntax of English accurately; inflections, endings, suffixes, prefixes One sign—one word	Complete representation of English elements	Seeing Essential English (SEE I) Signing Exact English (SEE II) Linguistics of Visual English (LOVE) Signed English Manual English
Fingerspelling	Letter-by-letter representation of English	Complete representation of English	Rochester Method Visible English

The concept of *Sign Language Continuum* was first proposed by Woodward (1973) as a way to view signing behavior among the American (United States) deaf population. This continuum suggests that any given person's signing is a combination of American Sign Language and Manual English. Each of these languages occupies separate and opposite ends of the continuum. It also suggests that there are some deaf persons who sign exclusively in American Sign Language, and others that sign exclusively in English gestures. It is believed that most deaf people in the United States fall in between these two extremes, signing a mixture of both American Sign Language and Signed English. Unfortunately, to date there has been no empirical research to support this concept since Woodward's publication of the theory.

American Sign Language represents the native language of the North American deaf population. As with any language, there are regional variations (as noted by Woodward, 1976), dialects, and even "accents" similar to those that appear in spoken communication systems. These variations account for *local signs*. Local signs are those signs used in a particular geographical region or group of deaf individuals.

For example, signs for names of towns and cities as well as for states may vary from state to state. Furthermore, many black deaf people in the South use signs quite different from white southerners.

Unfortunately, in the hurry for deaf educators and researchers to make up for years of persecution of the language used by deaf persons in North America and elsewhere, the acceptance of American Sign Language as a formal language has been based primarily upon emotion and not upon a great deal of research. Substantive research, however, has now begun and is being reported by Baker (1977), Padden (1978), Stokoe (1972), Woodward (1978), and others.

ASL or Ameslan is now thought of as a language of its own, with syntactic and grammatical rules. It is the fourth most commonly used language—after English, Spanish, and Italian in the United States. Ameslan has its own syntax which does not follow the rules of the English language.

Manual English represents the other end of the proposed continuum, opposite ASL. This system of communication is, linguistically speaking, English; it has been altered so that it can be expressed not only by vocal and written means, but also in gestural fashion. There is no single system of Manual English; various systems have been proposed, all of which seek to develop a way to express the English language in gestures and overt, visible behavior. At least four basic sign systems have been designed to represent English manually. Each includes the use of signed word affixes, structure words (at, and, it, so on) and other morphological variations of language. Each system follows English syntax, including English word order. Among the four are SEE_1, SEE_2, LOVE, and Signed English.

Signed English, however, is not directly related to this group. Signed English was created specifically for preschool children by a group at Gallaudet College (Bornstein, et al., 1975). This system uses some ASL signs without alteration, others with modifications. Rather than create signs for all English syntactic markers, this system creates signs for markers that occur frequently in the language. It follows English word order.

In addition to those systems which seek to express words or word parts manually, there is also *Fingerspelling,* which seeks to express a letter-for-letter relationship in a manual fashion. Fingerspelling is incorporated into Manual English and American Sign Language when an English word (often formal names for persons, places, etc.) must be expressed by the signer and there is no sign in that person's vocabulary to match the word.

The *Rochester Method* uses fingerspelling in an attempt to represent each letter of the spoken message with a specific handshape. This method is an attempt to provide the most complete representation of the English language.

Home signs are those that evolve out of the needs of deaf individuals and their families. They are agreed upon signs within a family unit and are not, in most cases, consistent from one place to another. Therefore, unless they are basically pantomime, the signs home will not be understood outside the family.

Childrenese is a system of signs which children invent and use among themselves at school and at play. This phenomenon may be considered a form of baby talk compared to ASL the way that hearing children initially use English incorrectly. These signs are frequently abandoned if the children are exposed to a formal sign system.

In tailoring a communication program for the needs of the multihandicapped hearing-impaired student, the teacher should keep in mind the continuum of sign language. Students who perform appropriate gestures on a consistent basis could be likened to using "school" or "home signs" on the sign language continuum. As in the Van Dijk approach, the movement from gestures to formal signs could parallel the sign language continuum to the next "sign-conceptual" level of functioning.

Teachers must seriously consider the home and school environment when outlining the child's language program. If the child's parents and peers will be mostly hearing-impaired individuals, then cultivation towards ASL should be seriously considered. If, however, the majority of the student's contacts will be with hearing individuals, then some degree of manual English skills should be involved in the training.

The severe or profoundly multihandicapped deaf-blind child needs to have a program consistent with his or her needs and level of intellectual functioning. If a sign language continuum used in conjunction with the Van Dijk approach for language development can be accepted and understood, it can assist the instructor in providing the most meaningful and dynamic approach towards developing communication skills in this population.

Bibliography

Baker, C., & Padden, C. *American Sign Language: A look at history, structure, and community.* Silver Spring, Md.: T. J. Publishers, Inc., 1978.

Baker, C. Regulators and turn-taking: American Sign Language discourse. In L. Friedman (Ed.), *On the other hand: New perspectives on American Sign Language.* New York: Academic Press, 1977.

Bornstein, H. et al. (Eds.). *The Signed English dictionary.* Washington, D.C.: Gallaudet College Press, 1975.

Halliday, M. A. K. Learning how to mean. In E. Lenneberg & E. L. Lenneberg (Eds.), *Foundations of language development: A multidisciplinary approach* (Vol. 1). New York: Academic Press, 1975.

Stokoe, W. C. Classification and description of sign languages. In T.A. Sebeok (Ed.), *Current trends in linguistics* (Vol. 12). The Hague: Mouton, 1972.

Van Dijk, J. The first steps of the deaf-blind child toward language. *Proceedings of the Conferences on the Deaf-Blind,* 1965. Boston: Perkins School for the Blind, 1965, 41–51.

Woodward, J. Facing and handling variation: American Sign Language phonology. *Sign Language Studies,* 1976, *10,* 43–51.

Woodward, J. Language continuum: A different point of view. *Sign Language Studies,* 1973, *2,* 81–83.

Woodward, J. Historical bases of American Sign Language. In P. Siple (Ed.), *Understanding language through sign language research.* Baltimore: University Park Press, 1978, 333–348.

The Development of Language in the Deaf-Blind Multihandicapped Child: Progression of Instructional Methods

Edwin Hammer

Dr. Edwin Hammer describes in great detail the work of Jan Van Dijk. Van Dijk urges educators of the deaf-blind to utilize experiences of movement, first to develop concepts in the minds of deaf-blind children, and eventually to develop modes of communication and imitation. Dr. Hammer notes that this sequence is a prerequisite of language development in any individual and a particularly crucial one for the deaf-blind.

Communication may be defined operationally as any way in which one person lets another person know an idea, a concept, a value, a judgment, or a feeling. It is a total process. Communication involves the internal feelings of a person. There is not reason to communicate until there are feelings or values to be communicated. Language, as a variety of communication, is rooted in feelings, emotions, and values. Because of these feelings, language represents an attempt to attach a symbol system to thinking so that affect may be expressed. Thus, language is a mode by which a person acts on the environment rather than being totally at the mercy of the environment and having the environs act on the person.

Language is the way in which the person learns what is permitted in society. It is the most important social experience. Without language, there is no society. It is only through the use of a common language that each generation is able to "bind time," that is, pass along what has happened so that the present generation benefits from past generations' knowledge, experiences, and emotions.

Language is also based on motor acts. It is true that language is embedded in affect and that it becomes the affiliational link with the society and culture of the person; yet neither the expression nor the relation to society is possible without the motor base which underlies the transmission. In the study of language acquisition in deaf-blind children, the work of Jan Van Dijk of the Netherlands stands as a prominent example of the level of understanding and practice. He has studied the motor base of language acquisition in deaf-blind children for over a decade, and his work provides an important framework in the study of language development and the study of instructional approaches to facilitate language use with deaf-blind children. His article, "The First Steps of the Deaf-Blind Child Towards Language" (Van Dijk, 1966), is one of the more important single publications in the literature on deaf-blind children. His movie, *Motor Development in Deaf-Blind Children* (Van (Van Dijk, 1965), is, in my opinion, the most logical presentation of the development of language in any single format. Even more important, his influence over others who work with deaf-blind children has had great impact in thinking, in practice, and in challenges to provide appropriate language opportunities for deaf-blind

Recently, Van Dijk presented his current efforts in the area of assessment of language in deaf-blind children. These studies (Van Dijk, 1977) show how truly dynamic Van Dijk is in his work. Even more relevant, these approaches offer greater insight into language development in sensorially impaired persons.

Van Dijk has provided a means to study language progression in deaf-blind persons by observing the motor base of language. (See Table 1.) To Van Dijk, the progression is from gross to fine, from general to specific, with the attachment of meaning to movement in an ever refining process that leads to expressive performance. In this model, the total body is the base for language learning. Movement becomes the means to experience the body as a unit. Language development in deaf-blind children, therefore, begins with awareness of the body and learning to move the body.

This approach has evolved over time from Van Dijk's work at St. Michielsgestel in the Netherlands. The basic premise is to structure the experiences of the deaf-blind child so that the body becomes the source for defining external reality. This does not differ so much from the experience and development of non-impaired children: rather, it seeks to be more specific in assuring the deaf-blind child's experiences and progression towards language performance. The progression starts where

Table 1
Language Development for Deaf-Blind Children: Presymbolic Levels

Level I	**Ego-Consciousness**
	Developing relationships towards the world and learning the "me" and the "not me."
Level II	**Motor Patterns for Concepts**
	Experiencing things of action, that objects are for doing, acting, and using.
Level III	**Development of Body Schema or Body Image**
	Learning that the body is a unit; that it is connected; that there are specific parts that may be used for specific things; that hands and feet are located at the ends of arms and legs; that the body has a certain size and shape.
	Substage
	Co-active movement: movement of the body in relation to a pattern. Non-representational reference: using a sculpted image to present parts of the body, movement of the body to repeat a pattern.
	Substage
	Imitation: learning to follow an example using the body.
Level IV	**Natural Gesture**
	Development of symbol consciousness, through de-contextualization (anticipation) and de-naturalization (slight movement that is indicative of full gesture).

Source: J. Van Dijk, The first steps of the deaf-blind child towards language. *Proceedings of the Conference on the Deaf-Blind, Refsnes, Denmark, July 1965.* Boston: Perkins School for the Blind, 1965, 47–51.

the child *is* in his or her language development and proceeds to the point where the child will go in language development.

For the most basic level, attempts are made to help the child differentiate the "me" and the "not me." The deaf-blind child may not be conscious that he or she exists separate from another. In this state, it is as if the child were an extension of another, and even more difficult, the other person does not always seem to be acknowledged as a person but rather as an object. The deaf-blind child may also react to himself or herself as an object. This often requires the encouraging of values in the child when none seem to exist, or when it is difficult for the adult observer to perceive whether the child values any substance. The instructional method that sometimes works with the deaf-blind child in helping the "me" emerge is to recognize the stimulus-hunger that is present and to reinforce behaviors to build a set that may be observed. This means that most programs of instruction in language development for deaf-blind children must utilize a reinforcement program to increase responses. However, after the responses have been increased so that there is a range of behavior to use, reinforcement may be confined to social praise or deferred gratification, rather than a strict operant program that still uses token systems to reward responses.

The next stage of instruction is to increase the movement of the deaf-blind child so that the body is experienced as a unit. Once the child has learned the range of movements that are possible, it is feasible to begin the next stage of not only moving, but also experiencing the body moving in space: walking, running, jumping, and carrying the body over various planes, textures, and objects. This stage entails movement of the body at different rates to experience fast and slow, to feel the pressure of the atmosphere on the front and lack of pressure on the back of the body, and to begin to place emphasis on the body being in certain directional planes. These moves evoke special feelings of joy in movement, elation at rate changes in movement, and fear of moving, especially for a totally blind person, in areas that are unknown or unseen.

Once the experiences of movement have been achieved, it is possible to vary the atmosphere to help the child experience directionality. Water, sand, corn meal, dried beans, or any substance that will give a contrast to the air in the environment may be used. An effective atmosphere seems to be a swimming pool or large container of water. This permits the child to experience the difference between the environment of air compared to the environment of water. This also lets the child experience spatial relations by feeling the difference in being "in" the water, "out" of the water, "over" the water, "under" the water, or "through" the water.

These spatial relations are experienced before the child has the words to attach to the concepts. The concepts exist for the child because they have been felt. With these experiences come some of the most important types of learning, not only spatial relations, but also positions in space. Top, bottom, in, out, around, and other spatial terms have been incorporated into body schema in a direct manner. These concrete experiences permit the development of language, and they also begin encouraging imitation. If the deaf-blind child is to follow someone else's action, it is extremely important for the child to know where his or her own body is in space, how the body relates to objects in space, and which directions are possible in moving through space.

Imitation, therefore, is the next stage in the development of language. To have the child imitate the actions of another person means to have the child move as someone else moves, to have hands, arms, and body in positions similar to those of another, and to integrate these body movements into a coherent pattern of placement. These patterns tell how the deaf-blind person perceives his or her body as a unit and how another body is located in relation to his or her body. Initially, these imitative movements are gross movements, a doing of what has been done by another. Imitation at this level is for the development of patterns and for the application of the range of motion that has been previously experienced. If the child is not imitating, then the activity reverts to the previous level so that the child is retained in a *process* development rather than a *skills* development sequence.

From imitation of body movements and placement, it is possible to begin to refine these movements and placement. The next stage is to have the child move his or her body to a representation of body movements. This may be done with pictures, with pipe-cleaner stick figures for children who cannot benefit from pictures, or with a doll. The child can trace the placement of a doll's body and repeat the pattern with his or her own body. This phase is, in my opinion, the most crucial stage in working with the deaf-blind child to develop expressive communications. It often seems a quantum leap from the movement of one's own body to positioning one's own body from cues on paper or on a doll. The key lies in the child's knowledge of his or her own body and its relation to the world outside the body *and* the emergence of natural gestures for events or actions in that world.

Natural gestures represent the refinement of this progression to the point of a beginning awareness of symbols, at least those symbols unique to the individual. These symbols do not have meaning to others, but begin to be shaped into meaningful symbols by the child engaging in two activities. One activity Van Dijk called *de-contextualization*. That is, the child seems to begin to anticipate an act and indicates this by attending or preparing to receive information or action. The second activity Van Dijk called *de-naturalization*. That is, the gesture that has been unique to the individual becomes influenced by the world in which the action takes place, and the gesture goes through a transformation into a standard or full gesture.

With the acquisition of nautral gestures and the shaping of these through experiences in the environment, the deaf-blind child moves from a presymbolic level of language development into a symbolic level of language development.

Symbolic language, in Van Dijk's model, is a further refinement of the motor/imitation/gesture progression. As the deaf-blind child acquires more experience in using a movement to represent an idea or concept, it is possible to introduce concrete examples of items that may be matched to pictures or other symbols. Van Dijk utilizes items in the child's environment as initial symbols to be applied and learned. A comb, a knife, a ball, a spoon—all were used to help the child begin to provide a full gesture for the object. The added learning that takes place here is that the child is using a motor pattern to show something in the child's regular experiences, such as during eating, dressing, or in specific play activities. This motor pattern is from the child's experiences.

In regard to this stage of the progression, Van Dijk called attention to the importance of memory in moving from the concrete to symbolic levels of language development. (See Table 2.) Recall is one component of memory, but memory is not simply recall. There are other components, such as organizing, classifying, sequencing, and storing information in a logical context for retrieval and use later. All of these activities seem to involve collecting patterns of sensations into groups, which may be called perceptions, which may be stored for further use. Memory requires the child to learn to utilize rhythm, for example, to make patterns, such as collections of sounds, vibrations, or movements that are expressed as symbols. Tempo also seems important in developing the sequential abilities that increase the

Table 2
Language Development for Deaf-Blind Children: Symbolic Levels

Level V	**Memory and Retrieval**
	Collecting patterns of sensory experiences from items by class, sequence, place, recall, rhythm, tempo, similarity, and difference.
Level VI	**Play Acting or Imaginative Play**
	Using symbols to help imagine a situation or repeat a previous experience or show a perceived situation; using symbols to show internal reality or inner thinking; using symbols in play settings to reflect external world.
Level VII	**Reversibility**
	Using concrete items (graphic or tactile representation of an object; full gesture or sign; drawing or picture) to show an object evoked by another using sign, gesture, concrete model, or picture.
Level VIII	**Consistent Expression**
	Using consistent modalities to express ideas in one-word statements; showing values through communication; expressing likes and dislikes.
Level IX	**Expansion**
	Vocabulary expanding; using specific signs or gestures or sounds; emergence of time as a distance conveyed by communication.
Level X	**Generative Communication**
	Re-grouping and re-combining signs, gestures, or sounds to make new patterns of communication; adding more than one sign or gesture or sound; making up new signs for new ideas or asking for new signs, gestures or sounds; seeking information and relaying this; language competence may emerge.

Source: E. K. Hammer, The development of language in the deaf-blind, multihandicapped child. *Monograph I: The multihandicapped hearing-impaired child*. Washington: Gallaudet College, June 21, 1977.

use of memory skills. A final component in the development of memory is the use of relationships: comparing data for similarities, analogies, or other devices which facilitate storage and retrieval. Again, these activities are experienced through motor components and become symbols by experience.

The symbolic process demands that the deaf-blind child perceive items as being "the same" or "not the same." Classification is used to compare objects that are presented in a concrete manner. From these representations, refinement takes place as the concrete gives way to recall. Remembering what was which becomes a symbol to use for grouping, comparing attributes, and sorting into logical categories. This progression follows from the actual item being compared to another actual item for sameness. Then comparison is possible to a symbol of the actual, either a graphic or tactile representation. Once the child has been able to compare the actual to a representation, it is possible to begin to use gesture to request the comparison. Thus, the sign or full gesture for the item is introduced as a companion to a comparison of the actual item or to a graphic or tactile representation. The sign may then be substituted for the graphic symbol, and in response to the sign or gesture, the child can give the actual item to the instructor. It is also possible to have the child give the representation to the examiner in response to the sign. (The child is not asked to provide the full gesture or sign at this time.) The child is responding to three variables available to him: request for an actual item, request for a graphic or tactile representation of the item, or request for a full gesture or sign for an item to be given to the instructor.

The introduction of the fourth variable follows. The item may now be presented in a graphic form constructed by the child or by the instructor. That is, the child draws a picture or makes a clay model of the item that is requested. At first, the child may draw around the item, then begin to make a clay mold of the item, and then later begin to model the clay after the item. Thus, the child has four options available in responding to a request for an item from everyday experiences: the item itself, the graphic representation of the item, the sign or full gesture, or a model of the item that has been constructed by the child in clay or in a drawing.

The next phase reverses the activities that have been undertaken. Instead of the teacher framing a request for items to the child, now the goal becomes a request from the child for the items. This naming is accomplished by giving the child the full gesture or sign for the activity. A request is made for the child to provide what is needed to complete the activity. For example, in dressing, the socks have been put on. What is missing? The child is to give the sign for shoe. It is also possible to have the child express the missing part in other ways, such as drawing the shoe, making a clay model of the shoe, showing the picture of a shoe as being what is missing. Thus, expressive skills as well as receptive skills are emerging, and importantly they are related to events in the child's daily experiences. A range of options becomes available to the child in how to express information. The symbol, in itself, does not have meaning for the child, but it is related to the meaning of the items in terms of use in the daily life of the child. From this, there is a way for the child to begin to operate on the external reality. These symbols, therefore, receive meaning as they become ways to operate on the environment.

When the child has begun to use the full gesture or sign or to respond in a meaningful way to the vibration for items, it is possible to begin to introduce sounds to the child as part of the sign or gesture system. This is to provide the child with another variable in expressing the symbol: through sign, gesture, graphic, or sound. Because of the dual impairments of the child, it is necessary to have as many channels of input as possible for all symbols. The deaf-blind person seems to need at least two sensory channels to receive information: one channel to carry the context cue and one channel to reinforce what has been received on the first channel.

When the child has learned the expressive gestures or sign for items in his or her environment, expansion of expression becomes a target. More abstract words that convey actions that the child has experienced in motor activities may be introduced: "go," "come," "up," "down," "in," "on," "over," and other action words are paired with labeled items to make two-word utterances. This type of learning may be utilized in symbolic play where the child is acting out what happened in life through drama. "Shoe," for example, now becomes an item or symbol that may be manipulated just as the total body was manipulated in the past. By using the item "shoe," it is possible to expand to "shoe on," or "shoe up." This is accompanied with imitative procedures. However, the imitation of two-word gestures or signs with sounds attached is the basis of knowing, acting upon, and relating a feeling or idea to the external reality. It is through this type of activity that language becomes internalized. That is, language becomes a part of the deaf-blind child's internal reality. The child experiences the movement in himself or herself, then acts upon this item as he or she acted upon himself or herself. In this manner, the child is beginning to express likes and dislikes, is beginning to build vocabulary, and is emerging as a participant in the surroundings.

The child may now begin to expand communication skills. At this point, it may be helpful to have a communication board, but not so much for the child as for the adults in the child's life to keep up with the words that have been used and learned to some degree. (This board is not to be confused with communications boards that have been used for expressive communication skills; this board is more for the benefit of those in the child's environment.) In knowing what the child has learned, how it is used, and what new words are being introduced, it is easier for the adults in the child's life to supply *consistent* language input to the child. A communication board may serve as a coordinating device for the adults to maintain this consistency.

Another device that may be used in helping the child expand language skills is an activity board. This board can be located in the living area in the school. It tells in sequence what activities are to be done. The child may use this board as a reference to tell what is happening next and to structure the day for himself or herself. The child may also signal that the next activity is to begin or indicate readiness for the next activity by getting the card from the activity board.

The child needs to be encouraged to group and regroup signs and sounds to form new ideas or express new needs. This action also indicates that new signs and sounds will be added to words that are expressed. This activity may include trial and error learning and then intuitive learning as the child begins to use expressive language skills to try to communicate new patterns of experiences. This will also take coordination on the part of the adults to assure a responsive atmosphere surrounding the child at this time. If expansion is to lead to increased communication, a supportive group of persons must respond to the deaf-blind child. Too often, this need seems to be overlooked; the reason language development is stressed is so that the deaf-blind person will have someone *to* whom to communicate feelings and ideas and *from* whom to receive communication. This component is just as important as any of the other components outlined in this presentation. From use, the deaf-blind child will have an opportunity to ask for information or to relay experiences. With this increased use, competence in the use of language may begin to emerge with the deaf-blind person. This, after all, is the goal of an instructional program for language development in deaf-blind children.

Bibliography

Hammer, E. The development of language in the deaf-blind, multihandicapped child: Progression of instructional methods. In E. Shroyer & D. Tweedie (Eds.), *Monograph I: The multihandicapped hearing-impaired child*. Washington, D.C.: Gallaudet College, 1977.

Van Dijk, J. The first steps of the deaf-blind child towards language. *Proceedings of the Conference on the Deaf-Blind, Refsnes, Denmark, July 1965*. Boston: Perkins School for the Blind, 1965, 47–51.

Van Dijk, J. Motor development in the education of deaf-blind children. *Proceedings of the Conference on the Deaf-Blind, Refsnes, Denmark, July 1965*. Boston: Perkins School for the Blind, 1965, 41–46.

18

The Language of Hearing-Impaired Mentally Retarded Children

Donald Moores

Dr. Donald Moores distinguishes between mentally retarded hearing-impaired children for whom language acquisition is a feasible goal and those for whom, for whatever reason, it is not. With the former, he says, we teach those intermediate skills necessary to "natural" acquisition of language. With the latter, he observes, we set limited goals and teach communication skills necessary to everyday functioning, as ends in themselves. Dr. Moores then reviews several modes of communication that may help a child attain those goals.

The ability to acquire and use language seems to be a defining characteristic of human beings. Children who do not suffer from severe physical, mental, or emotional handicaps and who grow up in an environment even minimally stimulating acquire language naturally and unconsciously through the auditory channel. Children who are deaf can acquire language just as naturally if they are exposed to manual communication on a daily basis.

In fact, when a child does not acquire language, we assume that there is a serious problem, either with the child or with the environment. There may be unnatural environmental conditions, as in the case of isolated or abused children. There may be profound emotional problems, such as those presently classified as autism or childhood schizophrenia.

The more severe the language problem—regardless of cause—the less natural the process of language acquisition. Thus we find ourselves moving away from finding the key towards "normalization." In other words, we begin to introduce specific teaching and training techniques to develop carefully defined skills which have been identified as necessary or desirable for everyday functioning. In many cases our goals may be limited. For example, rather than providing all children with tools by which language acquisition may be achieved primarily through their own efforts, in some cases we may have to strive for the development of communication adequacy restricted to a small set of circumstances and a limited subset of people. Obviously, the means by which such a restricted functional adequacy might be developed are significantly different from the means we might employ to foster linguistic mastery in a deaf child with no other handicaps.

I should stress that at present we have no clear picture of the relative incidence of mental retardation in the hearing-impaired population or of hearing impairment in the mentally retarded population. Even considering the difficulties in intellectual assessment of the hearing impaired, it is clear that many causes of deafness and mental retardation are related and that for this reason the deaf population exhibits a relatively high incidence of mental retardation (Moores, 1978; Vernon, 1969a, 1969b).

Studies of the incidence of deafness combined with mental retardation typically have come from two sources: (1) children enrolled in schools and classes for the deaf and (2) children and adults in institutions for the retarded. It is quite likely, as Power and Quigley (1971) have suggested, that those in schools and classes for the deaf primarily have represented the traditional category of educable mental retardation (EMR), and those in institutions for the retarded have tended to fall within the category of trainable mental retardation (TMR). However, it should be clear that societal trends are reducing institutional populations. We may expect to find deaf children with severe mental retardation in a much wider variety of settings, with an increasing number residing at home and receiving educational services through local or regional school districts.

The subject of this paper, then, is deaf children with significant mental retardation and not those traditionally classified as EMR. Many of those children classified as EMR may not have been retarded but misdiagnosed. Too often deaf children have been classified as retarded by professionals who had no knowledge of the communication problems faced by deaf individuals and by professionals who operated under the mistaken assumption that language and speech problems are symptoms of mental retardation.

Conditions for Language Intervention with the Hearing-Impaired Mentally Retarded

One of the most powerful recent developments in the area of language intervention has been the utilization of nonspeech communication systems, including manual communication (Moores, 1974, 1979; Wilbur, 1976), graphic systems (Clark & Woodcock, 1976) and expressive communication aids for nonvocal severely handicapped children (McDonald, 1979). Much of the recent growth of interest can be traced to evidence of the effectiveness of manual communication with deaf children of deaf parents and to the introduction of manual communication as a pedagogical tool in most programs for the deaf in the United States. At the same time, there have been several reports of success in the use of nonspeech systems with retarded children in a variety of settings.

In the current enthusiasm for manual communication and other nonvocal symbol systems, it is necessary to sound a note of caution. Although the evidence suggests that the use of nonvocal systems has been effective with at least some children, there is no evidence to indicate that, without modification, such systems can be introduced with all types of handicapping conditions. There has been a tendency to believe that if something is successful with one group of children, it will be successful with all children. Frequently, people not familiar with the problems of hearing-impaired retarded children assume that the effects of hearing loss and retardation are additive, when in fact they are not. The educational, psychological, and linguistic difficulties facing such children are qualitatively different from those of deaf children or retarded children. Because hearing-impaired mentally retarded children frequently have one or more additional handicaps—such as vision defects, heart problems, physical anomalies—it is dangerous to talk about the children without emphasizing the need for individualization of instruction.

In the past we have been influenced by implicit beliefs that to a large extent have determined our goals and even the specific techniques we have used. Perhaps the strongest unfortunate influence has been what may be identified as the press towards so called "normalcy." Related to this has been an emphasis on output or response modes, which has distracted us from consideration of the complete child within a particular environment.

Of course, the goal of normalcy, per se, is justifiable. The harm occurs when this goal is distorted or becomes the only objective established for a handicapped or multihandicapped individual. This may be noted in the worst abuses of the present mainstreaming movements where some individuals have distorted the concept of "least restrictive environment" to mean that mere placement of deaf, profoundly retarded, autistic, or multihandicapped children in contiguity with average children would tend to normalize the behavior and academic achievement of the handicapped. The second mistake, concentration on output only—in conjunction with "normalization"—leads to a misperception of the fundamental problem. It is clear, at least to me, that concentration on output—articulation—in the deaf child has had devastating effects on academic, linguistic, and psychological development.

In the case of manual communication, linguists and educators have come to accept sign systems as true languages in every sense of the word. In the past several years, evidence has accumulated to indicate that the use of manual communication at very early ages can have very positive effects on development (Moores, 1974, 1978; Wilbur, 1976, 1979). Substantial amounts of work have also been done on graphic modes and symbol system modes of communication (Clark & Woodcock, 1976; McDonald & Schultz, 1973). It is the purpose of this paper to consider different aspects of nonspeech systems in their application to hearing-impaired retarded children.

It must be emphasized that the nature of the communication system must depend on the nature of the child's deficits and upon the characteristics of the impairment. An alternative communication system might be introduced prior to, in coordination with, or independently of the vocal system, depending on the individual's characteristics and progress. There are several reasons why a nonvocal system might be selected (Moores, 1979):

- An alternate system may be used as part of a diagnostic procedure to determine patterns of functioning. The introduction of the system may be the first step in a clinical program which may later be generalized to other systems or other environments.
- A system may be the most effective means for providing factual information, for concept development, and for the understanding of a relationship.
- A system may provide the individual with a mechanism for expressing needs.
- A system may provide a basis for the establishment of functional language processes.

- A system may be used to develop, supplement, and/or strengthen oral language skills.
- An alternate system may provide some individuals their only effective means of communication.

Manual Communication

The use of manual communication has increased tremendously with deaf children, retarded children, and deaf retarded children, as well as with other categories such as autistic children. It is obvious that the manner of such communication—as well as the goals—will vary considerably across groups. For example, a deaf child of deaf parents may be exposed to a complete language system from birth and acquire mastery over language in a natural manner. Parents with normal hearing may learn a variant of sign language designed to approximate aspects of English grammar and then use it in coordination with speech with their deaf children in everyday home activities. Some may even master the Rochester Method, fingerspelling every letter of every word in coordination with speech. It is unrealistic to assume that children suffering from severe cognitive deficits in addition to hearing loss would benefit greatly from exposure to the Rochester Method (with its demands on perceptual and motor integration), or to the complete, sophisticated American Sign Language, or to one of its variants.

Rather, the use of manual communication will tend to be on a more restricted basis, usually developed with specific goals in mind. In fact, signs per se may not even be used. Webster, McPherson, Sloman, Evans, and Kucher (1973), for example, used a gesture approach to train a nonvocal autistic boy to follow and give instructions. Rutter (1968) reported that many autistic children respond appropriately to gestures or demonstration but not to the spoken word. Churchill (1972) successfully utilized a simplified sign language to teach an autistic child association. Baumtrog (1976) achieved some success in teaching signs to three autistic children but reported that understanding was not generalized outside the clinical situation because signs were not used consistently throughout the day.

Miller and Miller (1973) have used American Sign Language, body awareness exercises, and language training films to train 19 autistic children to use and understand signs related to designed activities or goals. Creedon (1973) has been involved in a program utilizing Total Communication (simultaneous speech and signing), with autistic children. Creedon reported improvement in socialization and play with resulting decreases in self-stimulation. Children's signs were first limited to teachers, and later expanded to include other adults and children. Like Miller and Miller, Creedon found that some of the children who first began to communicate by sign later attempted vocalization. The results suggest that rather than impeding attempts to develop vocal communication, signs may be an initiator of speech for some children.

Bricker (1972) used sign training effectively with severely language-delayed children by first training children through imitation and later shaping appropriate responses when the children were presented with specific stimuli. Hoffmeister and Farmer (1972) trained a group of institutionalized deaf retarded adults to develop a repertoire of functional signs to express needs related to everyday living.

An indication of the expansion of the use of manual communication with nonvocal handicapped individuals is provided by the results of a national survey of speech, hearing, and language services for the retarded (Fristoe, 1975), which reported that 10% of the respondents were using some form of nonvocal communication system. When manual communication was used, it typically was not the full fledged American Sign Language or one of the pedagogical systems. Instead, the number of signs and the grammatical complexity were controlled. A large portion of the respondents utilized vocabulary from American Sign Language, but not in all cases. Mayberry (1976) has discussed various types of manual communication systems and their appropriateness for use with nonverbal individuals of differing etiologies. She argues that success cannot be obtained simply by introducing a hitherto noncommunicating individual to signs.

It is clear that manual systems will be used with increasing frequency with deaf retarded individuals, but a clear pattern has not evolved, so there is some uncertainty over the forms such systems will take. Systems of manual communication seem to be uniquely suited for a wide range of abilities. The vocabulary may be as large as that of the English language or may be simplified or, again, may correspond to the English language. The available evidence suggests that manual communication does not inhibit the development of speech or language skills but may, in fact, act as a facilitator. It is hoped that creative and productive procedures will be developed and evaluated in the near future. With this evaluation may come answers to the generalizability of techniques from the clinical situation and a closer delineation of constraints inherent in a visual motor communication mode.

Graphic Communication

The graphic mode of communication would appear to be of much less potential benefit for deaf retarded children than the manual mode. Broadly defined, the graphic mode involves the use of written words, phrases, and sentences to communicate. The basic elements of this mode are the letters of the alphabet. Aside from fingerspelling, which represents a one-to-one correspondence with the 26-letter written alphabet, the graphic mode is distinct from manual communication.

Work with other categories of handicapped children suggests that graphic communication might be of some benefit to deaf retarded children. For example, McDonald and Schultz (1973) enabled cerebral palsied children to express their needs by providing pictures and printed words on a language board and allowing the children to point to appropriate pictures and words. Because of a reduction of the response demands, the children appeared more relaxed, and oral responses actually increased. For the most basic communication a child might be provided cards with the words "yes" and "no" printed on them to convey basic agreement or disagreement. Such a system might be useful when the children communicate with individuals who do not understand manual communication and who have recourse to no other means.

Utilizing Peck's (1971) system of functional communication, Marshall and Hegrenes (1972) worked with an autistic boy by allowing him access to a typewriter. He was led through the development of words and learned to point to correct cards on cue when the words were sequenced.

The use of graphic systems apparently has met with success only with a relatively small number of children. The major failing seems to be a lack of generalizability to nonclinical settings. The lack of generalizability is related to the use of cards. Deaf retarded children, who typically will not develop sophisticated spelling and reading skills, cannot be expected to write their own messages. However, the graphic mode might be quite useful for some deaf retarded children in limited situations where there simply is no alternative means of expressing needs or interacting with individuals outside of a clinical setting.

Symbol System Communication

The symbol system mode of communication refers to nonspeech systems which may use symbols varying in size, color, and so forth, in order to help the child receive and express messages. Much of the impetus for such systems has been traced by Wetherby (1978) to work on miniature linguistic systems over the past 60 years. Technically, miniature linguistic systems may not be considered complete systems in the same way as natural languages. For example, they tend to lack creativity, the means of generating a potentially infinite number of novel yet appropriate sentences. On the other hand, the systems tend to be very pragmatic, functional, and easily learned. Three symbol systems of potential usefulness with deaf retarded children will be reviewed here. They are the Non-SLIP, Rebus, and Bliss Symbol Systems.

NON-SPEECH LANGUAGE INITIATION PROGRAM (NON-SLIP) Non-SLIP was developed by Carrier and Peak (Carrier, 1974, 1976; Carrier & Peak, 1975) and is an extension of work originally done by Premack (1970, 1971). It has been used extensively with severely retarded children.

Non-SLIP consists of a nonspeech symbol system utilizing plastic chips as symbols. It is designed to teach the child a set of conceptual skills necessary to the acquisition of functional linguistic communication. Carrier and Peak operated under the assumption that, for many children, the complexity of the speech response system interferes with language acquisition (Schiefelbusch, Ruder, & Bricker, 1976). Using plastic forms as language constituents, the child may select and arrange units in ways to convey appropriate messages. Again, using training procedures based on Premack's work, McLean and McLean (McLean, 1973; McLean & McLean, 1974) trained two of three autistic children to a criterion of six three-element sentences utilizing plastic chips. The investigators assumed that it was effective to reduce the response requirements on the children and provide them with the elements of communication (plastic chips) rather than requiring them to generate utterances, either vocal or nonvocal, on their own. Although Schiefelbusch, et al. (1976) reported mixed success with such an approach, results to date suggest that many children who do not exhibit any language or communication ability when vocal responses are required can develop at least some demonstrable expressive and receptive skills when symbols are provided for them.

DeVilliers and Naughton (1974) developed a nonspeech training program which also was based on Premack's work. Reported success was minimal. This result may have been due in part to limited time devoted to training, which averaged only 15 minutes per child per week.

REBUS The Rebus System (Clark & Woodcock, 1976) uses ideographic symbols as a means of initiating reading instruction. It is utilized with a variety of children exhibiting a wide range of communication difficulties. It has been used also with nonhandicapped children as a mechanism for developing prereading skills while phasing into prereading of traditional orthography.

Clark, Moores, and Woodcock (1975a, 1975b) utilized the Rebus System to develop the Minnesota Early Language Development Sequence (MELDS). The MELDS program utilizes the vocal mode, a manual mode (signs from American Sign Language), and a symbol mode (Rebuses). The program consists of 120 lessons for the classroom or clinic and 120 lessons for the home. The experimental edition has been field-tested with deaf children, retarded children, and developmentally delayed children. With some modifications, it might be beneficial for some deaf retarded children.

THE BLISS SYMBOLS The Bliss System (Bliss, 1965; Clark & Woodcock, 1976; McDonald, 1979) probably is attracting more attention than any other nonspeech systems at present. Where the Non-SLIP symbols are completely arbitrary, the Rebus symbols and Bliss symbols are ideographic or concept based. The Rebus symbols, however, tend to show more of the influence of spoken English. For example, the same Rebus would be used for the words *can* in both strings, "A tin *can*" and "He *can*."

In terms of effectiveness of the different systems, there is very little evidence to support the use of one over the others. It is probable that each has different strengths and could be useful, depending on the needs of a particular child. It appears that the Rebus material is simpler to learn at first. Clark (1977) compared the use of learning of Non-SLIP, Rebus, Bliss, and traditional orthography. Traditional orthography was more difficult than any of the lothographic symbol systems. The Rebus System was easiest to learn, followed by Bliss and Non-SLIP. However, ease of initial learning should not be the sole criterion. For example, it appears that the Bliss System ultimately has more flexibility in that items can be combined and recombined in a potentially wider number of ways. Thus the teacher will have to make a choice. It seems to me that the choice will depend ultimately on where a particular child is at a particular point in time.

Summary

In essence we have four modes of communication at our disposal in working with deaf retarded children. These are:
1. The vocal mode,
2. The manual mode,
3. The graphic mode,
4. The symbol system mode.

It is highly likely that, at one time or other, each of these modes will be utilized, either separately or in coordination with others. In many cases, the goals will be more limited and will represent a deliberate choice to teach or develop specific skills. A large number of techniques and programs have been developed for use with a variety of handicapped children. With modification many of them should be appropriate for use with deaf retarded children.

Bibliography

Baumtrog, C. *The use of nonvocal symbol systems as a means of communication in autistic children*. Unpublished MA paper, University of Minnesota, 1976.

Bliss, C. *Semantography*. Sydney, Australia: Semantography Publications, 1965.

Bricker, D. Imitative sign training as a facilitator of word-object association with low functioning children. *American Journal of Mental Deficiency*, 1972, 76, 509–516.

Carrier, J. Application of functional analysis and a nonspeech response mode to teaching language. *American Speech and Hearing Association Monograph*, No. 18, 1974.

Carrier, J. Application of a nonspeech language system with the severely language handicapped. In L. L. Lloyd (Ed.), *Communication assessment and intervention strategies*. Baltimore: University Park Press, 1976.

Carrier, J., & Peak, T. *Non-SLIP*. Lawrence, Kans.: H & H Enterprises, 1975.

Churchill, D. The relation of infantile early autism and early childhood schizophrenia to developmental language disorders of childhood. *Journal of Autism and Childhood Schizophrenia*, 1972, 2, 182–197.

Clark, C. *A comparative study of young children's ease of learning words represented in the graphic systems of Rebus, Bliss, Carrier-Peak, and traditional orthography*. Unpublished doctoral dissertation, University of Minnesota, 1977.

Clark, C., Moores, D., & Woodcock, R. *The Minnesota Early Language Development Sequence: Teacher's manual*. University of Minnesota Research, Development, and Demonstration Center in Education of Handicapped Children, Development Kit #1, 1975 (a).

Clark, C., Moores, D., & Woodcock, R. *The Minnesota Early Language Development sequence: Parent's manual*. University of Minnesota Research, Development, and Demonstration Center in Education of Handicapped Children, Development Kit #2, 1975 (b).

Clark, C., & Woodcock, R. Graphic systems of communication. In L. L. Lloyd (Ed.), *Communication assessment and intervention strategies*. Baltimore: University Park Press, 1976.

Creedon, M. P. *Language development in nonverbal autistic children using a simultaneous communication system*. Paper presented at Society for Research in Child Development Meeting, Philadelphia, March 1973.

deVilliers, J., & Naughton, J. Teaching a symbol language to autistic children. *Journal of Consulting and Clinical Psychology*, 1974, *42*, 111–117.

Fristoe, M. *Language intervention systems for the retarded*. Decatur, Ala.: L. B. Wallace Developmental Center, 1975.

Hoffmeister, R., & Farmer, A. The development of manual sign in mentally retarded deaf individuals. *Journal of Rehabilitation of the Deaf*, 1972, *6*, 19–26.

Marshall, N., & Hegrenes, J. The use of written language as a communication system for an autistic child. *Journal of Speech and Hearing Disorders*, 1972, *37*, 258–261.

Mayberry, R. If a chimp can learn sign language, surely my nonverbal client can, too. *Journal of the American Speech and Hearing Association*, 1976, *18*, 223–229.

McDonald, E. Early identification and treatment of children at risk for development of intelligible speech. In R. Schiefelbusch (Ed.), *Nonspeech language and communication: Analysis and intervention*. Baltimore: University Park Press, 1979.

McDonald, E., & Schultz, A. Conversation boards for cerebral palsied children. *Journal of Speech and Hearing Disorders*, 1973, *38*, 73–88.

McLean, L. *Acquisition of a nonverbal language form by developmentally delayed, nonverbal children*. Unpublished doctoral dissertation, Peabody College, 1973.

McLean, L., & McLean, J. A language training program for nonverbal autistic children. *Journal of Speech and Hearing Disorders*, 1974, *39*, 186–193.

Miller, A., & Miller, E. Cognitive developmental training with elevated boards and sign language. *Journal of Autism and Childhood Schizophrenia*, 1973, *3*, 65–68.

Moores, D. Nonvocal systems of verbal behavior. In R. Schiefelbusch & L. Lloyd (Eds.), *Language perspectives: Acquisition, retardation, and intervention.* Baltimore: University Park Press, 1974.

Moores, D. *Educating the deaf: Psychology, principles, and practices.* Boston: Houghton Mifflin Co., 1978.

Moores, D. Alternate communication modes: Visual motor systems. In R. Schiefelbusch (Ed.), *Nonspeech language and communication: Analysis and intervention.* Baltimore: University Park Press, 1979.

Peck, B. Compendium of patterned language. *Journal of the American Speech and Hearing Association,* 1971, *10,* 2–3.

Power, D., & Quigley, S. *Problems and programs in education of multiply disabled deaf children.* Champaign, Ill.: University of Illinois Institute for Research on Exceptional Children, 1971.

Premack, D. A functional analysis of language. *Journal of Experimental Analysis of Behavior,* 1970, *14,* 107–125.

Premack, D. Language in chimpanzees? *Science,* 1971, *172,* 808–822.

Rutter, M. Concepts of autism: A review of research. *Journal of Child Psychology and Psychiatry,* 1968, *9,* 1–25.

Schiefelbusch, R., Ruder, K., & Bricker, W. Training strategies for language deficient children: An overview. In N. G. Haring & R. L. Schiefelbusch (Eds.), *Teaching special children.* New York: McGraw-Hill, 1976.

Vernon, M. *Multiply handicapped deaf children: Medical, educational and psychological considerations.* Washington, D.C.: Council for Exceptional Children Research Monograph, 1969 (a).

Vernon, M. Multiply handicapped deaf children: The causes, manifestations and significance of the problem. In H. Brelje & B. Wolff (Eds.), *The mentally retarded deaf child.* Portland, Oreg.: Lewis and Clark College, 1969 (b).

Webster, C., McPherson, H., Sloman, H., Evans, M., & Kucher, E. Communicating with an autistic boy by gesture. *Journal of Autism and Childhood Schizophrenia,* 1973, *3–4,* 337–346.

Wetherby, D. Miniature languages and the functional analysis of verbal behavior. In R. Schiefelbusch (Ed.), *Bases of language intervention.* Baltimore: University Park Press, 1976.

Wilbur, R. Nonspeech symbol systems. In R. Schiefelbusch (Ed.), *Nonspeech language and communication: Analysis and intervention.* Baltimore: University Park Press, 1979.

The Development of Language in the Mentally Retarded Hearing-Impaired Child: Instructional Methods

Kathleen Stremel-Campbell

For those teaching language to the mentally retarded hearing-impaired child, Ms. Kathleen Stremel-Campbell outlines assessment procedures and describes a particular curriculum which has achieved a measure of success with this population.

Considerations for Language Training

LaVeck (1972) states that six million people in our society evidence impaired behavior during some part of their lives because of subnormal intelligence. The majority of these people will display deficits or delays in their language and communication behavior. The language of mentally retarded children and youth will vary in accord with their handicapping conditions. Generally, the more severely handicapped children will demonstrate greater impairment in language functioning than trainable or educable children. However, the forms the language problems take, the relationship of language to intellectual functioning, and the relationship of language to other psychological and physiological factors cannot be specified for each group of mentally handicapped children. The language problems of mentally handicapped children must be defined for each individual child. Even though the skills and needs of these children may be similar, they will not be identical.

Public Law 94-142 mandates that all handicapped children have available a free, appropriate public education and related services to meet their needs. These needs can be determined for each individual child only from a careful assessment of the child, the environment, and his or her interactions within that environment. Language and communication will be a priority need in meeting the educational objectives for the majority of these children. The language and communication assessment cannot be complete without input concerning the child's socio-affective, sensorimotor, perceptual, and conceptual skills and needs.

We must specify a handicapped child's needs in specific objectives that are related directly to training. For instance, a goal stating that the child should verbalize spontaneously does not direct us in setting up a program for that child. The skills that the child already possesses must be assessed as well as the needs since we must have a starting point in our training program. Once the skills and needs are specified, small and sequential goals must be outlined for the child. The handicapped child has multifaceted needs and a pluristic approach must be taken to meet those needs.

Assessing the Language of the Mentally Retarded

There are several major factors that must be considered in assessing the language and communication of any mentally handicapped child. First, the acquisition of a language system is a complex process that is related to the student's cognitive-perceptual growth and his or her interactions in an environment of objects, events, and relations. Second, the handicapped child has a right to communicate in some form. Speech is the most effective and efficient means of communication for many people; however, many handicapped children may not have the potential or prerequisite skills for speech. Many of these children may require an alternate or augmentive mode of communication. Third, the child must utilize this language system for a reason. Halliday (1975) suggests that there is language as soon as there are *meaningful* forms of expression. With the normal child, this occurs at a time before words and structures are used to express meaning. Fourth, the semantic and grammatical components must be considered in assessing the child's language system. This assessment must include both oral (speech) and non-oral language systems. Fifth, the type of assessment utilized is important since the description of needs and skills will only be as accurate as the testing instrument.

COGNITIVE AND PERCEPTUAL SKILLS Miller (1977) stresses that cognitive-linguistic behaviors must be considered when developing a communication program for the severely handicapped or the young handicapped child. Early cognitive and perceptual skills may be viewed as skills that are prerequisite to initial language skills. The way the child perceives his or her environment and interacts with objects, events, people, and their relationships will influence his or her language. Since public schools are now responsible for the younger and more severely handicapped child, we must extend our communication assessment and training to the more basic aspects of prelinguistic functioning. Uzgiris and Hunt (1975) describe an approach to the assessment of psychological development in infancy. They view early achievements as a coherent sequence of order levels, and examine progress in different areas of intellectual functioning.

LANGUAGE MODALITY Traditionally, only speech has been utilized as a means of training severely handicapped students to express their wants, needs, feelings, and relationships. Training has often been a long and laborious process, at times achieving little, if any, measurable progress. Even though speech is our ultimate communication goal for children, this goal may be unrealistic for many children who do not have potential or do not have the oral mechanism necessary for speech. Only recently have supplementary means of nonspeech communication been explored and found effective with the nonvocal or severely handicapped student (Vanderheiden & Vanderheiden, 1977).

Presently, the most widely used nonvocal means of communication are manual signing and non-oral communication boards. The communication boards may vary in types of stimuli used (written words, Bliss symbols, and pictures) and the type of response required from the student (Vicker, 1974). The nonvocal communication strategies may also be used as a speech initiator or as part of a total communication plan for children who have the potential for speech. This type of initial communication training allows the child to communicate while he or she is learning sounds and oral words.

FUNCTION OF LANGUAGE Until recently, those concerned with language training tended to emphasize the training of structure and articulation skills before communication skills training. At times, we as language trainers assumed that if a child had acquired some form of language, communication would naturally follow.

Language is used to serve a variety of needs. The handicapped student uses language for three general purposes: (1) to express his or her wants and needs and to regulate other people, (2) to learn other skills and more language, and (3) to interact on a social basis with peers and adults. Bernstein (1971) stresses that in order for a child to succeed in the educational system, he or she must know how to use language as a means of learning and know how to use it as a means of social interaction. Halliday (1975) stresses the importance of investigating the functional use of language before the child utilizes words or structures for communication.

Halliday also provides a description of the developing functions of language. He characterizes utterances by five factors which may occur spontaneously: (1) the utterance itself; (2) the nonlinguistic features, such as gestures and facial expressions; (3) the context of the utterance (objects, people present); (4) another's response to that utterance; and (5) the speaker's response to the listener's responses.

Halliday's study of language development provides us with another list of the functions of child's language. He has divided the functions between *pragmatic*—influencing the behavior of others and satisfying needs—and *mathetic*—used for learning. The specific functions and their order of emergence are as follows:

Phase I (9–16½ months)
1. Instrumental—to satisfy own material needs;
2. Regulatory—to exert control over the behavior of others;
3. Interactional—to establish and maintain contact with those that matter;
4. Personal—to express individuality and self-awareness.

(Halliday found no indication of a developmental progression within the first four functions.)

Phase II (16½–18 months)
5. Heuristic—to explore the objective environment;
6. Imaginative—to create an environment of one's own;
7. Informative—to convey information.

The transition to the adult system in Phase II is characterized by a shift in the functional orientation and rapid advances in vocabulary, structure, and dialogue. During this phase, meanings are expressed by means of lexical items. Also, the use of words seems to enrich the existing functional patterns and the learning of vocabulary allows for functions to be combined. It is within this phase that the child begins to use structure or grammar, and the grammar allows different functions to be encoded together. The child also learns dialogue (the adoption and assignment of social roles) toward the end of Phase II.

It is important to assess the handicapped child's preverbal behavior to determine how he or she is obtaining wants, satisfying needs, and regulating the behavior of others. At times the child's needs may be fulfilled by the use of inappropriate behavior or stereotyped actions. However, if these behaviors are being used as some form of communication, they should be redirected and not extinguished.

SEMANTIC AND GRAMMATICAL RELATIONS According to Bloom (1970, 1974), a child's early language utterances result from the interaction of the child's developing cognitive perceptual organization and his or her linguistic and nonlinguistic experiences. Bloom analyzed these early utterances on the basis of the semantic relations. Miller and Yoder (1974) were among the first to stress the importance of the semantic relations in the early stages of a language training program. Brown (1973) suggests that the order in which structures are acquired will be related to the complexity of the semantic intent expressed and to the syntactic form which those semantic relations require for expression. After the semantic relations are acquired in training, the form (structure) of those utterances needs to become more complex if the handicapped child is to approximate the language system of the normal child more closely.

The assessment of grammar should include both vocabulary and structural assessment in receptive and expressive modes. Determining the type of vocabulary items that are used and knowing the frequency of use are important in developing a program for the child. However, vocabulary use has probably been overemphasized in the past. The vocabulary, or lexical items, cannot be assessed in isolation, but rather, the assessment must include their morphology and their relationship to one another in phrases and sentences. The types of structures that the child uses can be analyzed and compared to developmental norms in order to develop a sequential training model.

Additional questions must also be asked if the assessment is to determine the needs of the child effectively. If the child is using language at the one-word or multi-word level:
1. Are the forms used frequently?
2. Is the content meaningful?
3. Is the content appropriate to the situation?
4. Does the child have an opportunity to respond to the language of others?
5. Does the child have an opportunity to initiate language in the environment?

ARTICULATION The assessment of the mentally retarded child's articulation should be stressed only as it relates to language. In other words, the child should have something to say (content) and a way to say it (structure) before we concern ourselves with the articulation of the structure. However, once the child is trying to communicate, the signal must be clear enough to be understood in order for the communication act to be complete. Lillywhite and Bradley (1969) report that clinical observations show that retarded children make far more errors of omission than substitution or distortion; therefore, their speech is often unintelligible.

ASPECTS OF ASSESSMENT The assessment of the student's communication needs and skills is one of the most important parts of communication training. The assessment must measure the student's skill level to determine where within the communication curriculum the student should begin training. (Within this paper the point between what the student can do and cannot do will be defined as the "skill level.") Adequate assessment entails several considerations.

First, the behaviors within each component of speech, language, and communication must be assessed. For instance, if only the speech of the severely handicapped student is assessed, the results may show only that the student is untestable and may not show the student's actual skill level.

Second, the assessment should be directly related to training and provide more than an intelligence score or mental age. These scores may give us a general knowledge of the student's functioning, but they will not provide us with specific training goals.

Third, the assessment should show not only what the student cannot do (needs), but also what the student can do (skills). It is necessary to have a starting point in training if the student is to succeed and, in fact, if behaviors are to build.

Fourth, the assessment should be current. A specific time limit should be set for the completion of assessment and the initiation of training. Current assessment is necessary if the student's present level of functioning is to be determined.

Fifth, assessment must be continuous and constantly provide input into the training process. Additional information will be gathered during training, and this information should be used to modify the student's training program. For example, perhaps a student does not use any spontaneous vocalizations nor imitate any vowels or consonants during the formal assessment period. If spontaneous vocalizations are observed a month after training is initiated, the specific assessment tests should be re-administered and a specific observational system for recording spontaneous vocalizations should be introduced.

The types of assessment data needed will vary with the student's handicapping conditions, age, and educational history. The types of assessment that are currently available also vary according to the level, conditions, and sources of testing. Parental information, school records, and a medical history may be data that are used in selecting appropriate standardized and non-standardized tests. Information gained from standardized tests may compare one child to a representative sample of the normal population of that age range, and such tests may include developmental scales. Observation of specific behaviors may be necessary to determine generally under what conditions and at what frequency these behaviors occur. A general level of information is obtained from the tests that have been previously described. More specific assessment is required if educational placement and individual programming are to be undertaken.

The Communication Assessment Checklist developed at Project MESH (Model Education for the Severely Handicapped) offers an example of assessment from general to specific communication skills to set communication training goals and objectives. (See Appendix A.) Other standardized and non-standardized tests are used to supplement these tests. (See Appendix B for a resource list.) The MESH Communication Assessment Checklist is a screening test that provides the specialist with data that are used to select more precise tests. If possible, the checklist should be completed by the parent with the assistance of the communication trainer. The data from the checklist are analyzed, and from that analysis, tests are selected from the General Assessment Battery.

This battery of tests contains approximately 60 behaviors which are selected from the more critical behaviors listed on the checklist. It is divided into five major areas which correspond to the communication programs that are available: (1) Early Conceptual Assessment, (2) Prelanguage Assessment, (3) Early Language Assessment, (4) Early Intermediate Language Assessment, and (5) Late Intermediate Language Assessment.

The individual tests within each category are arranged in a hierarchy from easy to more difficult skills. Each test contains 10 to 20 items and gives a percentage score which is graphically plotted on the speech and language profile. Specific criteria are used to determine whether the student needs training in a particular area or whether further testing is necessary. The test results in the receptive component of Early Intermediate Language Training and certain pretests both help determine a feasible communication modality for the student. The later tests assess the grammatical aspects of language.

The general assessment battery is complete when the student performs fewer than 20% correct responses on five consecutive expressive tests and at chance level on five consecutive receptive tests. Then the percentage score of each test is plotted on a profile. Once a student has been tested, the general test scores are analyzed, and a number of pretests are selected to obtain additional information on the items in which the child should be trained. The pretests are administered to determine the specific programs in which the child will be trained and the stimulus conditions that are appropriate for initial training.

ASSESSMENT IN SUMMARY In determining the language of the mentally retarded, we must keep in mind an important principle. That is, the language needs and skills of the retarded child are the main point of assessment and not the fact that the child is retarded. In essence, our assessment procedures for nonretarded, deaf, multihandicapped, or language-delayed children should not differ from the assessment of the retarded. And the results of our assessment may differ just as much among retarded children as they would between a retarded and a nonretarded, language-delayed child. As more research data become available in the area of normal child development, hopefully we will be able to define more clearly the skill level of each individual child and develop an individualized program for that child.

Teaching Language and Communication to the Mentally Retarded Child

The assessment is effective only if the communication curriculum is directly related to that assessment. The content used within assessment is also used in teaching; however, content is only one aspect of developing a training program. A model communication curriculum is presented in Table 1. Even though this curriculum has been followed with several hundred retarded children, variations of the sequence may also be effective. The child may enter the curriculum at any point, depending on the assessment results. The child may be trained in many behaviors within each component concurrently with an adjacent behavior. Therefore, the order may be simultaneous as well as sequential.

EARLY CONCEPTUAL TRAINING Early Conceptual Training is the first program within the communication continuum. This program emphasizes the earlier developing skills that the student must learn in order to manipulate objects and interact with people. Since these skills may be prerequisites for the later training programs, the student must demonstrate these skills or be trained in these skills before entering the other programs.

Programs for conceptual training are similar to those in the academic and motor areas because they are prerequisite to a number of later skills. Training in these areas is specifically coordinated with the other content areas since many of these behaviors are prerequisites to academic work as well as language.

MODES OF COMMUNICATION Many severely and profoundly handicapped people may never acquire speech because of severe motor impairment. However, these students should receive training in order to communicate in a nonspeech mode. Therefore, one of the primary goals within the communication curriculum is developing a communication mode for each individual student. One oral program and three non-oral programs are included within the MESH Curriculum. They are the written program, the manual signing program, and the picture communicator. The nonverbal programs are ranked hierarchically in sequence according to their relationship to adult language systems and according to the extent to which they can be expanded.

The written program is the highest level in difficulty. If the student displays the prerequisite skills, written communication offers the advantages of being understood readily by adults and of being a permanent product. The written system may be limited at first, consisting of single word cards, but as the language content is expanded, the student learns semantic relations and syntax at the two- and then three-word level.

Certain advantages and disadvantages are inherent within the manual signing system just as they are in other non-oral systems. The primary advantage of the signing program is its feasibility for spontaneous use. Appropriate communicative features, such as facial expression and eye contact, can be maintained throughout the communication exchange. Also, transmission time is short. Thus, a manual signing system provides an efficient means of communication for student, trainer, and listener. However, for manual signing to be functional, the receiver has to be familiar with the system. Furthermore, the response topography has to be available to the student before the system can be utilized in an effective manner.

Initially, the need to train teachers and parents in a manual system may seem to be a disadvantage, but since manual sign language functions as a novel language system for the teachers and trainers, they may serve as better language trainers with the manual signs. Preliminary observational data collected in our classrooms showed that the teachers attended to the students' signs, prompted the correct signs, and expanded the signs significantly more than they attended to the oral correlates presented by the verbal students. The teachers became more aware of the students' language and communicated with them at their level of functioning.

The manual signing program is designed to serve three basic functions as a language system, a speech initiator, and a language facilitator. The first two components are designed specifically for the severely handicapped, nonverbal child. The third component, using manual signing as a language facilitator, is utilized primarily with the severely handicapped students who have some verbal language. It serves as a prompt to enhance the acquisition of the verbal elements.

The content and sequence of the signs are important issues in the development of the signing program. Special considerations are given to the vocabulary and syntactic components. Consequently, the following questions are asked:
1. From what signing system should the vocabulary be derived?
2. What syntax system should be used?
3. What signs should be selected for initial acquisition?
4. Should a normal language development sequence be used?

The following criteria should be taken into consideration when selecting initial sign vocabulary. Select signs that represent: (1) objects the student discriminates, (2) functional objects, (3) motivational objects, (4) noncategorical objects, and (5) variety in terms of touch/nontouch, two-handed/one-handed, symmetrical/asymmetrical, and similarity of signs.

The non-oral communicator is similar in design to the written program, with pictures being substituted for the written words. Small pictures representing the vocabulary (nouns, verbs, etc.) are used via a communication board or a mechanical system. This system presents some disadvantages because it may not be readily

Table 1
Project MESH Communication Curriculum

Mode				
Speech	Written	Manual Signing		Communicator
Vowel Imitation (referential)	Matching basic shapes	Handshaping sign		Object-Object Match
Consonant-Vowel/Vowel-Consonant Imitation	Matching word-nonword	Prompting with faded handshaping		Object-Picture Match
	Matching word-word dissimilar	Imitation of sign		Picture-Object Match
Consonant-Vowel-Consonant and Consonant-Vowel-Consonant-Vowel Imitation	Match word-word similar	Prompting with faded imitation		Picture-Picture Match
	Name discrimination	Noun production to Visual-Verbal		Large Picture Discrimination (Noun)
Prompted word imitation (prompts vary according to students)	Word to verbal-visual stimuli	Noun production to Visual		Small Picture Discrimination (Noun)
Word production with Question and Visual	Word to verbal stimuli (Noun)	Noun production to Verbal		Response Positioning
Word production without direct visual (What do you want)	Word to visual stimuli (Noun)			Response Accuracy
				Response Latency
Spontaneous production of noun	Use of Communication Board			Use of Communication Board

Early Conceptual Training

Attention to auditory and visual stimuli	Function of object	Joint activity		Picture discrimination
Following moving objects	Matching objects	Matching object to picture		Direction following
Reaching to grasp objects	Means-end	Matching picture to object		
Object permanence	Specific object placement	Object discrimination		

Table 1 (continued)

Early Language

Noun Expansion	Examples
a. Toys	ball
b. Clothes	shoe
c. Food	pop, cookie
d. Transportation	bus
e. Personal	comb
f. School	book
g. Furniture	bed
h. Places	home
i. Body parts	nose
j. Animal	dog
k. People	boy
l. Proper nouns	Joe

Verbs

	Examples
a. Action	eat
b. State	want

Verb Noun

	Examples		Examples
a. State-Object	want coat	Verb—Pron	take it
b. Action-Object	eat cookie	Prop Noun—Verb—Pron	Tim go home
c. Action-Location	go house	1st Pron(s)—Verb—Noun	I eat cookie
Noun-Verb		2nd Pron(s)—Verb—Noun	You drink milk
a. Person-Affected-State	I see	Noun—Verb—Pron (o)	Tim take it
b. Agent-Action	Tim eat	Noun—Verb—Noun	Man drive car
Noun-Noun		Noun—Verb—Adj	Boy get dirty
a. Possessive		Verb—Prop Noun—Noun	Give Tim cookie
b. Locators		Verb—1st Pron(o)—Noun	Give me ball
Verb—1st pron (o)	Tim cup	Verb—Noun—Noun	Put coat chair
Verb—2nd pron (o)	cup floor	Verb—Adj—Noun	Take two penny
Verb—Prop Noun	help me	Noun—Verb—Adj—Noun	Boy take two cookie
1st Pron (p)—Noun	see you	Prop Noun—Verb—Adj—Noun	Tim get red token
1st Pron (p)	push Tim	1st Pron(p)—Verb—Adj—Noun	I wash dirty pan
Adj—Noun	my shoe	2nd Pron(p)—Verb—Adj—Noun	You see brown dog
Verb—Adverb	mine	Prop Noun—Verb—Adverb—Noun	Doug sit down chair
	pretty dress	Noun—Verb—Adverb—Noun	Boy sit here chair
	sit here	1st Pron(s)—Verb—Adverb—Noun	I fall down floor
		2nd Pron(s)—Verb—Adverb—Noun	You sit down chair
		1st Pron(s)—Verb—Verb—Adverb	I want play here
		1st Pron(s)—Verb—Verb—Noun	I want play car
		2nd Pron(s)—Verb—Verb—Noun	You want get coat
		2nd Pron(s)—Verb—Verb—Adverb	You want get dirty
		1st Pron(s)—Verb—Verb—Adj	I want take two
		Prop Noun—Verb—Prep—Noun	Bonnie go get it
		Verb—Prep—Noun	Sit on chair
		Wh—Pron	What that?
		Wh—Adj	What new?
		Wh—Adv	What here?
		Wh—Noun	Where Bill?
		Wh—Noun—Verb	What boy get?
		Wh—Pron—Verb	What you doing?

Table 1 (continued)

Early Intermediate Language

	Examples	
Noun—Verb—Prep—Noun	Boy sleep on bed	Prop Noun—Verb—Prep—Art—Noun
Prop Noun—Verb—Prep—Noun	Bill drive to school	Noun—Verb—Part—Art—Noun
1st Pron(s)—Verb—Prep—Noun	I play with ball	Noun—Verb—Prep—3rd Pron—Noun
2nd Pron(s)—Verb—Prep—Noun	You get on chair	Noun—Verb—Part—3rd Pron—Noun
Noun—Verb—Part—Noun	Boy put on coat	Noun—Neg—Verb—Art—Adj—Noun
Prop Noun—Verb—Part—Noun	Tim put on shoe	Neg—Verb—Pron—Prep—Art—Noun
1st Pron(s)—Verb—Part—Noun	I turn on light	Neg—Verb—Part—Art—Noun
2nd Pron(s)—Verb—Part—Noun	You turn off light	Neg—Verb—Prep—Pron(p)—Noun
1st Pron(s)—Neg—Verb—Part	I don't want that	Variations with 3rd person objective pronouns
Neg—Verb—Pron—Prep	Don't put it on	Variations with 3rd person subjective pronouns
Neg—Verb—Pron—Noun	Don't take my car	Variations with 3rd person reflexive pronouns
Neg—Verb—Pron—Adverb	Don't put it here	
1st Pron—Verb (inf)—Verb—Prep—Noun	I want to play with ball	Copula (is/are)
		Modifier—Noun(Pronoun)—Copula—Adjective (Preposition—Modifier—Noun)
1st Pron—Verb (inf)—Verb—Prep—Pron	I want to play with you	Wh—Copula—Adjective (Preposition—Modifier—Noun)
		Modifier—Noun—Copula—Negative—Adjective (Preposition—Modifier—Noun)
1st Pron—Verb (inf)—Verb—Prep—Prop Noun	I want to play with Tim	Auxiliary (is/are)
Verb—Art—Noun	Get the ball	Modifier—Noun (Pronoun)—Auxiliary—Verbing—(Preposition)—Modifier—Noun
1st Pron—Verb—Art—Noun	I see the bus	
Prop Noun—Verb—3rd Pron(p)—Noun	Tim comb his hair	Wh—Auxiliary—Modifier—Noun (Pronoun)—Verbing
Verb—3rd Pron(p)—Noun	Get your coat	Modifier—Noun (Pronoun)—Auxiliary—Negative—Verbing—(Preposition)—Modifier—Noun (Pronoun)

available if the student initiates communication. If the student is not ambulatory, the communicator can be attached to the student's wheelchair. Students with poor motor control are trained to use a head stylus or touch plates for a response mode.

PRELANGUAGE The prelanguage oral program is designed to train a student with limited vocalizations to produce a set of nouns. The sounds that the student initially produces are paired with objects in order to give meaning to the student's vocalizations. Motokinesthetic techniques are then used to aid the student in emitting additional vowels and consonants. Shaping procedures are used to train the student to approximate more closely the phonetically correct word. For some students, signs are used as prompts. The student is trained to pair the sign with the word production rhythmically. The student is initially trained to produce words that are monosyllabic (pop) or repetitive bisyllabic (cracker), and contain vowel-consonant, consonant-vowel, consonant-vowel-consonant, and consonant-vowel-consonant-vowel combinations. The initial set of words are selected with these criteria: (1) words that are functional, (2) sounds that the student can imitate, and (3) phonemes that develop early.

EARLY LANGUAGE TRAINING The Early Language Training Program is designed to expand the student's vocabulary and to increase intelligibility. The semantic organization of the lexical items is refined, and additional examples of semantic functions are presented and expanded. Then, basic grammatical relations are taught while additional content words are incorporated within the basic structure. The student also learns to use the structures he or she has been taught to express a number of different language functions. A social communication system is introduced early within this program, so that a student is trained in social communication concurrently as well as horizontally.

EARLY INTERMEDIATE LANGUAGE TRAINING The length of the student's utterances is extended by expanding the classes of content words and by introducing function words. At this stage, the student learns to incorporate internal markers of questions and negation into his or her utterances. The student also learns to use optional pronouns and a variety of different utterances for the same communicative function.

Morehead and Ingram (1976) report that linguistically deviant children do not develop bizarre linguistic systems that are qualitatively different from normal children. These children develop a linguistic system that is quite similar to any other. Their linguistic deviance is characterized by a delay in the onset and a longer period of acquisition. Lackner (1976) states that retarded children of different mental ages do not develop language behavior differently from normal children, but present a delayed developmental sequence with a lower level of language skill. This data gives us more reason to utilize a normal developmental sequence in determining our training content and training sequence. However, these studies primarily used grammar as an index of similarity and difference. We must also determine whether the retarded child is using meaning and is communicating similarly to a normal child. There are some retarded children who present very bizarre language, but overall, these may be the exceptions and not the rule. For instance, a child may use grammatical utterances that are articulated perfectly with normal voice and intonation patterns. "That old cow stepped all over me and I'll take one of those and my grandmother came." These utterances are even meaningful within themselves, but they are disconnected discourse with no obvious referent. Other children may use grammatical sentences but at a rate of two utterances over a two-week period. The training program for these children would vary because, even though they have some language skills in common, their needs differ.

LANGUAGE TRAINING PROCEDURES Various behavioral procedures have been reported as effective in training the mentally retarded child to use language (Baer, Peterson, & Sherman, 1967). There is relatively little data that provides evidence that one specific set of procedures is more efficient or effective than another. The strategies and techniques that are selected for training will depend somewhat upon the specific behavior to be learned and upon the child requiring training. Many language programs utilize some sequence of imitation, comprehension, and production for training a child in a specific behavior. Comprehension training should assure that the child understands what it is he or she is to produce. Verbal imitation is often a means to get to production. Schedules may vary widely across programs as well as among different children.

Other strategies may also be included with a training component. Many programs employ telegraphic speech in parts of the training, using only specific content words in the stimulus presented to the child, such as "What you doing." This strategy reduces the amount of input to the child. Additional research is needed to determine whether various levels of telegraphic speech increase the child's language acquisition and to discover exactly how telegraphic inputs help the child. Waryas and Stremel-Campbell (1977) describe a training program utilizing a concurrent element of training in which the child may receive training on more than one language behavior during any session. The authors also used discrete (single-word) developmentally sequenced expansions of the child's utterance.

Initially language and communication training may need to be highly structured and somewhat isolated from other training. However, once the child has acquired the behavior, training should be integrated with other education programs to promote generalization of that behavior.

There are three important reasons for the close integration of these skills. First, certain cognitive, socio-affective, and perceptual skills may serve as prerequisite skills for the linguistic component of language. Training efforts in these areas may often be duplicated, but training should be purposefully duplicated or extended with specific objectives being outlined.

Second, the training of other skill areas, such as self-help and daily living skills, often requires a certain degree of receptive language, if the additional training is to be successful.

Third, these areas also suggest additional functional content for language. For instance, the handicapped student may have trouble labeling (with speech, signing, or communication boards) pictures of soap or a toothbrush. Unless the student is actively and functionally involved with these objects, the acquisition of that labeling behavior may progress very slowly. There are also some instances in which expression should be kept to a minimum, such as during certain vocational tasks where verbalizations may interfere with the rate or accuracy of performing a task. Care must be taken not to train a sequence of behaviors in isolation. Training should incorporate the language into other environments and utilize it with other trainers. If newly acquired language behavior is not directly related to the next behavior in which the child is trained, it must be maintained to prevent extinction.

Special Considerations for the Multihandicapped Hearing-Impaired Child

The multihandicapped hearing-impaired (MHHI) child needs special consideration in his or her placement and program. Initially, we must know the handicapping conditions that exist with the hearing impairment and the extent of those handicaps. Basically, we can divide handicapping conditions into four classes:
1. Hearing-impaired and mentally retarded;
2. Hearing-impaired and visually impaired;
3. Hearing-impaired and motorically impaired;
4. Hearing-impaired and emotionally disturbed.

A child may have one or more handicaps in addition to a hearing impairment. Each handicapping condition makes our programming more difficult, and we must realize that the child's progress will be slower than if the child were a normal hearing-impaired individual.

Manual signing may be employed as the language modality with all groups except those with motor impairment. Even with this group, we must determine whether they are candidates for signing or a communication board. Many retarded children who do not appear to have motor impairments may, in fact, be delayed in motor skills. We may actually be training children in motor movements and signs simultaneously. A child with vision and hearing impairments may also need special consideration in sign training. This section of this chapter will focus on manual sign training with hearing-impaired children who also display mental retardation, emotional problems, or delayed motor development.

Recently the Speech Pathology and Audiology Division of the American Association on Mental Deficiency (AAMD) surveyed signing programs. They sought to determine what type of sign system was used, when and why signing was initiated with an individual, how and where it was taught, and what assessment procedures were employed. The results of the survey indicated that signing is currently being used with a wide range of handicapping conditions. The results seemed to indicate that if the individual had sufficient manual dexterity, signing was preferred over other nonverbal systems. Even though the assessment procedures were limited to criteria for entry, the results indicated that persons who are involved in training children to use signs have different priorities for making decisions concerning program placement.

SELECTING A COMMUNICATION SYSTEM Once assessment is completed and the data are analyzed and discussed with the child's parents and teacher, a decision concerning program placement must be made. The parents and teacher must be made aware of the communication approaches that are available and of the criteria for entry into each program. Table 2 shows a matrix of skills involved in each program. The table also indicates where the skills can be utilized best. The table is simply a guide in matching the child's skills to the skills required in each program. In some cases, the nonverbal child may be a likely candidate for either manual signing or a communication board. In these cases, the trainer must decide which system would receive the most support from the environment. Also, some nonverbal children who initially do not vocalize may eventually learn to speak. We just cannot predict how long the training may take. Here, the child's age must be taken into account. All of these variables must be taken into account when selecting a communication program.

We must also decide whether the child has the basic skills that may be necessary for any language system. Many of the professionals working with severely handicapped children feel that early conceptual behaviors are prerequisite to language development. Even those people not prescribing a normal development sequence agree that mastery of certain skills may facilitate the acquisition of more difficult skills. Kahn (1975) found that seven out of eight children who had minimal language (at least 10 words) functioned at Piaget's Stage 6; eight other children who did not display language could not function at Stage 6. Kahn suggested that meaningful expressive language should begin with an assessment of cognitive skills. Uzgiris and Hunt (1975) have developed an assessment based on Piaget's six stages of cognitive development. Fieber (1977) also discusses the conceptual assessment and training strategies for the severely handicapped child.

Teaching a Nonverbal Communication System

There are several critical issues in training the multihandicapped hearing-impaired child to use manual signing. (The reader is referred to Vanderheiden and Vanderheiden [1976, 1977] for considerations in training children to communicate via

Table 2
Skills within Each Communication System

The child	Speech	Manual	Object Comm	Picture Comm	Bliss Comm	Abstract
Desires to communicate	●	●	●	●	●	●
Exhibits early conceptual behaviors	●	●	●	●	●	●
Has auditory discrimination	●					
Has visual discrimination		○	○	●	●	○
Is ambulatory	●	●				
Has at least minimal hand/arm dexterity		●	○			○
Uses gestures for communication	●	●				
Uses eye movement for communication				●	●	
Vocalizes	●					
Imitates gross motor movements		●				
Imitates vowels	●					
Imitates words	●					
Exhibits function of object	●	●	●	●	●	
Matches objects			●	●	●	●
Discriminates objects	●	●	●	●	●	●
Matches object to picture				●	●	●
Matches pictures				●	●	
Discriminates pictures				●	●	
Attends to gestures		●				
Attends to verbal messages	●					
Attends to pictures or written messages				●	●	
Has failed in oral program		●	●	●	●	●

● Program requires this skill.   ○ Less skill is adequate for the program.

communication boards.) Even though the emphasis will be directed towards signing, many of the considerations are pertinent to speech and other nonverbal programs as well. Basically, four areas need to be addressed in the development of a signing program:
1. Considerations in response topography;
2. Considerations in communication training;
3. Considerations in the language sequence and content selection;
4. Considerations in programming.

These considerations will vary according to the skills and needs of each hearing-impaired child. For instance, if a child is able to imitate most signs and demonstrates a fairly high receptive language, his or her training program will be different and less detailed than that of a child not demonstrating these skills.

RESPONSE TOPOGRAPHY

Motor movement Minimal arm and hand movements are necessary if the child is to succeed in a signing program. For those of us not skilled in motor assessment and training, it is difficult to specify what "minimal movements" consist of. Johnson (1977) has developed a motor assessment that can be used to determine whether the child is a candidate for signing. (See Table 3.) There are not yet data available which show that a child not demonstrating a certain motor movement cannot learn a sign which contains that configuration or movement. However, the trainer must realize that the specific motor movement and the sign are being taught concurrently; therefore, training will take longer for a child who lacks certain motor skills than for a child who has these motor movements within his or her repertoire. Also, a physical or occupational therapist should be consulted if the child exhibits motor impairments. If no other non-oral system is available for that child, a gross gesture system may be initiated so that the child can communicate while he or she is learning more precise movements.

The child's hand preference should also be determined before the signing program is initiated. The trainer must be consistent when he or she physically assists shaping with the child's dominant hand. The trainer must also decide the seating position before training is initiated. If the child is placed across the table, the mirror-image effect may confuse both the child and trainer. The child must also be placed in a position where the trainer can provide physical assistance.

Successive approximations If the child does not imitate signs correctly, other considerations arise. Will approximations of the signs be accepted? Exactly which approximations will be accepted? Often trainers accept general approximations without changing their approximation criterion. Unless consistent successive approximations are discriminately reinforced, the trainer may find herself or himself taking twice as long to "clean up" the child's signs as to teach acquisition. Another trap that is easy to fall into is not modeling the correct sign, but instead, modeling

Table 3
Fine Motor Assessment

Movement	Sample Implications
Purposeful reach	direct hand to correct position for signing
	direct hand to pick up and manipulate objects
Hands to midline	necessary to produce signs with cross midline position
Crude Palmer grasp	difficulty turning pages of picture book or picking up small objects
Bilateral hand movements	necessary to produce any two-handed signs
Raking grasp	incorporates use of thumb implications for manipulating objects and signs which involve thumb
Transfer object	implications for hands working together in two-handed signs or manipulating object
Neutral forearm position	necessary to hold container upright; necessary for some signs (cup, car)
Full Palmer grasp	implications for manipulating object
Pick up two objects (one in each hand)	use of both hands simultaneously
Hold and manipulate	implications for hands working together (cap off toothpaste, lid off chocolate)
Stimulated release	implications for placing objects
Lateral pincher	improved control of fingers
Pick up two objects with one hand	improved control of fingers
Reach into	implications for specific steps and signs (remove bread from bag, sign "pop")
Supination, wrist rotation	implications for specific steps and signs (sign "cup," "open," "book"; brush top teeth)
Wrist deviation	implications for specific steps and signs (turn on faucets, screw caps on and off; sign "shoe," "brake," "broom")
Voluntary release	able to place objects
Pincher grasp	improved control of fingers
Apply pressure to move object	implications for specific steps (pushing on faucet)
Point and poke with individual fingers	improved finger control; implications for signs requiring individual finger positions and manipulation of objects

J. Johnson (1977) Project Pride

the child's approximation. If this happens, the child cannot see or feel what the actual sign is. Using successive approximations in training involves consistently fading the stimulus support (physical assistance) and/or shaping the response to more closely approximate the goal (sign). Consistent fading is especially important for children who are reinforced by tactile stimulation. More aversive physical assistance may be used, but we must consider what it would do to the language process. Behaviorally, the signs could become associated with the aversive stimulus. A good rule to use in handshaping is: Give the child only the support he or she needs, and do it as quickly as possible.

More precise hand movements become necessary as the child learns more signs. Similar configuration of signs will begin to overlap as new signs are learned. We can accept approximations until they become confused receptively with other signs. Some children may require intense training in sign "formation" just as verbal children may require specific articulation training. An error analysis will determine which motor configurations, movements, or placement features are absent across signs.

A child initially learning signs must also learn when to use signs. Learning neutral hand positioning is an important part of signing topography. A child that displays stereotyped hand movements must realize that these movements have no meaning. If the trainer does not include neutral hand positioning in training, stereotyped movements may be reinforced as part of a sign, and suspect motor behaviors may occur.

The child must also learn that his or her hands are to be maintained in a neutral position until the trainer has completed a sign or cue to communicate. This protocol would also apply to a verbal child. We must teach the child that his or her verbal response cannot interfere with the cue. As trainers, we often repeat a sign for emphasis when we are signing. When the child begins to use repeated movements consistently, we realize that we have, in fact, taught the child an incorrect rule.

Multihandicapped hearing-impaired children also need to know whether or not a response is required. One procedure to follow is for the signer to maintain the position of his or her final sign when a sign response is required and to return his or her hands to the neutral position when no sign response is required.

Manual systems Wilbur (1976) discusses the manual systems that are available and the differences among sign systems. American Sign Language (ASL) utilizes a different syntax from that of English. Fristoe and Lloyd (1977) state that it is important to select what can be most easily learned and used by others in the environment. If the child is deaf and resides with other deaf or hearing-impaired people, ASL would probably be the best system. However, if the teacher or parent does not know any signs, a system should be selected that does not rely heavily on fingerspelling and is familiar to the trainer. Possibly one of the most important considerations is that only one sign text be used so that everyone is producing the sign in the same way. If some of the functional or motivational signs are too complex for the motor skills of the child, these signs may be modified to be less demanding. These modifications should be noted in the teachers' and parents' signing resource books.

COMMUNICATION TRAINING Regardless of the language system selected for a child, language cannot be taught as a chained, rote response. Rather, the language must be used in a communication function—he or she must have a reason to talk or sign. If the child does not currently attempt to communicate, he or she will probably not use signs to communicate. A sign is a symbol used to represent an object, action, relation, or idea. Part of manual sign training should include teaching the child that signs are to be used as communication. We can teach the child to produce signs, but this does not insure that the child will use them for communication. If the handicapped child is hearing impaired or has auditory processing problems, the manual signs will be taught as a receptive language system as well as an expressive language system. The child who does not have an oral receptive and expressive language may learn that signs represent objects and actions sooner than the child who understands that speech represents objects and actions. The child who demonstrates receptive language may learn a paired association between the sign and the word; however, the child's minimal vocalizations may inadvertently be used in place of signs instead of being paired with those signs. If a child has even minimal vocalizations, these should be paired with the signs.

There are other communication features that are specific to signing. A child who is initiating signs as communication must learn that he or she needs some method of getting a listener's attention. The people who participate as listeners must agree on which attention-getting devices they will accept. Many of the child's own devices, such as tugging and loud vocalizations, may become irritating, and the listener may actually tune-out the child's attempt to communicate. Once a child learns to communicate with signs, he or she must learn that one cannot communicate if one's hands are active in another task. Observations of normal adult signers show that they put an object down before signing, or sign before they reached for an object, or short-cut a two-handed sign by using one hand. Multihandicapped children must also learn that manipulation of objects should not interfere with their communication system.

There are also features of communication training that are not specific to sign training. As speakers, we have something to say, a way to say it, and a reason for saying it (Miller & Yoder, 1972). Our training should include more than teaching a labeling function. A child who learns only to label an object when it is paired with a specific verbal cue may not learn to communicate his or her wants and needs. This training must be extended to include arranging stimulus conditions so that the child will learn to ask for objects, regulate the behavior of others, give information, and so forth. Even though children initially talk about the "here and now," language is primarily necessary when the referent is not present. Therefore, we must not only teach the child to sign nouns, verbs, and relations, but the child must learn that these isolated signs can control the environment in a number of different ways

(Waryas & Stremel-Campbell, 1978). These functions will be discussed more extensively under Programming.

CONTENT SELECTION

Environment analysis Basically, our assessment should tell us where, syntactically and semantically, to begin teaching. The data from normal language development (Bloom, 1970; Bowerman, 1973; Brown, 1973; Schlesinger, 1974) provide guidelines for a language training sequence. Our assessment should also elicit data which determine what specific content should be selected for training. The content used in training is especially important in the initial acquisition and also for generalization. If the child's signs are not highly visible in the child's environment, the child will not have a chance to generalize them to other environments even if the child has reached learning criterion. The following procedures may be used in analyzing the child's communication and his or her interactions within the environment:
1. List child's communicative intentions;
2. Analyze other programmatic needs;
3. Record child's interactions with objects within other programs;
4. Record objects that the child voluntarily manipulates;
5. Record reinforcement preferences;
6. Record teacher verbalizations that require an obligatory response;
7. Record words that the child does use.

Response feature analysis Each sign has distinctive features which distinguish it from all other signs. Stokoe (1965) defines the signing features as configuration, placement, and movement. Signs also contain other aspects that must be considered in selecting content. More data on children with varying handicaps must be collected to determine which aspects may be important in initial sign acquisition. The iconicity of signs is probably over-rated as a critical feature of signs. Since adults have a wealth of information about their environment, signs are more iconic to an adult than to a handicapped child.

Other features of signs include touch and nontouch. A touch in signing may be defined as the active hand coming in contact with the base hand or another part of the body. Preliminary data on a limited number of severely handicapped children (Stremel-Campbell, Cantrell, & Halle, 1977) showed that touch signs were acquired more rapidly than nontouch signs. However, touch/nontouch was not a variable in acquisition with higher level children. Other variables will influence the data; for instance, if a nontouch sign is highly motivational, it may well be acquired before a touch, nonmotivational sign. Some children may acquire one-handed signs more rapidly than two-handed signs, especially if a motor impairment affects only one hand. Children who display good motor skills often seem to prefer two-handed signs over one-handed signs.

In many training programs, signs are taught within categories; that is, clothing items are taught, then foods, and so forth. Severely handicapped children may, in fact, make more errors within categories if these signs are included in the initial training. It is important that each child's data be analyzed to determine the most effective and efficient teaching strategies for that child. If a child interacts with objects, uses both hands to manipulate objects, demonstrates receptive nouns, and displays a conceptual base for language, we attempt to select an initial training set for that child. The following pairs of words would *not* be placed in the same set of initial training for these reasons:

comb—coat	phonetic similarity
school—paper	configural similarity
milk—pop	categorical similarity
kleenex—candy	iconic similarity and adult data

As children acquire more and more language, they must also learn these more complex discriminations. However, as children learn to communicate with signs and as their conceptual growth increases, they will be capable of learning these differences more rapidly. As children begin to learn verbs, additional nouns must be taught so that one verb can occur with at least two nouns. At this point, children must correctly produce nouns that are categorically similar.

Once the two-word semantic and syntactic combinations are added to training, we must make sure that children are not learning the combination as a one-word utterance. We have established a two-by-two rule in which any training verb has to occur initially with at least two nouns and that any noun has to occur with at least two verbs. If children do not generalize the taught verb to new, but untaught nouns, these additional combinations are taught.

PROGRAMMING There are various methods available that may be used in training. These procedures are not specific to signing because they may be used across a wide variety of training tasks. Basically, all procedures can be divided in two classes: error and errorless. Within each procedure there are differences in stimulus control, response definitions, consequences, and contingencies. Children may succeed or fail within a number of various procedures. However, our procedures and programming should allow children to reach the objectives that we, as trainers, have set.

Stimulus dimensions Different children require different degrees of stimulus control, and our assessment data should determine the requisite level. Initially, we list the program steps that may be included in a sign training program.

A. Materials
  1. Actual objects and events will be used.
  2. No less than two words and no more than five words will be taught in the initial training set.
  3. At least three different examples will be used.
B. Modes of training
  1. Physical Assist (PA)
  2. Imitation (I)

3. Production (P)
C. Conditions
   1. Verbal stimulus (noun) plus visual stimulus (object) (PA-I-P)
   2. Verbal stimulus (noun) (P)
   3. Visual stimulus plus question (P)
   4. Visual stimulus only (P)
   5. No visual stimulus immediately present (P)
   6. Vary trainer (P)
   7. Vary environment
   8. Vary communication functions from #2 to #7

Response dimensions If the child does not imitate simple manual signs, the trainer must decide whether approximations of signs will be taught and exactly what level of signs will be defined as correct or incorrect. Specific criteria should be set for acceptable approximations, and once the child has reached that level of competence, only closer approximations should be reinforced. During initial training, a table may be used as a base for some signs. Since the child must also learn to communicate standing up, the physical support must eventually be faded out.

An error analysis of the child's incorrect signs will provide us with information for program modifications. The following types of errors may occur, but strategies for dealing with all these errors will not necessarily be the same.
1. Substitute errors of other signs within the training set.
2. Configuration errors.
3. Movement errors.
4. Placement errors.
5. Categorical errors.
6. Semantic and syntactic errors. (Later in training, a child may use a noun when a verb sign is required.)

Consequence and contingency dimensions As trainers, we must remember that a consequence is a reinforcer only if it increases responses. Ideally, language should be reinforcing in and of itself. That is, if the child requests an object, he or she may get it; if he or she asks a question, it is answered. A child may initially be reinforced only by edibles, but for various reasons, we would like more natural consequences to reinforce the response. Many educational programs use social praise and tokens as consequences. If these consequences are also paired with the specific object or action, perhaps the child will learn that the sign or combination of signs is directly reinforced by the object or event to which that sign refers. Some of these objects may not be directly reinforcing to the child, but by chaining these objects to reinforcing events, they become reinforcing. For example, if a child enjoys going outside, he or she learns that one must sign "coat" before getting a coat and going outside. Other signs, such as "pop," may be highly motivational.

In one program, a variation of Touchette's (1971) temporal delay procedure is used. This procedure allows the child to make only a minimal number of errors. It also shows when the child is ready to imitate or produce the sign. Therefore, the trainer does not have to determine subjectively when the child is ready for the next level of training. Children may initially be taught signs that are more motivational or functional for them.

Once the child has learned to imitate an initial set of nouns, we decide which sequence of training to use across additional sets. Little data is available to show whether one sequence is better than another. However, the trainer should have a systematic sequence planned before training is initiated. Basically, two sequence types are available: (1) Imitation of Set I followed by Production of Set I, (2) Imitation of Set I followed by Imitation of Set II. Probes can be used to determine when a child can imitate new signs without direct training and when he or she is able to produce signs that have been learned in imitation training.

An arbitrary number of nouns needs to be selected for training before verbs are taught. Manual signing programs typically select 10 to 20 nouns before initiating verb training. The program should be set up so that the child will know whether a noun or verb response is required.

The training program must include procedures that teach communication functions. Variations in the stimulus arrangements are necessary if the child is to learn that the same sign or combination of signs can mean different things. A handicapped child should learn to communicate as speaker *and* listener with peers and adults that are in his or her environment. One novel stimulus arrangement focuses on communicative functions, both instrumental and regulatory. Two peers who are approximately at the same stage in the program train together; they exchange roles as speaker and listener in the regulatory function. Not only do they learn to regulate each other's behavior, but in order to do this, they must also learn to attend to and to discriminate one another's signs. Nouns, verbs, verb-noun structures, and so forth, can be taught in this manner.

Summary

Once the multihandicapped hearing-impaired child has been assessed, and data have been collected which help us determine the most appropriate program for a specific child, constant re-evaluation of placement and the program must be made. What should we consider failure? If a child has not made progress within six months or a year, do we select another communication system, or will programmatic changes be sufficient for progress? Here again, we can only look at each individual child's data to make these decisions. We need to know where within the program the child is not succeeding. Is he or she relying completely on physical assistance from the trainer? Is the child producing signs only under tight stimulus control? Is he or she using nouns and verbs but has trouble combining the two? Answers to these questions will help us determine the problem areas and possible solutions. The most important question that can be asked is whether people in the child's environment are using signs in communicating with the child and whether they are expecting the child to utilize signs in his or her communication attempts.

Bibliography

Baer, D. M., Peterson, R. F., & Sherman, J. A. The development of imitation by reinforcing behavioral similarity to a model. *Journal of Experimental Behavior,* 1967, *10,* 405–416.

Bernstein, B. (Ed.). *Class, codes, and control,* Vol. I: *Theoretical studies towards a sociology of language.* Primary Socialization, Language and Education Series. London: Routledge and Kegan Paul, 1971.

Bloom, L. Talking, understanding, and thinking. In R. Schiefelbusch & L. Lloyd (Eds.), *Language perspectives: Acquisition, retardation, and intervention.* Baltimore: University Park Press, 1974.

Bowerman, M. *Early syntactic development: A cross-linguistic study with special reference to Finnish.* New York: Cambridge University Press, 1973.

Brown, R. *A first language: The early stages.* Cambridge, Mass.: Harvard University Press, 1973.

Fieber, N. Cognitive skills. In N. Haring (Ed.), *Developing effective individualized educational programs for severely handicapped children and youth.* Washington, D.C.: Thomas Buffington, 1977.

Fristoe, M., & Lloyd, L. L. *The use of manual communication with the retarded.* Paper presented at Gattlinburg Conference on Research in Mental Retardation, March 1977.

Halliday, M. A. K. Learning how to mean. In E. Lenneberg & E. Lenneberg (Eds.), *Foundations of language development: A multidisciplinary approach* (Vol. 1). New York: Academic Press, Inc., 1975.

Johnson, J. Paper presented at the American Association for the Education of the Severely and Profoundly Handicapped, San Francisco, 1977.

Kahn, J. V. Relationship of Piaget's sensorimotor period to language acquisition of profoundly retarded children. *American Journal of Mental Deficiency,* 1975, *79,* 640–643.

Lackner, J. R. A developmental study of language behavior in retarded children. In D. Morehead & A. Morehead (Eds.), *Normal and deficient child language.* Baltimore: University Park Press, 1976.

LaVeck, G. D. Foreword. In R. L. Schiefelbusch (Ed.), *Language of the mentally retarded.* Baltimore: University Park Press, 1972, p. xiii.

Lillywhite, H. S., & Bradley, D. P. *Communication problems in mental retardation.* New York: Harper and Row, 1969.

McIntire, M. L. *Acquisition of American Sign Language.* Doctoral dissertation, Department of Linguistics, University of California, Los Angeles, 1975.

Miller, J. On specifying what to teach: The movement from structure to structure and meaning, to structure and meaning and knowing. In E. Sontag (Ed.), *Educational programming for the severely and profoundly handicapped*. Reston, Va.: CEC Division on Mental Retardation, 1977.

Miller, J., & Yoder, D. An ontogenetic language teaching strategy for retarded children. In R. Schiefelbusch & L. Lloyd (Eds.), *Language perspectives: Acquisition, retardation, and intervention*. Baltimore: University Park Press, 1974.

Morehead, D. M., & Ingram, D. The development of base syntax in normal and linguistically deviant children. In D. Morehead & A. Morehead (Eds.), *Normal and deficient child language*. Baltimore: University Park Press, 1976.

Schlesinger, I. Relation concepts underlying language. In R. Schiefelbusch & L. Lloyd (Eds.), *Language perspectives: Acquisition, retardation, and intervention*. Baltimore: University Park Press, 1974, 129–151.

Stremel-Campbell, K., Cantrell, D., & Halle, J. Manual signing as a language system and as a speech initiator for the nonverbal severely handicapped student. In E. Sontag (Ed.), *Educational programming for the severely and profoundly handicapped*. Reston, Va.: CEC Division on Mental Retardation, 1977, 335–347.

Stokoe, W. *A dictionary of American Sign Language on linguistic principles*. Washington, D.C.: Gallaudet Press, 1965.

Touchette, P. E. Transfer of stimulus control: Measuring the movement of transfer. *Journal of Experimental Analysis of Behavior*, 1971, *15*, 347–354.

Uzgiris, I., & Hunt, J. McV. *Assessment in infancy: Ordinal scales of psychological development*. Champaign, Ill.: University of Illinois Press, 1975.

Vanderheiden, G., & Vanderheiden, D. Communication techniques and aids for the non-vocal severely handicapped. In L. L. Lloyd (Ed.), *Communication assessment and intervention strategies*. Baltimore: University Park Press, 1976, 607–652.

Vanderheiden, D., & Vanderheiden, G. Basic considerations in the development of communicative and interactive skills for the non-vocal severely handicapped child. In E. Sontag (Ed.), *Educational programming for the severely and profoundly handicapped*. Reston, Va.: CEC Division on Mental Retardation, 1977, 323–334.

Vicker, B. *Nonoral communication system project*. Iowa City, Iowa: University Hospital School, The University of Iowa, 1974.

Waryas, C. Personal communication, 1977.

Waryas, C., & Stremel-Campbell, K. Grammatical training for the language-delayed child: A new perspective. In R. L. Schiefelbusch (Ed.), *Language intervention strategies*. Baltimore: University Park Press, 1978.

Wilbur, R. B. The linguistics of manual languages and manual systems. In L. L. Lloyd (Ed.), *Communication assessment and intervention strategies*. Baltimore: University Park Press, 1976, 423–501.

Appendix A
Communication Assessment Checklist

Name: _____ Parent: _____

Birthdate: _____ Examiner: _____

Age: _____ Date: _____

Additional Information (such as handicapping conditions)

1) _____

2) _____

Consistently Displays	Inconsistently Displays	Never Displays	Information Not Available			
				\multicolumn{2}{l}{**Section I: Nonlanguage Behaviors**}	Comments
				1.01	Is ambulatory.	
				1.02	Is toilet trained.	
				1.03	Establishes eye contact.	
				1.04	Maintains seat.	
				1.05	Accepts tactile and verbal reinforcers.	
				1.06	Accepts edible reinforcer.	
				1.07	Does not display stereotyped behaviors.	
				1.08	Does not drool.	
				1.09	Does not protrude tongue.	
				\multicolumn{2}{l}{**Section II: Prelanguage Behaviors**}	
				2.01	Attends to people.	
				2.02	Follows slowly moving objects with eyes.	
				2.03	Reaches out to grasp objects.	

Consistently Displays	Inconsistently Displays	Never Displays	Information Not Available		Comments
				2.04	Looks for objects no longer in sight (toys in a box, cookies in a jar, etc.).
				2.05	Imitates familiar gestures with object (combs hair when model is given).
				2.06	Demonstrates the function of objects (stirring with a spoon).
				2.07	Responds to pointing gestures (by looking at object or picking up object).
				2.08	Places objects in container or rings on stick.
				2.09	Imitates unfamiliar gestures without object (claps hands when model is given).
				2.10	Uses one object to obtain another that is out of reach.
				2.11	Matches objects.
				2.12	Shows objects to adults for joint attention.
				2.13	Initiates joint activity with adult (throws ball to adult to initiate playing ball).
				2.14	Waves "hi" and "bye."
				2.15	Shakes head "no" to indicate denial, refusal, or rejection.
				2.16	Shakes head "yes" to indicate acceptance.
				2.17	Uses facial gestures for means of expression.
				2.18	Matches object to picture.

Section III: Language Modalities

A. Speech—Perception & Reception

				3.01	Responds to loud non-standard speech sounds (as, turning in direction of horn or whistle).

Consistently Displays	Inconsistently Displays	Never Displays	Information Not Available			Comments
				3.02	Responds to loud speech sounds (as, turning in direction of shouting or loud talking).	
				3.03	Responds to normal speech.	
				3.04	Responds to name (by looking up or in speaker's direction).	
				3.05	Selects an object when name of object is given (as, "cup," "shoe," "dog," "ball").	
				3.06	Selects a picture when the name is given.	
				3.07	Demonstrates an action verb on command (as, "Sit" or "Go").	
				3.08	Follows simple directives (as, "Pick-up your sock," "Turn on the light," or "You go bathroom").	
				3.09	Ceases behavior when command is given (as, "No" or "Stop").	
				3.10	Selects colors when color name is given (as, "Give me blue").	
				3.11	Follows more complex commands (as "Hang up your coat and sit down").	
				3.12	(Continued reception subsumed under section V.)	
					A. *Speech—Expression*	
				3.13	Vocalizes with laughing, crying, grunts.	
				3.14	Imitates some vowels (as, /a/, /o/, /i/).	
				3.15	Produces some vowels without model.	
				3.16	Imitates some consonants (as, /b/, /p/, /r/, /c/).	
				3.17	Produces some consonants without the model.	
				3.18	Babbles and uses syllable combinations as "bada" with inflection.	

Consistently Displays	Inconsistently Displays	Never Displays	Information Not Available			Comments
				3.19	Imitates some words (as "Mama," "bye-bye").	
				3.20	Uses limited sounds with inflection to express meaning.	
				3.21	Single words are intelligible (can be understood easily).	
				3.22	Speech is intelligible.	
				3.23	Speech is intelligible only if topic is known (is not always understood).	
				3.24	Speech is loud enough to be easily understood.	
				3.25	Speech is slow enough to be easily understood.	
					B. Written Reception	
				3.01	Matches object to picture.	
				3.02	Matches picture to picture.	
				3.03	Sorts out written words vs. pictures.	
				3.04	Matches shapes (as, circles, shapes, and squares).	
				3.05	Matches identical written words when other stimuli differ in length and configuration (as, /show/, /a/, /bathroom/).	
				3.06	Recognizes some written words (as, own name).	
				3.07	Points to a written word when a verbal name is given ("Show me 'shoe' ").	
				3.08	Selects written word when picture is presented and no verbal stimulus is given.	
				3.09	Uses single word cards to communicate.	
				3.10	Can sequence letters to form a word.	

Consistently Displays	Inconsistently Displays	Never Displays	Information Not Available			Comments
				3.11	Can write his or her name.	
				3.12	Can write the alphabet.	
				3.13	Can write words in addition to own name.	
				3.14	Can write or print legibly.	
					C. Manual Signing Reception	
				3.01	Responds to gestures that represent objects or actions (as, "Wash hands").	
				3.02	Responds to one-word signs (as, "Go").	
					C. Manual Signing Expression	
				3.03	Does not resist handshaping.	
				3.04	Shows a definite hand preference.	
				3.05	Performs fine manipulation of objects during play or activities (as, turning a dial or knob).	
				3.06	Uses gestures representing objects or actions.	
				3.07	Imitates some manual signs.	
				3.08	Produces manual signs.	
					D. Non-oral Communicator Reception	
				3.01	Matches object to picture.	
				3.02	Matches picture to picture.	
					D. Non-oral Communicator Expression	
				3.03	Reaches past body midline.	

Consistently Displays	Inconsistently Displays	Never Displays	Information Not Available			Comments
				3.04	Responds to familiar pictures (with touch, stylus, or head movement).	
					E. Abstract Symbol Reception	
				3.01	Matches object to picture.	
				3.02	Matches picture to picture.	
				3.03	Matches simple shapes (as, circle, triangle, square).	
				3.04	Matches more complex shapes (rectangles, stars, etc.).	
				3.05	Matches size.	
				3.06	Matches color.	
				3.07	Matches a sequence of shapes (as, circle-circle, square-square, etc.).	
					E. Abstract Symbol Expression	
				3.08	Picks up flat objects (as, a wooden puzzle piece).	
				3.09	Gives object to adult when hand is held out.	
				3.10	Responds with symbol to verbal stimulus and pictures.	
				3.11	Responds with symbol to picture only.	
				3.12	Gives symbol to adult to receive an object.	
				Section IV: Functions of Language		
				A. Instrumental Function to obtain wants and needs		
				4.01	Child demonstrates inappropriate behavior (as, crying or throwing tantrums to obtain objects).	

Consistently Displays	Inconsistently Displays	Never Displays	Information Not Available			Comments
				4.02	Child gestures with prompt (prompt = adult saying, "What do you want?")	
				4.03	Child gestures without prompt.	
				4.04	Child gets object and gives it to adult with prompt (as, handing cup to adult when child wants milk).	
				4.05	Child gets object and hands it to adult without prompt.	
				4.06	Child uses speech utterance with prompt.	
				4.07	Child uses speech utterance without prompt.	
				4.08	Child uses other modality with prompt.	
				4.09	Child uses other modality without prompt.	
					B. Regulatory Function to regulate the behavior of others	
				4.01	Demonstrates inappropriate behavior.	
				4.02	Gestures with prompt.	
				4.03	Gestures without prompt.	
				4.04	Gets object and gives it to adult with prompt.	
				4.05	Gets object and gives it to adult without prompt.	
				4.06	Uses speech utterance with prompt.	
				4.07	Uses speech utterance without prompt.	
				4.08	Uses other modality with prompt.	
				4.09	Uses other modality without prompt.	

Consistently Displays	Inconsistently Displays	Never Displays	Information Not Available			Comments
				\multicolumn{2}{l|}{*C. Interactional Function to establish and maintain contact with those that matter*}	
				4.01	Demonstrates inappropriate behavior.	
				4.02	Touches or maintains close body contact.	
				4.03	Gestures at objects to gain adult's attention.	
				4.04	Uses speech utterance.	
				4.05	Uses other modalities.	
				\multicolumn{2}{l|}{*D. Personal Function to express individuality and self-awareness*}	
				4.01	Demonstrates inappropriate behavior.	
				4.02	Makes personal contact.	
				4.03	Gestures at objects.	
				4.04	Uses speech utterance.	
				4.05	Uses other modalities.	
				\multicolumn{2}{l|}{*E. Heuristic Function to explore the objective environment*}	
				4.01	Demonstrates inappropriate behavior.	
				4.02	Notices novelties, but does not indicate to adult.	
				4.03	Indicates novelties and known objects to adults.	
				4.04	Uses speech utterance.	
				4.05	Uses other modalities.	
				4.06	Uses other modalities.	

The Development of Language in the MR/HI Child: Instructional Methods

Consistently Displays	Inconsistently Displays	Never Displays	Information Not Available			Comments
					F. Imaginative Function to create an environment of one's own	
				4.01	Demonstrates inappropriate behavior.	
				4.02	Uses objects for imaginative functions.	
				4.03	Uses speech with imaginative functions.	
				4.04	Uses other modalities to express imagination.	
					G. Information Function to convey information by speech or other modality	
				4.01	Responds to "wh" question.	
				4.02	Responds to a command.	
				4.03	Responds to a statement.	
				4.04	Responds to a response.	
				4.05	Initiates language to convey information.	
					Section V: Grammar	
				5.01	Uses one-word noun utterances (as, "Mama").	
				5.02	Uses one-word verb utterances (as, "Go").	
				5.03	Uses question inflections (such as "Outside?" with a final rising inflection).	
				5.04	Uses two-word, subject-verb utterances (as, "I go," "Mama come").	
				5.05	Uses two-word, verb-object utterances (as, "Want drink," "Go home").	
				5.06	Uses external negation (as, "No ball" or "No, I want that").	

Consistently Displays	Inconsistently Displays	Never Displays	Information Not Available			Comments
				5.07	Uses size adjectives (as, "Big ball" or "Little cup").	
				5.08	Uses color adjectives (as, "Red shoe").	
				5.09	Uses three-word, subject-verb-object utterances (as, "I want cookie," "Mama get cup").	
				5.10	Uses adverbs (as, "Go fast").	
				5.11	Gives at least one-word responses to questions (as, "What do you want?" or "Where are you going?").	
				5.12	Uses "wh" questions (as, "What," "Who," etc.).	
				5.13	Uses prepositions in two or more word utterances (as, "Put in box," "Turn off light").	
				5.14	Uses four- to six-word sentences.	
				5.15	Uses internal negation (as, "I not want that").	
				5.16	Uses internal, contracted negation (as, "Don't").	
				5.17	Uses articles (a, the, some) in phrases or sentences.	
				5.18	Uses third person pronouns (his, her, them, he, she, they).	
				5.19	Uses plural markers with nouns (as, "Cups" or "Dogs").	
				5.20	Uses copula and auxiliary verbs in sentences (as, is, are, was).	
				5.21	Uses possession marker (as, "Jim's car").	
				5.22	Uses more complex questions (as, "Can I . . ." or "Do you . . .").	
				5.23	Uses past tense markers with verbs (as, "spilled" or "combed").	
				5.24	Uses seven- to ten-word sentences.	

Consistently Displays	Inconsistently Displays	Never Displays	Information Not Available			Comments
				5.25	Can carry on conversations using three or more sentences.	
				5.26	Uses variation in types of language structures.	
				5.27	Uses language structures fairly frequently (if opportunity is presented).	
				5.28	Uses language structures to express relevant meaning.	

Appendix B
Assessment

Assessment in Infancy-Ordinal Scales of Psychological Development
    Uzgiris and McV. Hunt
    University of Illinois Press
    Chicago, Illinois

BCP Observation Booklet
    VORT Corporation
    P.O. Box 11132
    Palo Alto, California

A Developmental Approach Toward Assessing Communication Behavior in Children
    Jon Miller
    Waisman Center on MR and Human Development
    Madison, Wisconsin

Houston Test for Language Development
    Margaret Crabtree
    Houston Test Company
    Box 35152
    Houston, Texas

Minimum Objective System for Pupils with Severe Handicaps
   Center for Special Education
   University of Vermont
   Burlington, Vermont

Pennsylvania Training Model—Individual Assessment
   Ellen Somerton
   123 Foster Street
   Harrisburg, Pennsylvania

Sequenced Inventory of Communication Development
   D. Hendrick, E. Prather, and A. Tobin
   University of Washington Press
   Seattle and London

TARC Assessment Inventory for Severely Handicapped
   W. Sailor and B. J. Mix
   H & H Enterprises
   Box 3342
   Lawrence, Kansas

Strategies for Teaching Language- and/or Learning-Disabled Hearing-Impaired Children

Ann Rutledge Powers
Ann Reilly Harris

To assist teachers of the hearing impaired as they work with increasing numbers of language-disabled and learning-disabled students, Dr. Ann Powers and Ms. Ann Harris offer a variety of suggestions. They insist that a thorough knowledge of normal language development provides the basis for working with disabled students. They describe traditional materials and current improvements for teaching language, and they append an annotated list of published resources dealing with language and learning disabilities.

The number of hearing-impaired children who exhibit language and/or learning difficulties above and beyond those which have been traditionally attributed to hearing loss appears, at least on the surface, to be increasing rather rapidly. Educators of the hearing impaired are finding themselves in the position of having to search for methods which will facilitate learning in this puzzling group of children. In the majority of cases, the methods which have traditionally been used with the hearing impaired do not seem to be appropriate for the hearing-impaired child with language and/or learning disabilities. This chapter focuses on possible teaching strategies which may have some utility for hearing-impaired children with language and/or learning disabilities.

Before we discuss teaching strategies, we must establish the basic framework from which the various methods and strategies will be approached. It is thought that the prerequisites for effective teaching of the hearing-impaired child with language and/or learning disabilities should include a basic understanding of:
1. Normal child development with particular emphasis on linguistic and cognitive development (Menyuk, 1976);
2. Various curricula used with hearing-impaired children;
3. Various approaches used in teaching language acquisition in the developmentally disabled child; and
4. Language and/or learning problems in hearing-impaired children.

Normal Child Development

Currently it is possible to present teachers who are preparing to work with hearing-impaired children with a fairly sound foundation in normal child development. Theories of cognitive development have been provided by psychologists such as Piaget and Bruner. Piaget's theory, in particular, has provided the framework for a wealth of research and numerous curricula in both normal and abnormal child development. In addition, the work of other child psychologists, such as Burton White (1978), provides both parents and teachers with significant information regarding the importance of a stimulating, nonrestrictive environment for infants and preschool children.

There has been an increase in research on normal language development. Chomsky's *Syntactic Structures* (1957) prompted a new era in child language study, and the amount of research in language development has been phenomenal during the last two decades. Among the more recent texts in language development is *Language Acquisition* (de Villiers & de Villiers, 1978), which presents a thorough discussion of normal language acquisition and its relationship to language acquisition in the developmentally disabled child. Another recent text on normal language development has been written by Bloom and Lahey (1978). The text provides students of language development with a comprehensive background in which linguistic and cognitive development are well integrated and are related to language disorders. In a brief but pertinent article, Menyuk (1976) has discussed the relationship of cognitive and linguistic development as it pertains to the hearing-impaired child. These references represent but a limited sample of the material which is available on normal child development. However, it is imperative that teachers of the hearing impaired be knowledgeable in the areas of normal linguistic and cognitive development inasmuch as the knowledge of normal developmental patterns provides a basis for understanding abnormal development.

Curricula for the Hearing Impaired

During the last few years several language curricula for use with the hearing impaired have emerged. Several of the curricula are the result of new information on normal language and cognitive development. Among the more recently developed curricula are: *Apple Tree* (Caniglia, et al., 1972); *Sentences and Other Systems* (Blackwell, et al., 1978); and *Language Development and Intervention with the Hearing Impaired* (Kretschmer & Kretschmer, 1978).

The Apple Tree curriculum focuses on the teaching of ten sentence patterns in a sequential and spiraling fashion through the use of five fundamental teaching steps. The steps include: comprehension, manipulation, substitution, production, and transformation.

In contrast, only five basic sentence patterns are central to the curriculum used at the Rhode Island School for the Deaf (Blackwell, et al., 1978). The five sentence patterns are presented in a conceptually based framework which includes exposure, recognition, comprehension, and production.

Kretschmer and Kretschmer (1978) have integrated linguistic and cognitive development in the guidelines which they present for a developmentally based language program for the hearing impaired. In addition to being familiar with recently developed curricula, the effective teacher of hearing-impaired children should be aware of techniques and methods which have been used with the deaf through the years. The Fitzgerald Key (Fitzgerald, 1929), which was preceded by the Wing

Symbols (Wing, 1887) and the Barry Five Slates (Barry, 1899), continues to be used with success in numerous programs throughout the country. It is interesting to note that the Key and *Pugh's Steps in Language Development* (1947) have been suggested as useful methods for some language-disordered children (Myers & Hammill, 1969). In describing the Key, Kretschmer and Kretschmer (1978) indicate that although Fitzgerald stressed the use of the Key in "a language learning atmosphere, allowing for constant exposure to language experiences like those encountered by normally hearing children," in the majority of the classrooms in which the Key has been used, the critical association between language development and experience has not occurred (Kretschmer & Kretschmer, 1978, p. 215). Instead, users have focused on the Key for developing the structure of language.

Another traditional method for teaching language to the hearing impaired is the Natural Language Approach (Groht, 1958), which stresses the importance of helping the hearing-impaired child learn concepts through language. The importance of developing language in meaningful situations based upon the interests and the needs of the child was emphasized by Groht. Although Groht's theory is based upon a viable premise, there is a major weakness in her approach in that she did not provide clearly delineated steps for the development of language. Consequently, the intent of the Natural Language Approach has been lost in many instances. It must be noted that the approach does have considerable value in the development of the idea of communication in both hearing-impaired and multihandicapped hearing-impaired children, if it is used properly.

Patterning, as another means of developing language in the hearing impaired, has been discussed by d'Arc (1958) and Buckler (1968). Patterning has been described as drawing "upon the strength of structured language approaches . . . while encouraging natural experiences in keeping the content of patterns in line with the developmental needs of the child" (Kretschmer & Kretschmer, 1978, p. 217-18). The approach appears to be very effective in the development of language in hearing-impaired youngsters who present no additional problems in learning.

The preceding discussion of language curricula is representative of only a few of the traditional and contemporary approaches which are available. It is suggested, however, that teachers of the hearing impaired be proficient in the use of more than one language method.

Learning Disabilities Approaches

Recently from the field of learning disabilities has come a considerable number of theories which have provided numerous teaching strategies for a variety of learning problems. Perusal of general texts in the area of learning disabilities (Myers & Hammill, 1976; Lerner, 1976) suggests no less than 20 different approaches to various types of learning problems. The task of becoming knowledgeable about the numerous strategies suggested for use with language- and/or learning-disabled children is a formidable one indeed. Although it is not realistic to expect teachers of the hearing impaired to be proficient in the use of the many approaches available for children with learning disabilities, it is imperative that teachers be aware of the term *language- and/or learning-disabled* and of the sources from which they may obtain suggestions for working with children who present language and/or learning problems.

Language- and/or Learning-Disabled Hearing-Impaired Children

Hearing-impaired children with additional language and/or learning difficulties present an enigma to the vast majority of their teachers. Only recently have the unique problems of the hearing-impaired child with language and/or learning disabilities been included as a part of the curriculum in teacher preparation programs. Most teachers continue to be bewildered by the nebulous problems presented by these children. There is a dearth of published information concerning hearing-impaired children with language and/or learning disabilities. At the present time, it appears that educators of the hearing impaired need to combine the knowledge which they have about hearing-impaired youngsters with information about language and learning difficulties. There is also a significant need for applied research concerning effective methods for use with these children.

The following section presents a brief summary of some of the methods which have been developed for children with language and/or learning disabilities.

MILDRED MCGINNIS One of the first approaches developed for children who did not acquire language via traditional methods used with the deaf was the Association Method (McGinnis, 1963). The method was developed to aid the language-delayed hearing-impaired child or the asphasic child. It aimed to develop specific skills and associate those skills which are necessary to the understanding and expression of oral communication. The five major principles of the approach stand in contrast to the more traditional methods of teaching language to the deaf. The five principles are:
1. Words are taught using a phonetic or elemental approach.
2. Each sound is learned by emphasizing precise production.
3. The correct production of an individual sound is associated with the appropriate Northampton symbol.
4. Expression is the basis for language development, and understanding follows production.
5. Systematic sensorimotor association is used.

Because the principles are not in agreement with those used in the majority of language methods for the hearing impaired, there has been considerable controversy surrounding the Association Method as a viable approach to language learning. It must be noted, however, that there are children who continue to profit from the approach or variations of the approach. McGinnis described the Association Method in depth in *Aphasic Children* (1963).

EDNA MONSEES Monsees (1972) has developed an approach for working with language learning problems. The approach utilizes various concepts from the Association Method along with some ideas based on the multisensory approach suggested by Fernald (1943). Monsees has integrated structured language methods for teaching the hearing impaired with her experiences in working among language-delayed children. Concepts and procedures from operant conditioning and programmed learning are also evident in her approach. The linguistic aspect of the curriculum is based upon descriptive linguistics and transformational generative grammar. The curriculum consists of two components: linguistic content and teaching methodology. Monsees' structured language method represents a viable approach for some children who have language and/or learning problems and who are hearing impaired.

HORTENSE BARRY Barry described her approach to teaching children with a variety of learning problems in *The Young Asphasic Child: Evaluation and Training* (1961). Barry's approach is similar to Monsees' in that it is eclectic. However, Barry did not advocate an elemental or phonetic approach in the teaching of words, as has been done by McGinnis (1963) and Monsees (1972). As expressive language is developed through a whole word approach in meaningful situations, Barry suggested that the Fitzgerald Key be used for structure. In the initial chapter of her book, Barry made a statement which is still pertinent today. She wrote, "No one specific method, no one set of tools, no one simple approach is or can be the solution to so complex a problem" (Barry, 1961, p. 1). As is indicated by the title of her book, Barry dealt with both assessment and training. Included in the suggestions for training is a discussion of the physical environment thought to be most conducive to learning for asphasic children. An uncluttered, nonstimulating environment was suggested by Barry. It should be noted that the efficacy of nonstimulating environments for learning-disabled children has been questioned (Cruickshank, et al., 1961). Barry has made suggestions for training psychomotor dysfunctions and perceptual impairments including: impaired body image; impaired visual, tactile, and auditory perceptions; figure-ground disturbances and spatial disorganization; and impaired motor functioning. Barry's framework for evaluation and training involves inner, receptive, and expressive language, and is similar to that suggested by Myklebust (1955).

DORIS JOHNSON AND HELMER MYKLEBUST *Learning Disabilities: Educational Principles and Practices* (Johnson & Myklebust, 1967) provides a description of one theory of learning disabilities along with teaching suggestions for a wide variety of learning problems. Because Myklebust's theory of learning disabilities evolved from his work in the areas of deafness, childhood aphasia, and speech and language pathology, many of the teaching suggestions provided by Johnson and Myklebust are useful for hearing-impaired children with language and/or learning disabilities. The concept of differential diagnosis utilizing a multidisciplinary approach is central to Myklebust's theory of learning disabilities (Myklebust, 1954). Even though empirical evidence is incomplete concerning Johnson and Myklebust's concept of psychoneurological learning disabilities, the educational suggestions do have relevance for language- and/or learning-disabled hearing-impaired children. Educational strategies are provided for the following categories of learning problems: disorders of auditory language, disorders of reading, disorders of written language, disorders of arithmetic, and nonverbal disorders of learning. Myklebust supports a synthetic approach to the teaching of words, an approach similar to that of Barry. The analytic or elemental approach suggested by McGinnis is incompatible with Johnson and Myklebust's methods. It must be noted, however, that each approach has had its successes and failures.

SUMMARY OF LEARNING DISABILITIES STRATEGIES Since the publication of Johnson and Myklebust's text in 1967, numerous books have appeared which suggest teaching strategies for children with language and/or learning disabilities. Table 1 includes a summary of a number of texts on learning disabilities. The texts are listed by author(s). The types of learning and/or language problems for which suggestions are provided in a particular text are indicated by a "●" in the appropriate column. The intent of the table is to provide teachers of hearing-impaired children with language and/or learning disabilities a list to which he or she may refer for suggestions for teaching strategies for specific types of language and learning problems.

Suggestions for Selecting Strategies for Hearing-Impaired Children with Language and/or Learning Disabilities

In order to select appropriate educational procedures to be used with a hearing-impaired child with language and/or learning disabilities, the teacher must be aware of the child's strengths and weaknesses in learning as well as his or her developmental levels. In order for this to be done effectively, the teacher must have, as indicated previously, a firm foundation in normal child development. Although the focus of the present chapter is on teaching strategies rather than assessment of language and/or learning problems, it is essential that the evaluative and teaching processes interface with one another in practice. Only when a child's learning style is ascertained and accommodated in a developmental perspective is the teacher able to select appropriate strategies for the child.

Table 1
Summary of Educational Strategies for Learning-Disabled Children

	Bush & Giles (1977)	Gardner (1974)	Guszak (1972)	Hammill & Bartel (1978)	Johnson & Myklebust (1967)	Kephart (1971)	Kirk & Kirk (1971)	Kirk, Kliebhan & Lerner (1978)	Kozloff (1974)	Lerner (1976)	Mann & Suiter (1974)	Slingerland (1971)	Stephens (1977)	Valett (1967)	Wallace & Kauffman (1973)	Wallace & McLoughlin (1975)	Wiig & Semel (1976)
Gross Motor	•			•		•			•	•	•			•	•	•	
Fine Motor	•			•		•			•	•	•			•	•	•	
Body Movement				•	•	•			•	•				•	•		
Memory General		•		•					•								
Auditory	•			•			•	•		•	•	•	•	•	•		•
Visual	•						•	•		•	•	•	•	•	•		
Listening to Oral Language	•			•	•			•	•	•	•		•	•	•	•	•
Spoken Language	•			•	•	•			•	•			•	•	•	•	•
Written Language				•	•					•			•		•	•	
Spelling	•			•	•					•	•		•	•	•	•	
Arithmetic	•			•	•					•			•	•	•	•	
Behavior Strategies	•	•		•	•				•	•	•		•	•	•	•	
Modality Processing Visual	•			•	•	•	•	•			•	•	•	•	•	•	
Auditory	•			•	•		•	•		•	•	•	•	•	•	•	•
Tactile	•			•		•						•		•			
Cross Modal	•				•				•		•	•		•			•
Reading Recognition	•		•	•	•					•	•	•	•	•	•	•	
Reading Comprehension			•	•	•					•	•		•	•	•	•	
Reading Fluency			•													•	
Cursive Handwriting			•							•		•				•	
Left-handed Writing										•					•	•	
Typewriting										•						•	
Teaching Activities				•	•					•	•	•	•	•	•	•	

In many instances when a strategy from the field of learning disabilities is selected it may be necessary for some modification to be made in order for the strategy to be effective with the hearing-impaired child. Once the strategy has been implemented, it is critical that the teacher assess the effectiveness of the strategy in an objective manner. Strategies which are found to be effective should be utilized as long as the child is making progress. However, when no progress is evident, it is necessary to reevaluate the information which is available concerning the child and to find additional strategies which might be beneficial to the child. The process of evaluation of learning strategies, selection and utilization of teaching strategies, and evaluation of the effectiveness of the strategies must be continuous.

The number of hearing-impaired children who have additional problems in language and/or learning is unknown. One of the major difficulties in determining how many hearing-impaired children have language and/or learning problems rests, at least to some degree, in a lack of agreement on the definition of terms (Moores, 1978). Cursory observation and comments frequently made by teachers of the hearing impaired tend to lead one to believe that a relatively large percentage of hearing-impaired children have language, learning, and/or behavior problems. Rather than accepting that a large number of hearing-impaired children are language-disabled, learning-disabled, or behavior-disordered, it is proposed that educators of the hearing impaired take a more developmental perspective on the children with whom they work. Educators in general have tended to segregate the various components of the educational process so that the special educator has not been familiar with the responsibilities of the regular educator, and vice versa. More specifically, special educators have heretofore kept the various categories of exceptionality separate for educational purposes. It has been refreshing to see the gradual diminishment of barriers among the disciplines in recent years. With educators of the hearing impaired operating from a developmental perspective and benefiting from the new openness among disciplines, more hearing-impaired children should have a positive educational experience.

In the last few years, several language curricula for use with the hearing impaired have surfaced. These curricula hold promise for alleviating some of the language and/or learning problems seen in hearing-impaired children. One approach which appears to have possibilities for a wide range of hearing-impaired children is that presented by Kretschmer and Kretschmer (1978). In discussing the rationale and guidelines for developing a language-oriented learning program for hearing-impaired children, Kretschmer and Kretschmer have stated:

. . . despite the evidence that children with hearing loss can be fluent language users, too many continue to be described as having language learning disorders. Impoverished experience and lack of attention to developmentally oriented intervention strategies account for the majority of performance problems with English forms and functions exhibited by deaf children.

(Kretschmer & Kretschmer, 1978, p. 234)

Krestchmer and Kretschmer emphasize the importance of helping the hearing-impaired child acquire the deep structure of language. This approach attempts to go beyond surface structure as is done in linguistically based approaches. In designing language learning experiences to assist the hearing-impaired child in acquiring the deep structure of language, Kretschmer and Kretschmer present a discussion of five principles described by Libergott and Swope (1976). The first principle indicates that ". . . cognitive development is felt to structure language learning, so it could be said that children profit most from new information when they are ready to assimilate the information" (Kretschmer & Kretschmer, 1978, p. 237). It is imperative that the teacher take into account the child's level of cognitive development in providing experiences to facilitate language acquisition. In far too many cases, one of two things occurs in what are supposed to be language learning experiences. In some instances, the acquisition of syntactic rules becomes the goal of a lesson, and the child leaves the experience with no intuitive sense of the language rule. In other instances, an idea which the teacher finds appealing becomes the focus of the lesson with little attention given to the linguistic and cognitive needs of the individual children in the class. It is possible to target individual linguistic and cognitive goals and to integrate such goals into meaningful language learning experiences.

The second principle discussed by Libergott and Swope (1976) indicates that representation is developed as a "result of the differentiation of meaning from symbol and symbol from content" (Kretschmer & Kretschmer, 1978, p. 256). The child's ability to represent becomes apparent toward the end of the sensorimotor period of cognitive development, according to Piaget (1952), and it can be observed in the child's play behavior. If the child is unable to relate receptively and expressively to the linguistic symbols of his or her environment, then it is necessary to provide the child with appropriate experiences which will aid in the development of representation. Teachers of the hearing impaired need to be astute observers of children's play behaviors. Information obtained from such observation provides the teacher with considerable information about the child's cognitive development. The teacher must sequence learning tasks developmentally so as to assure that basic skills have been established prior to exposing the child to experiences at a higher level of cognitive development.

The third principle stresses the importance of symbolizing through the use of actions as a foundation for language acquisition. Although the statement appears trite, it is necessary that language be taught in as natural a manner as possible.

Sedentary activities or activities that involve static materials such as pictures or drawings may not be sufficient in the beginning stages to illustrate the dynamic aspects of language learning to deaf children, particularly those with an impoverished symbolist experience or intellectual limitations . . . . Language learning apart from language context, whether sandbox, bathroom, breakfast table, or family gathering, may yield some surface structure performance in children, but its usefulness may carry no farther than the classroom door.

(Kretschmer & Kretschmer, 1978, p. 257)

The fourth principle states that "... new content should first be expressed through old forms, and new forms should first encode old content" (Ibid). As in the case of the third principle, this idea may appear to be rather mundane. Yet it seems to be overlooked in many classrooms. Perhaps a more consistent application of this principle in designing language learning experiences would help to reduce what seem to be learning difficulties in a significant number of children.

The fifth principle stresses the importance of social interaction in stimulating cognitive and linguistic growth. It has been well documented that social interaction is critical to normal language acquisition (Snow, 1972; Bloom & Lahey, 1978; de Villiers & de Villiers, 1978). Educators of the hearing impaired need to keep the importance of social interaction in mind as they attempt to aid the hearing-impaired child in language acquisition. The current interest and immediate needs of the child must be foremost in the mind of the teacher in helping the child acquire a feel for language. As suggested by Groht, group lessons or activities can facilitate language development through social interaction. Unfortunately, her ideas concerning the development of language in the deaf have rarely been actualized. Groht's philosophy of language development for normal hearing-impaired children has also been used successfully with multihandicapped hearing-impaired children.

It seems apparent that all five of the principles suggested by Libergott and Swope (1976) for use in planning language learning experiences have applicability with hearing-impaired children with language and/or learning disabilities. Although the principles are not new to either the field of learning disabilities or the education of the hearing impaired, the test of their significance rests in the ability of educators to use them effectively with children.

Kretschmer and Kretschmer (1978) have expanded upon Groht's ideas about language development in the deaf through the use of conversation. They believe "... that only when children internalize symbols as well as the way of organizing those symbols will they truly have a self-generated command of English." (1978, p. 263) The importance of the use of vocabulary in sentences rather than in isolation is emphasized and is seen as necessary to the communication process. The traditional approaches of vocabulary teaching used with the hearing impaired are refuted by Kretschmer and Kretschmer.

Communication exchanges provide opportunity for rule induction, as well as for spontaneous or delayed imitation, which may play a role in language acquisition for some children ... Unless the deaf child sees language within the context of dialogue, however, it is uncertain whether he will ever learn it for functional use outside the classroom. It has been the author's experience that many students with an apparent lack of meaningful knowledge about English sentences will respond favorably to experience-dialogue techniques.
(Kretschmer & Kretschmer, 1978, p. 260)

In attempting to apply what Kretschmer and Kretschmer have proposed, teachers of the hearing impaired can benefit from the work of Holland (1975) and Lahey and

Bloom (1977) in deciding upon words for a child's core lexicon or basic vocabulary. Holland stated that ". . . language is not labeling, or matching pictures to words, or repeating what someone else says. It is instead an active, dynamic, interpersonal interchange and should be treated as such." (p. 518) Holland suggests a basic or core lexicon of approximately 35 words which are of interest to the child and which may then be used in developing basic sentence patterns. Lahey and Bloom suggest the following guidelines in developing a first lexicon:
1. Use of child language as the model to be taught;
2. Consideration of what is important to the child;
3. Use of objects and events that are present and happening;
4. Stress on communication as the overall goal.

In addition, Lahey and Bloom provide guidelines for what should not be included in a first lexicon. Among the types of words which should be excluded from a first lexicon are internal states, affirmation by "yes," pronouns, colors, and opposites. These guidelines obviously contrast to what has frequently occurred in classrooms for the hearing impaired.

It appears that teachers of the hearing impaired have an increasing number of options available to them in working with language- and/or learning-disabled hearing-impaired children. The increased knowledge in the area of normal language development and its application in curricula for the hearing-impaired child appears to have considerable utility for children with additional language and/or learning problems. In addition, the vast number of teaching strategies for learning-disabled children provide teachers with a menu of ideas for the hearing-impaired child with language and/or learning disabilities.

Summary

In summary, we offer the following suggestions. First, teachers of hearing-impaired children with language and/or learning disabilities can use normal child development as their reference in determining language and/or learning problems in hearing-impaired children. Normal child development must provide the basis for both the evaluation and teaching of language- and/or learning-disabled hearing-impaired youngsters. Second, teachers need to explore the various curricula available for use with children who have hearing impairments in order to determine possible teaching strategies. Some of the recent curricular developments designed for the hearing impaired appear to have definite possibilities for helping with hearing-impaired children with language and/or learning disabilities. Third, teachers need to be aware of the numerous strategies available for use with children who have various types of learning problems. A table which summarizes various categories of strategies for learning disabilities has been included in this chapter. Finally, the nebulous nature of the problems surrounding language- and/or learning-disabled hearing-impaired children has been presented, and options for helping such children have been offered.

Bibliography

Auxter, D. Learning disabilities among deaf populations. *Exceptional Children,* 1971, *37,* 573–578.

Barry, H. *The young aphasic child: Evaluation and training.* Washington, D.C.: Volta Bureau, 1961.

Barry, K. *The Five Slate System: A system of objective language teaching.* Philadelphia: Sherman and Company, 1899.

Blackwell, P., Engen, E., Fischgrund, J. E., & Zaracadoolas, C. *Sentences and other systems: A language and learning curriculum for hearing-impaired children.* Washington, D.C.: The Alexander Graham Bell Association for the Deaf, Inc., 1978.

Bloom, L. (Ed.). *Readings in language development.* New York: John Wiley and Sons, Inc., 1978.

Bloom, L., & Lahey, M. *Language development and language disorders.* New York: John Wiley and Sons, Inc., 1978.

Brannon, A. C., et al. *The hearing impaired/mentally retarded: A survey of state institutions for the retarded.* Lubbock, Tex.: Research and Training Center in Mental Retardation, Texas Technological University, 1975.

Bryan, T. H., & Bryan, J. H. *Understanding learning disabilities.* Port Washington, New York: Alfred Publishing Co., Inc., 1975.

Buckler, Sister M. Expanding language through patterning. *The Volta Review,* 1968, *70,* 89–96.

Bush, W. J., & Giles, M. T. *Aids to psycholinguistic teaching* (2nd ed.). Columbus, Ohio: Charles E. Merrill Publishing Co., 1977.

Caniglia, J., Cole, N. J., Howard, W., Krohn, E., & Rice, M. *Apple Tree.* Beaverton, Oreg.: Dormac, Inc., 1972.

Chomsky, N. S. *Syntactic structures.* The Hague: Mouton, 1957.

Combs, A. W. *Educational accountability: Beyond behavioral objectives.* Washington, D.C.: Association for Supervision and Curriculum Development, 1972.

Cruickshank, W., Bentzen, F. A., Ratzeburg, F. H., & Tannhauser, M. *A teaching method for brain-injured and hyperactive children.* Syracuse: Syracuse University Press, 1961.

d'Arc, Sister J. The development of connected language skills with emphasis on a particular methodology. *The Volta Review,* 1958, *60,* 58–65.

de Villiers, J. G., & de Villiers, P. A. *Language acquisition.* Cambridge, Mass.: Harvard University Press, 1978.

Faas, L. A. *Learning disabilities: A competency based approach.* Boston: Houghton Mifflin Co., 1976.

Fernald, G. M. *Remedial techniques in basic school subjects.* New York: McGraw-Hill, 1943.

Fitzgerald, E. *Straight language for the deaf.* Staunton, Va.: McClure Company, 1929.

Gardner, W. I. *Children with learning and behavior problems: A behavior management approach*. Boston: Allyn and Bacon, Inc., 1974.

Groht, M. *Natural language for deaf children*. Washington, D.C.: The Alexander Graham Bell Association for the Deaf, Inc., 1958.

Guszak, F. J. *Diagnostic reading instruction in the elementary school*. New York: Harper and Row, 1972.

Hammill, D. D., & Bartel, N. R. *Teaching children with learning and behavior problems* (2nd ed.). Boston: Allyn and Bacon, Inc., 1978.

Healey, W. C., et al. *The hearing-impaired mentally retarded: Recommendations for action*. Department of Health, Education, and Welfare, Social and Rehabilitation Service, Rehabilitation Services Administration, Division of Developmental Disabilities, 1975.

Holland, A. L. Language therapy for children: Some thoughts on context and content. *Journal of Speech and Hearing Disorders*, 1975, 40, 514–523.

Johnson, D. J., & Myklebust, H. R. *Learning disabilities: Educational principles and practices*. New York: Grune and Stratton, 1967.

Kaufman, R. A. *Educational system planning*. Englewood Cliffs, N.J.: Prentice-Hall, 1972.

Kephart, N. C. *The slow learner in the classroom* (2nd ed.). Columbus, Ohio: Charles E. Merrill Publishing Co., 1971.

Kirk, S. A., & Kirk, W. D. *Psycholinguistic learning disabilities*. Champaign, Ill.: University of Illinois Press, 1971.

Kirk, S. A., Kliebhan, Sister J. M., & Lerner, J. W. *Teaching reading to slow and disabled learners*. Boston: Houghton Mifflin Co., 1978.

Kozloff, M. A. *Educating children with learning and behavior problems*. New York: John Wiley and Sons, Inc., 1974.

Kretschmer, R. R., Jr., & Kretschmer, L. W. *Language development and intervention with the hearing impaired*. Baltimore: University Park Press, 1978.

Lahey, M., & Bloom, L. Planning a first lexicon: Which words to teach first. *Journal of Speech and Hearing Disorders*, 1977, 42(3), 340–350.

Lerner, J. W. *Children with learning disabilities: Theories, diagnoses and teaching strategies*. Boston: Houghton Mifflin Co., 1976.

Libergott, J., & Swope, S. Learners' needs: Speech and language disabilities. In F. Withrow and C. Nygren (Eds.), *Language materials and curriculum management for the handicapped learner*. Columbus, Ohio: Charles E. Merrill Publishing Co., 1976.

Mann, L., Goodman, L., & Wiederholt, J. L. *Teaching the learning disabled adolescent*. Boston: Houghton Mifflin Co., 1978.

Mann, P. H., & Suiter, P. *Handbook in diagnostic teaching: A learning disabilities approach*. Boston: Allyn and Bacon, Inc., 1974.

McGinnis, M. A. *Aphasic children*. Washington, D.C.: The Volta Bureau, 1963.

Menyuk, P. Cognition and language. *Volta Review*, 1976, 78(6), 250–257.

Monsees, E. K. *Structured language for children with special language learning problems*. Washington, D.C.: Children's Hearing and Speech Center, Children's Hospital of the District of Columbia, 1972.

Moores, D. F. *Educating the deaf: Psychology, principles, and practices*. Boston: Houghton Mifflin Co., 1978.

Morehead, D. M., & Morehead, A. E. (Eds.). *Normal and deficient child language*. Baltimore: University Park Press, 1976.

Myers, P. I., & Hammill, D. D. *Methods for learning disorders* (2nd ed.). New York: John Wiley and Sons, Inc., 1976.

Myklebust, H. R. *Auditory disorders in children*. New York: Grune and Stratton, 1954.

Myklebust, H. R. Training aphasic children. *Volta Review*, 1955, *57*, 149–157.

Peterson, B., & Schoenmann, S. *Building blocks for developing basic language*. Beaverton, Oreg.: Dormac, Inc., 1977.

Piaget, J. *The origins of intelligence in children*. New York: W. W. Norton and Co., 1952.

Pugh, B. *Steps in language development*. Washington, D.C.: The Volta Bureau, 1947.

Simmons-Martin, A., & Calvert, D. R. (Eds.). *Parent-infant intervention: Communication disorders*. New York: Grune and Stratton, 1979.

Slingerland, B. H. *A multisensory approach to language arts for specific language disability children: A guide for primary teachers*. Cambridge, Mass.: Educators Publishing Service, 1971.

Snow, C. E. Mothers' speech to children learning language. *Child Development*, 1972, *43*, 549–565.

Stephens, T. M. *Teaching skills to children with learning and behavior disorders*. Columbus, Ohio: Charles E. Merrill Publishing Co., 1977.

Stewart, L. G. *Serving hearing-impaired developmentally disabled persons*. Tucson: The Rehabilitation Center, College of Education, The University of Arizona, 1977.

Streng, A. H. *Syntax, speech, and hearing*. New York: Grune and Stratton, 1972.

Unruh, G. G. *Responsive curriculum development*. Berkeley: McCutchan Publishing Corp., 1975.

Valett, R. E. *The remediation of learning disabilities: A handbook of psychoeducational resource programs*. Belmont, Calif.: Fearon Publishers, 1967.

Van Hattum, R. J. *Developmental language programming for the retarded*. Boston: Allyn and Bacon, Inc., 1979.

Wallace, G., & Kauffman, J. M. *Teaching children with learning problems*. Columbus, Ohio: Charles E. Merrill Publishing Co., 1973.

Wallace, G., & McLoughlin, J. A. *Learning disabilities: Concepts and characteristics* (Rev. ed.). Columbus, Ohio: Charles E. Merrill Publishing Co., 1978.

White, B. L. *The first three years of life*. New York: Avon Books, 1978.

Wiig, E. H., & Semel, E. M. *Language disabilities in children and adolescents.* Columbus, Ohio: Charles E. Merrill Publishing Co., 1976.

Wing, G. The theory and practice of grammatical methods. *American Annals of the Deaf,* 1887, *32*, 84–89.

Index

American Annals of the Deaf, 1, 39
American Association on Mental Deficiency (AAMD), Speech Pathology and Audiology Division of, 224–225
American Sign Language (ASL), 120, 229
 continuum of, 189–191
 local signs of, 189–190
 teaching language with, 204–205, 207
Anoxia, 16
Aphasia/Aphasoid disorders, 2, 14, 18–20, 22, 53, 63, 135, 252–254
Apple Tree (language curriculum), 250
Arthur Point Scale of Performance Tests, 115
 subtests of, 115
Articulation
 assessment of, 214–215
 distortion, omission and substitution of, 215
 effects of, in the deaf child, 203
Assessment of preverbal behavior, 214
Association Method, 252–253
Attention, 164–166, 180
Attentional processes, 167
Attention/Hyperactivity problems, 62
Autism, 201, 203–204, 206–207
 assessment of, 115
Automaticity, 166

Babbidge Report, 2
Baby, interaction of, with environment, 106
Barry Five Slates, 251
Basic lexicon, 259
Behavioral Characteristics Progression (BCP), 152
Behavior management strategies, 39, 53–59, 159
Behavior systems, 96
Bender-Gestalt Test, 21, 128
Bill of Rights for handicapped children, 37. *See also* Public Law 94-142
Blindness. *See* Visual disorders
Bliss Symbol System, 207–208, 212
Body awareness exercises, 204
Body image, development of, 194–195
Body language, 185–186

Body movement, use of, with deaf-blind, 194–195
Body schema, development of, 187, 194–195
Boehm Test of Basic Concepts, 116
Brain damage, 53, 113, 135
Bureau of Education for the Handicapped, 6
 Regional Centers for the Deaf-Blind, 95

CAID (Convention of American Instructors of the Deaf), 1–2
Callier-Azusa Scale, 99, 114
Cattell and Merrill Palmer Scale, 114
CEASD (Conference of Executives of American Schools for the Deaf), 1
Centers and Services for Deaf-Blind Children, 2
Central Institute for the Deaf, 20
Central nervous system pathology, 15–17, 24
Cerebral palsy
 as an additional handicap, 95, 120
 complications resulting from, 21–23
 developmental delays as a result of, 104
 etiologies of, 13–16, 18–19, 63
 figure-ground discrimination affected by, 142
 graphic communication used with children with, 205–206
Child development, normal stages of, 108
Childhood schizophrenia, 201
Children
 basic needs of, 103–105
 developing independence in, 103, 105
 developmental lags in, 104
 parent/parent-substitute of, 103
Childrenese (a sign system), 191
Cognitive deficits, 204
Cognitive development, 250, 257–258
 Piaget's six stages of, 225
Cognitive goals, 257
Cognitive-perceptual growth, 212
Cognitive-perceptual organization, development of, 214
Cognitive skills, 212, 223, 225
Cognitive theory, 164–165

Communication
  American Sign Language, accents, dialects, and regional variations of, 189–191
  Ameslan, 190
  assessment of skills and needs, 215–217
  augmentative/alternative mode of, 212
  body language, 185, 188–189
  Childrenese, 191
  close body contact in, 187
  coactive stage of, 188
  cohesive stage of, 187
  contextual clues in, 118
  comprehensive or total, 32
  discrete functions of, 185, 187
  expressive aids, 202
  expressive skills, 198
  facial expressions in, 185, 188–189, 218
  fingerspelling, 188–191
  gesture system of, 187
  graphic mode of, in cerebral palsied children, 205–206
  graphic systems of, 202–203
  home signs, 190–191
  imitation level of, 188
  interaction with the environment, as a result of, 185–187, 212, 231
  internal feelings, 193, 200
  manual, development of, 157–158, 202–205, 208
  Manual English, 189–191
  manual expressive, 31, 38
  manual receptive, 31
  manual signing system of, 218, 225, 229
  modes of, 201, 208, 211–248
  of the MHHI, 185–191
  nonspeech systems of, 202–203, 205–208
  nonvocal symbol systems of, 202–205
  operational definition, 193
  oral expressive, 31–32, 38, 186
  oral receptive, 31–32
  pantomime, 188
  play as a means of, 118
  programs for severely handicapped, 212
  receptive skills, 114, 198
  repetition, 118
  rocking behavior as a means of, 187
  self-expression, 114
  Signed English, 189–191
  sign system, 186–187
  skills and goals for HI/MR, 118, 150
  Symbol Systems of, 206–208
  training goals of, 216. *See also* Appendix B, 247–248
  Van Dijk approach, 185–191, 193–200
  visual clues, 118
  vocal, 207–208
Communication Assessment Checklist (developed at Project MESH [Model Education for the Severely Handicapped]), 216–217. *See also* Appendix A, 237–247
Communication board, 202, 212, 218, 224–227
Communication strategies, development of, 185–191
Communication training, 230
Comprehension training, 223
Concept formation, as a curriculum component, 153
Conceptual behaviors, 225
Conceptualization, 164–166, 171, 180
Conceptual skills, acquisition of language through, 206
Conceptual skills and needs, 211
Conceptual training, 217
Context specificity, 166
Coping behavior, 124
  identification of, 126
Core lexicon, 259
Cortical inhibition, 113
CREED (Cooperative Research Endeavors in the Education of the Deaf) Curriculum, 162–176. *See also* Appendix A, 180–182
  behavioral objectives, construction of, 163
  educational diagnosis, redirection of attention to, 162
  educational tasks of, 164
  hierarchies of skills, 163–164, 171
  learner analysis, 176
  Piaget's influence on, 162–163
  subcomponents of, 162
  successful learners, 165–167, 175
  teacher administered tests, 163
  teacher involvement, 163, 176
  unsuccessful learners, 166–167, 171
Cue removal, 156
Cues, differentiation of, 167
Curriculum, definition of, 124

Curriculum guides, titles of, 119
Curriculum Research and Development Center in Mental Retardation of New York University, 153

Daily evaluation, 151–152
Daily living skills, 224
Deaf
  genetic syndromes of, 11, 63
  play patterns of, 75–76
  postlingually, 62–63
  prelingually, 63
  teachers of, 40–41
Deafness
  major etiologies of, 3, 11–25
    genetics/heredity, 3, 11, 17, 21
    meningitis, 3, 11, 15–16, 18, 20–23
    prematurity, 3, 11, 14–18, 20–23, 63
    Rh factor, 3, 11–12, 16, 20–23, 65
    rubella, 3, 11–14, 18, 20–23, 63
  primary handicap of, with the learning disabled/hearing impaired, 135
De-contextualization, 196
Deferred gratification, 187
De-naturalization, 196
Denver Developmental Scales, 99
Developmental Activities Screening Inventory (DASI), 114
Developmental Test of Visual Perception, 137–138
  subtests of, 137
Deviant behavior, 53
  contributing causes of, 53
  elimination/reduction of, suggested procedures for, 53–57
  examples of, 53–54
  overcorrection procedure, 53
Diagnostic Screening Forms for the Detection of Brain Injury in Deaf Children, administration of, 21
Discriminating features, patterns of, 170
Due process, 47–49

Early Intermediate Language Training Program, 222–223
Early Language Training Program, 222
Echolalia, 62
Edible reinforcement, 233

Education
  definition of, 95
  free, appropriate public, 44, 48, 211
  IEP (Individualized Education Program), 45–49
  Local Education Agencies (LEA), responsibilities of, 45
  placement tests, 45–47, 49
  related services, 44–45
  State Education Agencies (SEA), responsibilities of, 44–45
Educational placement/services, 37–41
  referrals, 37
  transfers from MHHI programs, 37–39
  transfers from "regular" HI programs, 37
Educational programming with the hearing impaired/mentally retarded, 148–160
  assessment of daily procedures, 151–152
  diagnosis and prescription of, 150–151
  instructional objectives of, 152
  parents involvement in, 150–152
  placement, 148–150
  structure in the daily schedule of, 152–153
Educational tasks, 164
Education for All Handicapped Children Act, 44–45. *See also* Public Law 94-142
Education of the Handicapped Act (EHA), 44
Education, U.S. Office of, Bureau for the Education of the Handicapped, 43
Ego-consciousness, 186
Emotional control, developing skills of, 156
Emotionally disturbed children, 2–3, 13, 15–16, 22–24, 39, 95, 103, 113, 120, 124–135, 151, 201, 224, 256
  activities for, 127
  curriculum planning for, 126
  definition of, 124, 126
  examination by specialists of, 127
  identification and prescription, Richard: A case study of, 127–133
  identification information, 127
  incidence of, in schools for the deaf, 125–126
  psychological evaluations of, 127
  support systems for, 131, 134
  TLC of, 125
Environment
  acting on by use of language, 193
  interactions within, 211

perception of, 212
structured, 101
Environmental disadvantage, 135
Epilepsy, 13–16
Equilibration, 170–171
Experiential deprivation, 154
remediation of, 154–156
Eye contact, 56–57, 118, 218
use of edible reinforcer in establishing, 56

Facial expressions, in communication, 185, 188–189, 218
Family counseling and involvement, 158
Feedback mechanism, 64
Fetus, insult to, by the rubella virus, 63
Figure-ground discrimination
assessment of, 141–143
complexity of stimulus, 143
definition of, 141
identifying difficulties in, 142
remediation of deficits, 142–143
Figure-ground disturbances, 253
Fingerspelling, 188–191, 204–205, 229
Rochester Method of, 190, 204
Fitzgerald Key, 250–251
Formal signs, 191
Free, appropriate public education, 44, 48, 211
Frostig Developmental Test of Visual Perception, 137–138
Functional linguistic communication, 206
Functional signs, 205
Function of language, 213

Gallaudet College, 2, 190
Department of Education, Teacher Training Program, MHHI specialization, 2
Office of Demographic Studies, 2–3, 40
Gesture
action-bound, 121
body, use of, 120–121
facial, use of, 120–121
natural system of, 120–121, 187–188, 194, 196, 204
use of, 113–114, 120–121, 186–188, 190–191, 196–199, 213, 227
vocalization in conjunction with, 121
Goldman Fristoe Test of Articulation, 116
Goodenough-Harris Drawing Test, 115

Grammar, beginnings of use of, 213–214
Grammatical relations, 222–223, 253
Graphic communication, 205–206, 208
Graphic/tactile representation, 198–199
Gross motor development, 180

Handicapped child, multifaceted needs of, 211
Hearing aids, training in use and care of, 158
Hearing impaired
definition of, 124
intellectual assessment of, 201
language skills of, delay in acquisition of, 104
mental retardation coupled with, 202
Hearing Impaired/Mentally Retarded, 29–35
assessment of, 113–117
bio-psycho-social factors in diagnosis of, 114
communication system for, 224–234
curriculum for, 113–120
definitions of, 31, 34
degree of severity of, 31–33
diagnostic instruments of, 113
education of, 113–122
evaluation of, 30, 34–35
gesture with, use of, 113–114, 120–121
hearing loss assessment of, 33–34
imitative behavior of, 114, 120
identification of, 30–31, 34–35
total programming for, 33–35
vocational adjustment of, importance of family involvement in, 120
Vocational Rehabilitation (VR) for, 32–33
Hearing loss
assessment of, in HI/MR, 33–34
audiometry, puretone, 34
Heart malformations, 95, 203
Home signs, 190–191
Hiskey Nebraska Test of Learning Aptitude, 116
Hyperactivity/attention problems, 62

Iconicity of signs, 231–232
Ideographic symbols, 207
Illinois School for the Deaf, 2
Impaired perceptions, 253
Independent functioning, 95, 102–103, 117
Independent living, 153

IEP (Individualized Education Program), 70, 100–102, 116–117, 216–217
  documentation of, 101
  evaluation of, 101
  implementation of, 101
  personalization of, 119
  program planning of, 117
Individualization, 119–120
  need for, 203
In-Seat behavior, teaching of
  eye contact, importance of, 56–57
  imitative activities of, 57
  reinforcements of, appropriate, 56–59
  sitting, approximation of, 56
Inservice training, emphasis of, 157–158
Intellectual functioning, 211
Interactions in the environment, influence on language of, 185–187, 212, 231
Interdisciplinary team, 134
Internalization of symbols, 258
Intervention, early
  importance of, 105, 113–122
  strategies of, 120–122

Junior high school, 47
  curriculum, components of, 153
  educational programming at, 150

Kernicterus, 14

Language
  assessment of, 211–212
  definition of, 193
  dysfunction, 63
  function of, 213
  internalization of, 199
  motor base of, 194
  social interaction, as a means of, 213
  symbol system, as a, 193
Language acquisition, 201, 206, 257
  lack of, in abused/isolated children, 201
  linguistic goals of, 257
  linguistic growth, 258
  natural, 201
  normalization of, 201
  symbolizing through actions, importance of, 257
  tools for, 201
Language development, 20, 118–119, 193–196
  assessment procedures of, 211
  assistance in, 158–159
  grammar, assessment of, 214
  imitation, use of, 196
  mathetic functions of, 213–214
  pragmatic functions of, 213–214
  receptive vocabulary, 119
  semantic relations, importance of, 214, 222
  systematic reinforcement in, 187
  through movement, 185–186, 195–196
  through patterning, 251
Language Development and Intervention with the Hearing Impaired (language curriculum), 250
Language disability, 24
Language modality, nonvocal strategies as a speech initiator, 212–213
Language problems, 62
Language system(s)
  acquisition of, 211–212
  non-oral, 212
  oral, 212
  utilization of, 212
Language training procedures, 223–224
Language training sequence, 231
Learning disabilities/disorders, 15–16, 39, 63, 249–259
  definition of, 85
  developmental deficits, age-related, 85
  remedial techniques with, 85
Learning Disabilities: Educational Principles and Practices, 253–255
Learning disabled
  assessment of, 115
  deficits in, remediation strategies for, 85–94
    auditory discrimination, 86
    body balance, 85–86
    figure-ground discrimination, 90
    haptic discrimination, 89
    hyperexcitability, 87
    mathematical comprehension, 93
    monitoring, 90–91
    reading comprehension, 92–93
    rehearsal, 87–88
    visual-auditory-haptic coordination, 91–92
    visualization, 89–90

visual pursuit, 85
writing, 93–94
developmental function deficits
  communication, 92–94
  memory, 86–88
  re-cognition, 88–90
  sensory orientation, 85–86
  synthesis, 90–92
teaching strategies
  prerequisites for effective teaching, 249
  suggestions for, 254–259
treatment of, use of drugs in, 87
Learning-Disabled/Hearing-Impaired (LDHI), 61–71
analysis, functional, 70
analysis, task, 70
assessment
  formal, 67–68
  implications of, 70–71
  informal, 68–69
  teacher's role in, 61–71
characteristics and terminology of, 65–67
child abuse, 64
developmental/functional age, consideration of, 67
diagnosis of, 64–65
DPT (diagnostic-prescriptive teaching), 70–71
dysfunctioning, age-related, 66–67
environmental factors of, 64
etiology of, 62–63
evaluation of, psycho-educational, 62
identification of, 61–65
physiological conditions of, 64
tests for, categories of, 69–70
  diagnostic evaluation, 70
  formative evaluation, 70
  placement evaluation, 69
Learning problems/learning disabilities, 135
  in deaf children, 135–136
  psychoneurological definition of, 136
Least restrictive environment, 203
Leiter International Performance Scale, 115
Lexical items, 213–214, 222
  morphology of, 214
Lexington School for the Deaf, 170
Linguistic concepts, 186
Linguistic development, 250
Lothographic symbol systems, 208

LOVE (Linguistics of Visual English), 189–190

Mailman Center for Child Development, 113, 115, 120
Mainstreaming movements, abuses of, 203
Malpractice, educational, 125
Manual communication, forms of, 204–205
Manual English, 189–191
Manual signing as the language modality, 224
Manual signing program, functions of, 217–218
Manual signing system, 217–218
  response topography of, 217
  syntactic components of, 218
  vocabulary components of, 218
Manual sign training, 230–235
  as an expressive language system, 230
  as a receptive language system, 230
Meier's table (assessment tool), 114
"Me-not-me" concept, development of, 186–187, 194–195
Mental age, 115
Mental handicap. *See* Mental retardation
Mental retardation, 2–3, 13–14, 16, 18, 22, 29–35, 53, 75–83, 95, 103–104, 113–122, 135, 201–204, 211, 224, 256
  EMR (Educable Mental Retardation), 202, 211
  TMR (Trainable Mental Retardation), 202, 211
Memory, 164–165, 173–175, 180, 197
  information, organization of, 173, 197–198
  "metamemory"/"metacognition", 173
  repetition, 174–175
  short- and long-term, 173–175
  time and space, limitations of, 175
Memory problems, 62
Metropolitan Readiness Test, 140
  Letter Recognition, subtest of, 140
Minnesota Early Language Development Sequence (MELDS), 207
Modes of communication, 201, 208, 211–248
Monsees' Structured Language Method, 253
Mother/child relationship, reciprocal or interactive, 106
Motor Development in Deaf-Blind Children (movie), 193

Motor-Free Test of Visual Perception, 138, 142, 144
Motor functioning, impaired, 253
Motorically impaired, 224
Motor/imitation/gesture progression, 185–191, 196–197
Motor movement, 227
Motor problems, 62
Movement experiences, building sensory concepts with, 187
Multihandicapped
  behaviors of, 96
  definition of, 95
  early intervention with, 95–102
  independent functioning, level of, 96
  individual educational plan, development of, 98–99
  individualized needs of, 95–96
  observation of, 98–100
    evaluation with developmental scales, 99
    informal, 100
    specific behavior areas, 99
  optimal development of, 108
  parents of, 103–108
    demands of, 103–105
    expectations of, 103–105
    guilt of, 104, 107–108
  planning long- and short-term goals for, 100
  teaching team approach with, 98
  total child approach with, 96–98
Multihandicapped/Hearing Impaired
  behavior management strategies for, 53–59
  definition of, 3
  degree of severity of, 3
  deviant behavior of, 53
  distribution of, 22–23
  educational placement of, 37–41
  etiologies of, 11–12
  identification of, 2, 39–41
  prevalence of, 3–5
  recognition of the needs of, 2
  types of multiple handicaps, 11–25

National Advisory Committee on Handicapped Children (1968), 135
Native language, 158
Natural Gesture Language System, 120–122
Natural Language Approach, 251

Nonspeech communication system, 202, 212–213
Non-speech Language Initiation Program (Non-SLIP), 206–207
Nonspeech mode of communication, 217–218
Nonverbal communication, 120–121
Nonverbal communication system, teaching of, 225–235
Nonvocal symbol systems, 202, 212, 218, 225
  communication boards, 212, 224–227
Normal child development, 249–254
  abnormal development, as a basis for understanding, 250, 259
Normalcy/normalization, 203
Normal language acquisition, 258
Normal language development, 249–250

One-to-one instruction, 151
Orthography, traditional, 207–208
Orthopedic defects, 21–22, 63, 95

Pantomime, 188–189
Paralysis, 15
Parents
  confidentiality with, 47
  counseling of, 44–45
  due process of, 47–49
  emotions of, unacknowledged, 107
  expectations of, 150, 159
  external/referral services for, 106–107, 120
  guilt of, 158
  increased militancy of, 37
  internal feelings, dealing with, 107
  involvement, importance of, 105–108, 158–160
  litigation involving, 4–5
  native language of, 47–48
  participation of, in IEP process, 46
  professionals' help/counseling for, 106
  role in assessment, 216
  rights of, under Public Law 94-142, 44, 47
Peer tutors, 151
Perception
  assessment and remediation of deficits, 137–145
    figure-ground discrimination, 141–143
    spatial relations, 143–145
    visual, 137–139

visual discrimination, 139–141
  definition of, 136–137
  internal cognitive process of, 137
  selective process of, 137
Perceptually handicapped, assessment of, 115
Perceptual-motor, as a curriculum component, 153
Perceptual-motor difficulties, 138, 153, 182
Perceptual-motor dysfunction, 135–136, 152
Perceptual problems, 62, 120, 137
  in hearing-impaired children, 135–147
Perceptual skills, 211–212, 223
Physical handicaps, 201–203
Physical problems, 95, 103, 113
Play behavior, cognitive development in, 257
Play in the hearing-impaired/mentally retarded
  anger and aggressiveness in, 78–79
  auditory stimulation in, 78
  behavior modification in, 79
  crawling and creeping, 80–81
  creative play skills, development of, 82
  developmental teaching approach of, 79
  development of skills, 79–83
  deviant behavior, channeling of, 78
  fantasy play, as a means of expression, 82
  grasping objects, 80
  group play, sharing in, 83
  imitative play, opportunities of, 82
  individual, 79–80
  language, paired with movement, 78–79
  manipulating objects in, 80
  one-to-one basis, teaching on a, 80
  parallel, 83
  patterns of, 75–77
    chronological age in, 76–77
    mental age in, 76–77
  recreation and physical education, 75–83
  socialization system, development of, 83
  structured, 78
  utilizing sensory modalities in, 78
  visual exploration, 80
  walking and running, developing skills of, 81
Prelanguage oral program, 222
Prelinguistic functioning, 212
Prenumber skills, 119
Prereading skills, 119
Prerequisite skills
  for classroom learning, 180–181

  for speech, 212
Preverbal behavior, assessment of, 214
Prevocational training, 156
Psychological development in infancy, assessment of, 212
Psychomotor dysfunctions, 253
Psychoneurological learning disabilities, concept of, 254
Psychoses/psychological disturbances, 21–22, 24
Public Law 94-142, 2, 5, 37, 40–41, 70–71
  assessment procedures, 211
  due process under, 47–48
  effects of, 44
  IEP, as mandated by, 45–47
  implications of, 43, 49
  limits of, 124–125
  overview of, 44–45
  personnel development under, 47
  purpose of, 47–48
Public Law 91-230, 2
Public Law 93-380, 5
Pugh's *Steps in Language Development*, 251

Rebus System, 207
Referral services, 106–107, 126, 142
Reinforcement, to increase responses, 195
Reinforcers, primary and secondary, 54–59
Response topography, 227, 229
Rhode Island School for the Deaf, curriculum used at, 250
Rochester Method, 190, 204
Role models, 150, 155
Routine, daily, 101
Rubella
  children, 12–14, 104
  epidemic of 1943, 13
  epidemic of 1964–65, 12–14, 63
  multiple handicaps as a result of, 18–25
Rules in the home, establishment of, 159

St. Joseph's School for the Deaf in New York, 172
Schema, theory of, 170–171, 176
Schools for the deaf/multihandicapped hearing impaired, 1, 29
  American Asylum for the Deaf and Dumb in Hartford, Connecticut, 1

Schools (*continued*)
  California School for the Deaf
    at Berkeley, 1
    at Riverside, 2, 17–18, 20
SEE$_1$ (Seeing Essential English), 189–190
SEE$_2$ (Signing Exact English), 189–190
Self-help, 101, 104–105, 115, 117–118
Self-help skills, 149, 150–154, 156, 159, 224
Sensorimotor input, 211
Sensorimotor integration, 180
Sensory deficits, in hearing and vision, 95
Sensory impairments, 186
Sensory input, 185, 199
Sensory isolation, 186
Sensory stimulation, 100–101
Sentences and Other Systems, 250
Sequential goals, 211
Services available for hearing-impaired/
    mentally retarded, 30, 32, 34
  lack of, 40–41, 43
  for MHHI, 43–49
Signed English, 189–191
Sign language
  American Sign Language, 204, 229
  assessment of motor skills for teaching, 227
  attention getting devices in, 230
  communication training through, 230–235
  continuum, 185, 188–191
  hand preference with, 227
  motor configurations, 229, 231
  neutral hand position, meaning of, 229
  systems, 188–189, 203
  transference of gesture to sign symbol, 188
Signs
  distinctive features of, 230–232
  formal, 188, 191
Social behavior, 149
  skills of, 156
Social communication system, 222
Social development, assistance in, 158–159
Social interaction, 153, 155, 173, 258
Social learning, as a curriculum component, 153–154
Social Learning Curriculum (SLC), 153–154, 158
Socio-affective skills, 211, 223
Spatial deficits, remediation of
  letter forms, spatial manipulation of, 145
  three-dimensional objects, use of, 144
  two-dimensional objects, use of, 144
  visual cues, use of, 145
Spatial disorganization, 253
Spatial relations, 143–145
  assessment of, 143
  concepts, acquisition of, 143
  definition of, 143
  experience of, for language development, 195–196
  reconstruction, 144
  visual functioning, implications of, 143
Specialized information, help with comprehension of, 108
Specialized tasks, 108
Specific objectives, directly related to training, 211
Speech, as an unrealistic goal with MR/HI, 212
Speechreading, 158
  visual reinforcement in, 121
Stanford Achievement Test (SAT), 128
Stanford Achievement Test Battery, 135
Structuring the environment, 181
Subnormal intelligence, 211
Support staff members, 150–151
Symbolic hand movements/signs, 188
Symbol system communication, 206–208
  Bliss Symbols, 207–208
  Non-Speech Language Initiation Program (Non-SLIP), 206–208
  Rebus System, 207–208
Syntactic rules, acquisition of, 257

Task analysis, 175–176
Task specificity, 166, 171
Teaching
  concept development, 57–58
  working independently, 58–59
Teaching language and communication, 217–234, 252
Teaching the deaf, 1, 2
  personnel development, 47
Telegraphic speech, 223
Templin-Darly Tests of Articulation, 116
Testing procedures
  administration of, 47–49
  evaluation of, 47–49
  placements from, 45–49

Texas Technological University, Research and Training Center in Mental Retardation at, 30
Time-Out
 alternative behaviors in, 55
 appropriate use of, 54–55
 consistency in use of, 54
 eliminating inappropriate behaviors in, 55
 placement in, reasons for, 55
Topeka Association for Retarded Citizens Test (TARC), 115
Total communication, 204
Total praise reinforcement system, 187

Uneven skills, 62
U.S. Office of Education: Bureau of Education for the Handicapped (BEH), 48, 148
Usher's Syndrome, 17
Utterances
 characterizations of, 213, 232
 semantic relations of, 214, 223
Uzgiris-Hunt tool of assessment, 115

Verbalization, spontaneous, 211
Vineland Social Maturity Scale, 115
Visual analysis, 164–166, 168, 169, 171, 180
 multisensory input of, 168
Visual discrimination, 135, 139–141
 activities for, 140
 assessment of, informal, 140
 color, 141
 definition of, 139
 distinctive features of, 139–141
 remediation of, 140–141
 spatial memory, 139
 stimulus of, 139
 texture of, 141
 theory of differentiation of, 139
Visual disorders, 2, 3, 13–16, 20–22, 63, 95, 104, 135, 202, 224
Visual motor communication mode, 205
Visual perception
 assessment of, 137–139
 difficulties of, 138
Visual-perceptual difficulties, in the deaf child, 139
 assessment of, 139
 remediation of, 139

Visual-perceptual objects, manipulation of, 145
Vocalizations, 204, 230
 signs, as a facilitator of, 205
 signs, as an initiator of, 204

Waardenburg Syndrome, 17
Water, movement through, 187, 195
Wechsler Adult Intelligence Scale (WAIS), Performance Scale IQ, 128
Wing Symbols, 251

FLAGLER COLLEGE LIBRARY
KING STREET
ST. AUGUSTINE, FLORIDA 32084